OBSTETRICS
by Ten Teachers

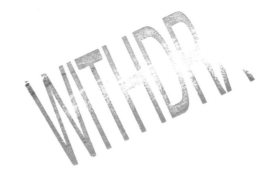

OBSTETRICS

by Ten Teachers

19th edition

Edited by

Philip N Baker BMEDSCI BM BS DM FRCOG FRCSC FMEDSCI

Dean of the Faculty of Medicine and Dentistry,
University of Alberta, Edmonton, Canada

Louise C Kenny MBCHB (HONS) MRCOG PHD

Professor of Obstetrics and
Consultant Obstetrician and Gynaecologist
The Anu Research Centre,
Cork University Maternity Hospital,
Department of Obstetrics and Gynaecology,
University College Cork,
Cork, Ireland

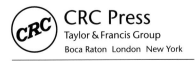

CRC Press
Taylor & Francis Group
Boca Raton London New York

CRC Press is an imprint of the
Taylor & Francis Group, an **informa** business

CRC Press
Taylor & Francis Group
6000 Broken Sound Parkway NW, Suite 300
Boca Raton, FL 33487-2742

© 2011 by Taylor & Francis Group, LLC
CRC Press is an imprint of Taylor & Francis Group, an Informa business

No claim to original U.S. Government works

Printed and bound in India by Replika Press Pvt. Ltd.

Visit the Taylor & Francis Web site at
http://www.taylorandfrancis.com

and the CRC Press Web site at
http://www.crcpress.com

This book is dedicated to my younger daughter, Sara (PNB)
And to my sons, Conor and Eamon (LCK)

Instructions for the Companion Website

This book has a companion website available at:
http://www.hodderplus.com/obsgynaebytenteachers

To access the image library included on the website, please register using the following access details:

Serial number: srfp326lw7ty

Once you have registered, you will not need a serial number but can log in using the username and password that you will create during your registration.

Contents

The Ten Teachers

Philip N Baker BMEDSCI BM BS DM FRCOG FRCSC FMEDSCI

Dean of the Faculty of Medicine and Dentistry, University of Alberta, Edmonton, Canada

Griffith Jones MRCOG FRCSC

Assistant Professor, Division of Maternal–Fetal Medicine, University of Ottawa, Ottawa, Canada

Lucy Kean MA DM FRCOG

Consultant Obstetrician and Subspecialist in Fetal and Maternal Medicine, Department of Obstetrics, City Campus, Nottingham University Hospitals, Nottingham, UK

Louise C Kenny MBCHB (HONS) MRCOG PHD

Professor of Obstetrics and Consultant Obstetrician and Gynaecologist, The Anu Research Centre, Cork University Maternity Hospital, Department of Obstetrics and Gynaecology, University College Cork, Cork, Ireland

Alec McEwan BA BM BCH MRCOG

Consultant in Obstetrics and Subspecialist in Fetal and Maternal Medicine, Department of Obstetrics, Nottingham University Hospitals, Nottingham, UK

Gary Mires MBCHB MD FRCOG FHEA

Professor of Obstetrics and Undergraduate Teaching Dean, School of Medicine, University of Dundee, UK

Keelin O'Donoghue MB BCH BAO MRCOG PHD

Senior Lecturer and Consultant Obstetrician and Gynaecologist, The Anu Research Centre, Cork University Maternity Hospital, Department of Obstetrics and Gynaecology, University College Cork, Cork, Ireland

Janet M Rennie MA MD FRCP FRCPCH DCH

Consultant and Senior Lecturer in Neonatal Medicine, Elizabeth Garrett Anderson and Obstetric Hospital, University College London Hospitals, London, UK

Clare Tower MBCHB PHD MRCOG

Clinical Lecturer and Subspecialty Trainee in Fetal and Maternal Medicine, Maternal and Fetal Health Research Centre, St Mary's Hospital, University of Manchester, UK

Sarah Vause MD FRCOG

Consultant in Fetal and Maternal Medicine, St Mary's Hospital, Manchester, UK

Preface

Obstetrics by Ten Teachers is the oldest and most respected English language textbook on the subject. As editors we fully appreciate the responsibility to ensure its continuing success.

The first edition was published as *Midwifery by Ten Teachers* in 1917, and was edited under the direction of Comyns Berkley (Obstetric and Gynaecological Surgeon to the Middlesex Hospital). The aims of the book as detailed in the preface to the first edition still pertain today:

This book is frankly written for students preparing for their final examination, and in the hope that it will prove useful to them afterwards, and to others who have passed beyond the stage of examination.

Thus, whilst the 19th edition is written for the medical student, we hope the text retains its usefulness for the trainee obstetrician and general practitioners. The 19th edition continues the tradition, re-established with the 18th edition, of utilizing the collective efforts of ten teachers of repute. The ten teachers teach in medical schools that vary markedly in the philosophy and structure of their courses. Some adopt a wholly problem-based approach, while others adopt a more traditional 'subject-based' curriculum. All of the ten teachers have an active involvement in both undergraduate and postgraduate teaching, and all have previously written extensively within their areas of expertise. Some of the contributors, such as Gary Mires, have been at the forefront of innovations in undergraduate teaching, and have been heavily involved in developing the structure of courses and curricula. In contrast, other teachers are at earlier stages in their career: Clare Tower is a clinical lecturer, closely involved in the day-to-day tutoring of students. The extensive and diverse experience of our ten teachers should maximize the relevance of the text to today's medical students.

This 19th edition has been extensively revised and in many places entirely rewritten but throughout the textbook we have endeavoured to continue the previous editors' efforts to incorporate clinically relevant material.

Finally, we echo the previous editors in hoping that this book will enthuse a new generation of obstetricians to make pregnancy and childbirth an even safer and more fulfilling experience.

Philip N Baker
Louise C Kenny
2011

Commonly used abbreviations

2,3-DPG	2,3-diphosphoglycerate
3D	three-dimensional
AC	abdominal circumference
aCL	anti-cardiolipin antibodies
ACR	American College of Rheumatology
ACTH	adrenocorticotrophic hormone
AFI	amniotic fluid index
AIDS	acquired immunodeficiency syndrome
AP	anteroposterior
APH	antepartum haemorrhage
APS	antiphospholipid syndrome
ARM	artificial rupture of membranes
ASBAH	Association for spina bifida and hydrocephalus
BMI	body mass index
BMR	basal metabolic rate
BPD	biparietal diameter
bpm	beats per minute
BPP	biophysical profile
BV	bacterial vaginosis
CBG	cortisol-binding globulin
CDC	Communicable Disease Center
CEMACH	Confidential Enquiry into Maternal and Child Health
CEMD	Confidential Enquiries into Maternal Death
CF	cystic fibrosis
CKD	chronic kidney disease
CMACE	Centre for Maternal and Child Enquiries
CMV	cytomegalovirus
CNST	Clinical Negligence Scheme for Trusts
CPD	cephalopelvic disproportion
CPR	cardiopulmonary resuscitation
CRH	corticotrophin-releasing hormone
CRL	crown–rump length
CRM	clinical risk management
CSE	combined spinal–epidural
CT	computed tomography
CTG	cardiotocograph
CTPA	computed tomography pulmonary angiogram
CVS	chorion villus sampling
DCDA	dichorionic diamniotic
DDH	developmental dysplasia of the hip
DHA	docosahexaenoic acid
DHEA	dihydroepiandrosterone
DIC	disseminated intravascular coagulation
DVT	deep vein thrombosis

eAg	e antigen
ECG	electrocardiogram
ECT	electroconvulsive therapy
ECV	external cephalic version
EDD	estimated date of delivery
EEG	electroencephalography
EFM	external fetal monitoring
EFW	estimate of fetal weight
EIA	enzyme immunoassay
ERCS	elective repeat Caesarean section
FBS	fetal scalp blood sampling
FEV1	forced expiratory volume in 1 second
fFN	fetal fibronectin
FGR	fetal growth restriction
FHR	fetal heart rate
FL	femur length
FRC	functional residual capacity
fT4	free T4
FVS	fetal varicella syndrome
G6PD	glucose 6-phosphate dehydrogenase
GBS	group B streptococcus
GDM	gestational diabetes mellitus
GFR	glomerular filtration rate
GMH-IVH	germinal matrix-intraventricular haemorrhage
GnRH	gonadotrophin releasing hormone
GP	general practitioner
HAART	highly active antiretroviral therapy
HbF	fetal haemoglobin
HBIG	hepatitis B immunoglobulin
HBsAG	hepatitis B surface antigen
HBV	hepatitis B virus
HC	head circumference
hCG	human chorionic gonadotrophin
HCV	hepatitis C virus
HDFN	haemolytic disease of the fetus and newborn
HELLP	haemolysis, elevation of liver enzymes and low platelets
hGH	human growth hormone
HIE	hypoxic–ischaemic encephalopathy
HIV	human immunodeficiency virus
hPL	human placental lactogen
HSV	herpes simplex virus
IBD	inflammatory bowel disease
IDDM	insulin-dependent diabetes mellitus
Ig	immunoglobulin
IGF	insulin-like growth factor
IgG	immunoglobulin G
INR	international normalized ratio
IOL	induction of labour
IRT	immunoreactive trypsin

ITP	thrombocytopenic purpura
IU	international units
IUGR	intrauterine growth restriction
IVC	inferior vena cava
IVF	*in vitro* fertilization
LA	lupus anticoagulant
LDH	lactate dehydrogenase
LIF	leukaemia inhibitory factor
LLETZ	large loop excision of the transformation zone
LMP	last menstrual period
LMWH	low molecular weight heparin
MAS	meconium aspiration syndrome
MCA	middle cerebral artery
MCADD	medium chain acyl coenzyme A dehydrogenase
MCDA	monochorionic diamniotic
MCMA	monochorionic monoamniotic
MI	myocardial infarction
MMR	maternal mortality ratio; measles, mumps and rubella vaccine
MRI	magnetic resonance imaging
MSLC	Maternity Services Liaison Committee
MSU	midstream specimen of urine
NCT	National Childbirth Trust
NHS	National Health Service
NHSLA	NHS Litigation Authority
NICE	National Institute for Health and Clinical Excellence
NIDDM	non-insulin-dependent diabetes mellitus
NIPE	newborn and infant physical examination
NK	natural killer
NO	nitrous oxide
NYHA	New York Heart Association
OGTT	oral glucose tolerance test
PAI	plasma activator inhibitor
PAPP-A	pregnancy associated plasma protein-A
PBC	primary biliary cirrhosis
PCA	patient-controlled analgesia
pCO_2	partial pressure of carbon dioxide
PCR	polymerase chain reaction
PE	pulmonary embolism
PEP	polymorphic eruption of pregnancy
PG	pemphigoid gestationis
PH	pulmonary hypertension
pO_2	partial pressure of oxygen
PPH	postpartum haemorrhage
PPHN	persistent pulmonary hypertension of the newborn
PPROM	preterm prelabour rupture of membranes
PT	prothrombin time
PTCA	percutaneous transluminal coronary angioplasty
PTH	parathyroid hormone
PTL	preterm labour

PTU	propylthiouracil
PVL	periventricular leukomalacia
RA	rheumatoid arthritis
RCOG	Royal College of Obstetricians and Gynaecologists
RDS	respiratory distress syndrome
REM	rapid eye movement
SANDS	Stillbirth and Neonatal Death Society
SARS	severe acute respiratory syndrome
SCD	sickle cell disease
SFH	symphysis–fundal height
SGA	small for gestational age
SLE	systemic lupus erythematosus
SROM	spontaneous rupture of the membranes
SSRI	selective serotonin reuptake inhibitors
T3	tri-iodothyronine
T4	thyroxine
TAMBA	Twins and Multiple Birth Association
TCA	tricyclic antidepressant drugs
TENS	transcutaneous electrical nerve stimulation
TOF	tracheo-oesophageal fistula
tPA	tissue plasminogen activator
TPHA	*T. pallidum* haemagglutination assay
TRH	thyrotrophin releasing hormone
TSH	thyroid stimulating hormone
TTN	transient tachypnoea of the newborn
TTTS	twin-to-twin transfusion syndrome
UFH	unfractionated heparin
UTI	urinary tract infection
VACTERL	Vertebral, Anal, Cardiac, Tracheal, (O)Esophageal, Renal and Limb
VBAC	vaginal birth after Caesarean
VDRL	Venereal Diseases Research Laboratory
VKDB	vitamin K deficiency bleeding
VTE	venous thromboembolic disease
VWF	von Willebrand factor
VZIG	varicella zoster immunoglobulin
VZV	varicella zoster virus
WHO	World Heath Organization

CHAPTER 1

OBSTETRIC HISTORY TAKING AND EXAMINATION

Lucy Kean

OVERVIEW

Taking a history and performing an obstetric examination are quite different from their medical and surgical equivalents. Not only will the type of questions change with gestation but also will the purpose of the examination. The history will often cover physiology, pathology and psychology and must always be sought with care and sensitivity.

Etiquette in taking a history

Patients expect doctors and students to be well presented and appearances do have an enormous impact on patients, so make sure that your appearance is suitable before you enter the room.

When meeting a patient for the first time, always introduce yourself; tell the patient who you are and say why you have come to see them. If you are a medical student, some patients will decide that they do not wish to talk to you. This may be for many reasons and, if your involvement in their care is declined, accept without questioning.

Some areas of the obstetric history cover subjects that are intensely private. In occasional cases there may be events recorded in the notes that are not known by other family members, such as previous terminations of pregnancy. It is vital that the history taker is sensitive to each individual situation and does not simply follow a formula to get all the facts right.

Some women will wish another person to be present if the doctor or student is male, even just to take a history, and this wish should be respected.

Where to begin

The amount of detail required must be tailored to the purpose of the visit. At a booking visit, the history must be thorough and meticulously recorded. Once this baseline information is established, many women find it tedious to go over all this information again. Before starting, ask yourself what you need to achieve. In late pregnancy, women will be attending the antenatal clinic for a particular reason. It is certainly acceptable to ask why the patient has attended in the opening discussion. For some women it will be a routine visit (usually performed by the midwife or general practitioner), others are attending because there is or has been a problem.

Make sure that the patient is comfortable (usually seated but occasionally sitting on a bed).

It is important to establish some very general facts when taking a history. Asking for the patient's age or date of birth and whether this is a first pregnancy are usually safe opening questions.

At this stage you can also establish whether a woman is working and, if so, what she does.

Dating the pregnancy

Pregnancy has been historically dated from the last menstrual period (LMP), not the date of conception. The median duration of pregnancy is 280 days (40 weeks) and this gives the estimated date of delivery (EDD). This assumes that:

- the cycle length is 28 days;
- ovulation occurs generally on the 14th day of the cycle;

- the cycle was a normal cycle (i.e. not straight after stopping the oral contraceptive pill or soon after a previous pregnancy).

The EDD is calculated by taking the date of the LMP, counting forward by nine months and adding 7 days. If the cycle is longer than 28 days, add the difference between the cycle length and 28 to compensate.

In most antenatal clinics, there are pregnancy calculators (wheels) that do this for you (Figure 1.1). It is worth noting that pregnancy-calculating wheels do differ a little and may give dates that are a day or two different from those previously calculated. While this should not make much difference, it is an area that often causes heated discussion in the antenatal clinic. Term is actually defined as 37–42 weeks and so the estimated time of delivery should ideally be defined as a range of dates rather than a fixed date, but women have been highly resistant to this idea and generally do want a specific date.

Almost all women who undergo antenatal care in the UK will have an ultrasound scan in the late first trimester or early second trimester. The purposes of this scan are to establish dates, to ensure that the pregnancy is ongoing and to determine the number of fetuses. If performed before 20 weeks, the ultrasound scan can be used for dating the pregnancy. After this time, the variability in growth rates of different fetuses makes it unsuitable for use in defining dates. It has been shown that ultrasound-defined dates are more accurate than those based on a certain LMP and reduce the need for post-dates induction of labour. This may be because the actual time of ovulation in any cycle is much less fixed than was previously thought. Therefore, the UK National Screening Committee has recommended that pregnancy dates are set only by ultrasound. The crown–rump length is used up until 13 weeks + 6 days, and the head circumference from 14 to 20 weeks. Regardless of the date of the LMP this EDD is used. It is important that an accurate EDD is established as a difference of a day or two can make a difference in the risk for conditions such as Down's syndrome on serum screening. In addition, accurate dating reduces the need for post-dates induction of labour.

In late pregnancy, many women will have long forgotten their LMP date, but will know exactly when their EDD is, and it is therefore more straightforward to ask this.

Taking the history

Social history

Some aspects of history taking require considerable sensitivity, and the social history is one such area. There are important facts to establish, but in many cases these can come out at various different parts of the history and some can almost be part of normal conversation. It is important to have a list of things to establish in your mind. It is here more than anywhere that some local knowledge is helpful, as much can be gained from knowing where the patient lives. However, be careful not to jump to conclusions, as these can often be wrong.

The following facts demonstrate why a social history is important:

- Women whose partners were unemployed or working in an unclassifiable role had a maternal mortality rate seven times higher than women whose partners were employed according to the Confidential Enquiry into Maternal and Child Health 2003–2005 (CEMACH).

- Social exclusion was seen in 18 out of 19 deaths in women under 20 in the 1997–1999 Confidential Enquiries into Maternal Death (CEMD) (one

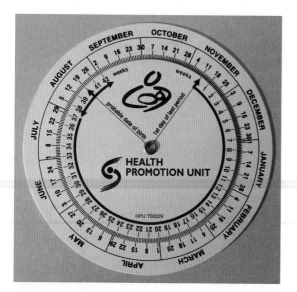

Figure 1.1 Gestation calculator

homeless teenager froze to death in a front garden).

- Married women are more likely to request amniocentesis after a high-risk Down's syndrome screening result than unmarried women. Husbands clearly have a strong voice in decision making.
- If a woman is unmarried, her partner cannot provide consent for a post-mortem after stillbirth.
- Domestic violence was reported in 12 per cent of the 378 women whose deaths were reported in 1997–1999.

Enquiry about domestic violence is extremely difficult. It is recommended that all women are seen on their own at least once during pregnancy, so that they can discuss this, if needed, away from an abusive partner. This is not always easy to accomplish. If you happen to be the person with whom this information is shared, you must ensure that it is passed on to the relevant team, as this may be the only opportunity the woman has to disclose it. Sometimes younger women find medical students and young doctors much easier to talk to. Be aware of this.

Smoking, alcohol and illicit drug intake also form part of the social history. Smoking causes a reduction in birthweight in a dose-dependent way. It also increases the risk of miscarriage, stillbirth and neonatal death. There are interventions that can be offered to women who are still smoking in pregnancy (see Chapter 8, Antenatal obstetric complications).

Complete abstinence from alcohol is advised, as the safety of alcohol is not proven. However, alcohol is probably not harmful in small amounts (less than one drink per day). Binge drinking is particularly harmful and can lead to a constellation of features in the baby known as fetal alcohol syndrome (see Chapter 8, Antenatal obstetric complications).

Enquiry about illicit drug taking is more difficult. Approximately 0.5–1 per cent of women continue to take illicit drugs during pregnancy. Be careful not to make assumptions. During the booking visit, the midwife should directly enquire about drug taking. If it is seen as part of the long list of routine questions asked at this visit, it is perceived as less threatening. However, sometimes this information comes to light at other times. Cocaine and crack cocaine are the most harmful of the illicit drugs taken, but all

have some effects on the pregnancy, and all have financial implications (see Chapter 8, Antenatal obstetric complications).

By the time you have finished your history and examination you should know the following facts that are important in the social history:

- whether the patient is married or single and what sort of support she has at home (remember that married women whose only support is a working husband may be very isolated after the birth of a baby);
- generally whether there is a stable income coming into the house;
- what sort of housing the patient occupies (e.g. a flat with lots of stairs and no lift may be problematic);
- whether the woman works and for how long she is planning to work during the pregnancy;
- whether the woman smokes/drinks or uses drugs;
- if there are any other features that may be important.

Previous obstetric history

Past obstetric history is one of the most important areas for establishing risk in the current pregnancy. It is helpful to list the pregnancies in date order and to discover what the outcome was in each pregnancy.

The features that are likely to have impact on future pregnancies include:

- recurrent miscarriage (increased risk of miscarriage, fetal growth restriction (FGR));
- preterm delivery (increased risk of preterm delivery);
- early-onset pre-eclampsia (increased risk of pre-eclampsia/FGR);
- abruption (increased risk of recurrence);
- congenital abnormality (recurrence risk depends on type of abnormality);
- macrosomic baby (may be related to gestational diabetes);
- FGR (increased recurrence);
- unexplained stillbirth (increased risk of gestational diabetes).

The method of delivery for any previous births must be recorded, as this can have implications for planning in the current pregnancy, particularly if there has been a previous Caesarean section, difficult vaginal delivery, postpartum haemorrhage or significant perineal trauma.

When you have noted all the pregnancies, you can convert this into the obstetric shorthand of parity. This is often confusing. Remember that:

- *gravida* is the total number of pregnancies regardless of how they ended;
- *parity* is the number of live births at any gestation or stillbirths after 24 weeks.

In terms of parity, therefore, twins count as two. Thus a woman at 12 weeks in this pregnancy who has never had a pregnancy before is gravida 1, parity 0. If she delivers twins and comes back next time at 12 weeks, she will be gravida 2, parity 2 (twins). A woman who has had six miscarriages and is pregnant again with only one live baby born at 25 weeks will be gravida 8, parity 1.

The other shorthand you may see is where parity is denoted with the number of pregnancies that did not result in live birth or stillbirth after 24 weeks as a superscript number. The above cases would thus be defined as: para 0^0, para 2^0 (twins), para 1^6.

However, when presenting a history, it is much easier to describe exactly what has happened, e.g. 'Mrs Jones is in her eighth pregnancy. She has had six miscarriages at gestations of 8–12 weeks and one spontaneous delivery of a live baby boy at 25 weeks. Baby Tom is now 2 years old and healthy'.

Past gynaecological history

The regularity of periods used to be important in dating pregnancy (see Dating the pregnancy p. 1). Women with very long cycles may have a condition known as polycystic ovarian syndrome. This is a complex endocrine condition and its relevance here is that some women with this condition have increased insulin resistance and a higher risk for the development of gestational diabetes.

Contraceptive history can be relevant if conception has occurred soon after stopping the combined oral contraceptive pill or depot progesterone preparations, as again, this makes dating by LMP more difficult. Also, some women will conceive with an intrauterine device still *in situ*. This carries an increase in the risk of miscarriage.

Previous episodes of pelvic inflammatory disease increase the risk for ectopic pregnancy. This is only of relevance in early pregnancy. However, it is important to establish that any infections have been adequately treated and that the partner was also treated.

The date of the last cervical smear should be noted. Every year a small number of women are diagnosed as having cervical cancer in pregnancy, and it is recognized that late diagnosis is more common around the time of pregnancy because smears are deferred. If a smear is due, it can be taken in the first trimester. It is important to record that the woman is pregnant, as the cells can be difficult to assess without this knowledge. It is also important that smears are not deferred in women who are at increased risk of cervical disease (e.g. previous cervical smear abnormality or very overdue smear). Gently taking a smear in the first trimester does not cause miscarriage and women should be reassured about this. Remember that if it is deferred at this point, it may be nearly a year before the opportunity arises again. If there has been irregular bleeding, the cervix should at least be examined to ensure that there are no obvious lesions present.

If a woman has undergone treatment for cervical changes, this should be noted. Knife cone biopsy is associated with an increased risk for both cervical incompetence (weakness) and stenosis (leading to preterm delivery and dystocia in labour, respectively). There is probably a very small increase in the risk of preterm birth associated with large loop excision of the transformation zone (LLETZ); however, women who have needed more than one excision are likely to have a much shorter cervix, which does increase the risk for second and early third trimester delivery.

Previous ectopic pregnancy increases the risk of recurrence to 1 in 10. It is also important to know the site of the ectopic and how it was managed. The implications of a straightforward salpingectomy for an ampullary ectopic are much less than those after a complex operation for a cornual ectopic. Women who have had an ectopic pregnancy should be offered an early ultrasound scan to establish the site of any future pregnancies.

Recurrent miscarriage may be associated with a number of problems. Antiphospholipid syndrome increases the risk of further pregnancy loss, FGR and pre-eclampsia. Balanced translocations can occasionally lead to congenital abnormality, and cervical incompetence can predispose to late second and early third trimester delivery. Also, women need a great deal of support during pregnancy if they have experienced recurrent pregnancy losses.

Multiple previous first trimester terminations of pregnancy potentially increase the risk of preterm delivery, possibly secondary to cervical weakness. Sometimes information regarding these must be sensitively recorded. Some women do not wish this to be recorded in their hand-held notes.

Previous gynaecological surgery is important, especially if it involved the uterus, as this can have potential sequelae for delivery. In addition, the presence of pelvic masses such as ovarian cysts and fibroids should be noted. These may impact on delivery and may also pose some problems during pregnancy. A previous history of sub-fertility is also important. Four deaths occurred in CEMACH 2003–2005 of women with ovarian hyperstimulation syndrome following IVF. Donor egg or sperm use is associated with an increased risk of pre-eclampsia. The rate of preterm delivery is higher in assisted conception pregnancies, even after the higher rate of multiple pregnancies has been taken into account. Women who have undergone fertility treatment are often older and generally need increased psychological support during pregnancy.

Legally, you should not write down in notes that a pregnancy is conceived by IVF or donor egg or sperm unless you have written permission from the patient. It is obviously a difficult area, as there is an increased risk of problems to the mother in these pregnancies and therefore the knowledge is important. Generally, if the patient has told you herself that the pregnancy was an assisted conception, it is reasonable to state that in your presentation.

Medical and surgical history

All pre-existing medical disease should be carefully noted and any associated drug history also recorded. The major pre-existing diseases that impact on pregnancy and their potential effects are shown in the box (also see Chapter 12, Medical diseases complicating pregnancy).

Previous surgery should be noted. Occasionally surgery has been performed for conditions that may continue to be a problem during pregnancy, such as Crohn's disease. Rarely, complications from previous surgery, such as adhesional obstruction, present in pregnancy.

Psychiatric history is important to record. These enquiries should include the severity of the illness,

---

Major pre-existing diseases that impact on pregnancy

- Diabetes mellitus: macrosomia, FGR, congenital abnormality, pre-eclampsia, stillbirth, neonatal hypoglycaemia.
- Hypertension: pre-eclampsia.
- Renal disease: worsening renal disease, pre-eclampsia, FGR, preterm delivery.
- Epilepsy: increased fit frequency, congenital abnormality.
- Venous thromboembolic disease: increased risk during pregnancy; if associated thrombophilia, increased risk of thromboembolism and possible increased risk of pre-eclampsia, FGR.
- Human immunodeficiency virus (HIV) infection: risk of mother-to-child transfer if untreated.
- Connective tissue diseases, e.g. systemic lupus erythematosus: pre-eclampsia, FGR.
- Myasthenia gravis/myotonic dystrophy: fetal neurological effects and increased maternal muscular fatigue in labour.

---

care received and clinical presentation, and should be made in a systematic and sensitive way at the antenatal booking visit. A good question to lead into this is 'Have you ever suffered with your nerves?'. If women have had children before, you can ask whether they had problems with depression or 'the blues' after the births of any of them. Women with significant psychiatric problems should be cared for by a multidisciplinary team, including the midwife, GP, hospital consultant and psychiatric team.

Drug history

It is vital to establish what drugs women have been taking for their condition and for what duration. You should also ask about over-the-counter medication and homeopathic/herbal remedies. In some cases, medication needs to be changed in pregnancy. For some women it may be possible to stop their medication completely for some or all of the pregnancy (e.g. mild hypertension). Some women need to know that they must continue their medication (e.g. epilepsy, for which women often reduce their medication for fear of potential fetal effects, with detriment to their own health).

Very few drugs that women of childbearing age take are potentially seriously harmful, but a few are, and it is always necessary to ensure that drug treatment is carefully reviewed. Pre-pregnancy counselling is advised for women who are taking potentially harmful drugs such as sodium valproate.

Family history

Family history is important if it can:

- impact on the health of the mother in pregnancy or afterwards;
- have implications for the fetus or baby.

Important areas are a maternal history of a first-degree relative (sibling or parent) with:

- diabetes (increased risk of gestational diabetes);
- thromboembolic disease (increased risk of thrombophilia, thrombosis);
- pre-eclampsia (increased risk of pre-eclampsia);
- serious psychiatric disorder (increased risk of puerperal psychosis).

For both parents, it is important to know about any family history of babies with congenital abnormality and any potential genetic problems, such as haemoglobinopathies. If any close family member has tuberculosis, the baby will be offered immunization after birth.

Finally, any known allergies should be recorded. If a woman gives a history of allergy, it is important to ask about how this was diagnosed and what sort of problems it causes.

Identifying risk

By the time you have finished the history, you will have a general idea of whether or not the pregnancy is likely to be uncomplicated. Of course, in primigravid women, the likelihood of later complications can be difficult to predict, but even here some features such as a strong family history of pre-eclampsia may be present.

Examination

Basic principles of infection control

Hospital acquired infection has been a major problem for some groups of patients. While the incidence among the obstetric population is small, adherence to the principles of infection reduction are vital. In any clinical setting you must remove any wristwatches or rings with stones. You should have bare arms from the elbow down. You should ensure that you use alcohol gel when moving from one clinical area to another (e.g. between wards) and always wash hands or use gel before and after any patient contact. The patient should see you do this before you examine them so that they are confident that you have done so.

Before moving on to examine the patient, it is important to be aware of what you are aiming to achieve. The examination should be directed at the presenting problem, if any, and the gestation. For instance, it is generally unnecessary to spend time defining the presentation at 32 weeks unless the presenting problem is threatened preterm labour.

Maternal weight and height

The measurement of weight at the initial examination is important to identify women who are significantly underweight or overweight. Women with a body mass index (BMI) [weight (kg)/height (m^2)] of <20 are at higher risk of fetal growth restriction and increased perinatal mortality. This is particularly the case if weight gain in pregnancy is poor. Repeated weighing of underweight women during pregnancy will identify that group of women at increased risk for adverse perinatal outcome due to poor weight gain. In the obese woman (BMI >30), the risks of gestational diabetes and hypertension are increased. Additionally, fetal assessment, both by palpation and ultrasound, is more difficult. Obesity is also associated with increased birthweight and a higher perinatal mortality rate.

In women of normal weight at booking, and in whom nutrition is of no concern, there is no need to repeat weight measurement in pregnancy.

Height should be measured at booking to assist with BMI assessment. Other than this, it is only relevant in pregnancy when fetal overgrowth or undergrowth is suspected, as customized charts have significant advantages in the case of very tall or short women, leading to more accurate diagnosis of growth restriction or macrosomia. Short women are significantly more likely to have problems in labour, but these are generally unpredictable during pregnancy. Shoe size is unhelpful when height is known. Height alone is the best indicator of potential problems in labour, but even this is not a useful predictor. On no account should you give women the impression that their labour will be unsuccessful because they are short. Were this always the case, the genes for being short would have disappeared from the population long ago.

Blood pressure evaluation

The first recording of blood pressure should be made as early as possible in pregnancy. Hypertension diagnosed for the first time in early pregnancy (blood pressure >140/90 mmHg on two separate occasions at least 4 hours apart) should prompt a search for underlying causes, i.e. renal, endocrine and collagen-vascular disease. Although 90 per cent of cases will be due to essential hypertension, this is a diagnosis of exclusion and can only be confidently made when other secondary causes have been excluded. Blood pressure measurement is one of the few aspects of antenatal care that is truly beneficial. It should be performed at every visit.

Measure the blood pressure with the woman seated or semi-recumbent. Do not lie her in the left lateral position, as this will lead to under-reading of the blood pressure.

Use an appropriately sized cuff. The cuffs have markings to indicate how they should fit. Large women will need a larger cuff. Using one too small will over-estimate blood pressure. If you are using an automated device and the blood pressure appears high, recheck it with a hand-operated device that has been recently calibrated (every clinic should have one).

Convention is to use Korotkoff V (i.e. disappearance of sounds), as this is more reproducible than Korotkoff IV. Deflate the cuff slowly so that you can record the blood pressure to the nearest 2 mmHg. Do not round up or down. If the Vth sound is heard to near zero, give the values for the IVth and Vth sounds.

Urinary examination

Screening of midstream urine for asymptomatic bacteriuria in pregnancy is of proven benefit. The risk of ascending urinary tract infection in pregnancy is much higher than in the non-pregnant state. Acute pyelonephritis increases the risk of pregnancy loss/premature labour, and is associated with considerable maternal morbidity. Additionally, persistent proteinuria or haematuria may be an indicator of underlying renal disease, prompting further investigation.

At repeat visits, urinalysis should be performed. This is the other proven beneficial aspect of antenatal care. If there is any proteinuria, a thorough evaluation with regard to a diagnosis of pre-eclampsia should be undertaken. A trace of protein is unlikely to be problematic in terms of pre-eclampsia, and may point to urinary tract infection. However, if even a trace of protein is seen persistently, further investigation should be undertaken.

General medical examination

In fit and healthy women presenting for a routine visit there is little benefit in a full formal physical examination. Where a woman presents with a problem, there may be a need to undertake a much more thorough physical examination.

Cardiovascular examination

Routine auscultation for maternal heart sounds in asymptomatic women with no cardiac history is unnecessary. Flow murmurs can be heard in approximately 80 per cent of women at the end of the first trimester. Studies suggest that women coming from areas where rheumatic heart disease is prevalent and those with significant symptoms or a known history of heart murmur or heart disease should undergo cardiovascular examination during pregnancy.

Breast examination

Formal breast examination is not necessary; self-examination is as reliable as a general physician examination in detecting breast masses. Women should, however, be encouraged to report new or suspicious lumps that develop and, where appropriate, full investigation should not be delayed because of pregnancy. The risk of a definite lump being cancer in the under 40s is approximately 5 per cent, and late-stage diagnosis is more common in pregnancy because of delayed referral and investigation. Nipple examination is not a good indicator of problems with breastfeeding and there is no intervention that improves feeding success in women with nipple inversion.

Abdomen

To examine the abdomen of a pregnant woman, place her in a semi-recumbent position on a couch or bed.

Women in late pregnancy or with multiple pregnancies may not be able to lie very flat. Sometimes a pillow under one buttock to move the weight of the fetus a little to the right or left can help. Cover the woman's legs with a sheet and make sure she is comfortable before you start. Always have a chaperone with you to perform this examination.

Think about what you hope to achieve from the examination and ask about areas of tenderness before you start.

Inspection

- Assess the shape of the uterus and note any asymmetry.
- Look for fetal movements.
- Look for scars (women often forget to mention previous surgical procedures if they were performed long ago). The common areas to find scars are:
    - suprapubic (Caesarean section, laparotomy for ectopic pregnancy or ovarian masses);
    - sub-umbilical (laparoscopy);
    - right iliac fossa (appendicectomy);
    - right upper quadrant (cholycystectomy).
- Note any striae gravidarum or linea nigra (the faint brown line running from the umbilicus to the symphysis pubis) – not because they mean anything, but because obstetricians like to see that students notice these.

Palpation

Symphysis–fundal height measurement

First, measure the symphysis–fundal height (SFH). This will give you a clue regarding potential problems such as polyhydramnios, multiple pregnancy or growth restriction before you start to palpate.

Feel carefully for the top of the fundus. This is rarely in the midline. Make a mental note of where it is. Now feel very carefully and gently for the upper border of the symphysis pubis. Place the tape measure on the symphysis pubis and, with the centimetre marks face down, measure to the previously noted top of the fundus. Turn the tape measure over and read the measurement. Plot the measurement on an SFH chart – this will usually be present in the hand-held notes. If plotted on a correctly derived chart, it is apparent that in the

late third trimester the fundal height is usually approximately 2 cm less than the number of weeks. It is always important to use the chart where one is available (Figure 1.2). Encourage women to ask to have their abdomen measured rather than just palpated at every visit and for the results to be plotted on the chart.

Fetal lie, presentation and engagement

Before you start to palpate, you will have an idea about any potential problems. A large SFH raises the possibility of:

- macrosomia;
- multiple pregnancy;
- polyhydramnios.

Rarely, a twin is missed on ultrasound!

A small SFH could represent:

- FGR;
- oligohydramnios.

After you have measured the SFH, palpate to count the number of fetal poles (Figure 1.3). A pole is a head or a bottom. If you can feel one or two, it is likely to be a singleton pregnancy. If you can feel three or four, a twin pregnancy is likely. Sometimes large fibroids can mimic a fetal pole; remember this if there is a history of fibroids.

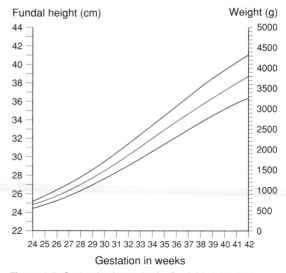

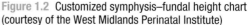

Figure 1.2 Customized symphysis–fundal height chart (courtesy of the West Midlands Perinatal Institute)

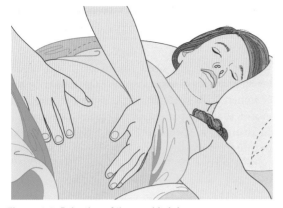

Figure 1.3 Palpation of the gravid abdomen

Now you can assess the lie. This is only necessary as the likelihood of labour increases, i.e. after 34–36 weeks in an uncomplicated pregnancy.

If there is a pole over the pelvis, the lie is longitudinal regardless of whether the other pole is lying more to the left or right. An oblique lie is where the leading pole does not lie over the pelvis, but just to one side; a transverse lie is where the fetus lies directly across the abdomen. Once you have established that there is a pole over the pelvis, if the gestation is 34 weeks or more, you need to establish what the presentation is. It will be either cephalic (head down) or breech (bottom/feet down). Using a two-handed approach and watching the woman's face, gently feel for the presenting part. The head is generally much firmer than the bottom, although even in experienced hands it can sometimes be very difficult to tell. As you are feeling the presenting part in this way, assess whether it is engaged or not. If you can feel the whole of the fetal head and it is easily movable, the head is likely to be 'free'. This equates to 5/5th palpable and is recorded as 5/5. As the head descends into the pelvis, less can be felt. When the head is no longer movable, it has 'engaged' and only 1/5th or 2/5th will be palpable (see Figure 1.4). Do not use a one-handed technique, as this is much more uncomfortable for the woman.

Do not worry about trying to determine the fetal position (i.e. whether the fetal head is occipito-posterior, lateral or anterior). It makes no difference until labour begins, and even then is only of importance if progress in labour is slow. What is more, we do not often get it right, and women can be very worried if told their baby is 'back to back'.

If the SFH is large and the fetal parts very difficult to feel, there may be polyhydramnios present. If the SFH is small and the fetal parts very easy to feel, oligohydramnios may be the problem.

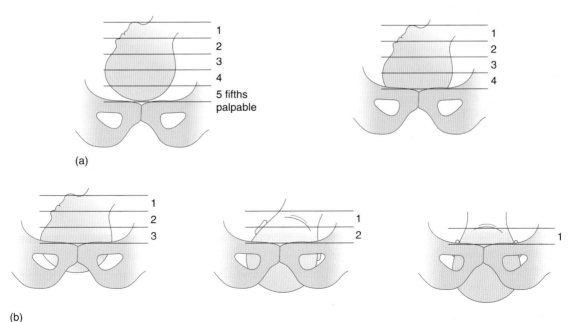

(a)

(b)

Figure 1.4 Palpation of the fetal head to assess engagement

Auscultation

If the fetus has been active during your examination and the mother reports that the baby is active, it is not necessary to auscultate the fetal heart. Very occasionally a problem is detected by auscultation, such as a tachyarrhythmia, but this is rare. Mothers do like to hear the heart beat though and therefore using a hand-held device can allow the mother to hear the heart beat. If you are using a Pinard stethoscope, position it over the fetal shoulder (the *only* reason to assess the fetal position). Hearing the heart sounds with a Pinard takes a lot of practice. If you cannot hear the fetal heart, *never* say that you cannot detect a heart beat; always explain that a different method is needed and move on to use a hand-held Doppler device. If you have begun the process of listening to the fetal heart, you must proceed until you are confident that you have heard the heart. With twins, you must be confident that both have been heard.

Pelvic examination

Routine pelvic examination is not necessary. Given that as many as 18 per cent of women think that a pelvic examination can cause miscarriage, and at least 55 per cent find it an unpleasant experience, routine vaginal examination if ultrasound is planned has few advantages beyond the taking of a cervical smear. Consent must be sought and a female chaperone (nurse, midwife, etc. – never a relative) present (regardless of the sex of the examiner). However, there are circumstances in which a vaginal examination is necessary (in most cases a speculum examination is all that is needed). These include:

- excessive or offensive discharge;
- vaginal bleeding (in the known absence of a placenta praevia);
- to perform a cervical smear;
- to confirm potential rupture of membranes.

A digital examination may be undertaken to perform a membrane sweep at term, prior to induction of labour.

The contraindications to digital examination are:

- known placenta praevia or vaginal bleeding when the placental site is unknown and the presenting part unengaged;

- prelabour rupture of the membranes (increased risk of ascending infection).

Before commencing the examination, assemble everything you will need (swabs etc.) and ensure the light source works. Position the patient semi-recumbent with knees drawn up and ankles together. Ensure that the patient is adequately covered. If performing a speculum examination, a Cusco speculum is usually used (Figure 1.5). Select an appropriate size.

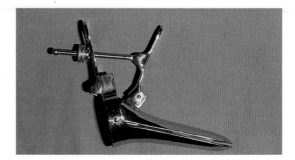

Figure 1.5 A Cusco speculum

Proceed as follows:

- Wash your hands and put on a pair of gloves.
- If the speculum is metal, warm it slightly under warm water first.
- Apply sterile lubricating gel or cream to the blades of the speculum. Do not use Hibitane cream if taking swabs for bacteriology.
- Gently part the labia.
- Introduce the speculum with the blades in the vertical plane.
- As the speculum is gently introduced, aiming towards the sacral promontory (i.e. slightly downward), rotate the speculum so that it comes to lie in the horizontal plane with the ratchet uppermost.
- The blades can then slowly be opened until the cervix is visualized. Sometimes minor adjustments need to be made at this stage.
- Assess the cervix and take any necessary samples.
- Gently close the blades and remove the speculum, reversing the manoeuvres needed to insert it. Take care not to catch the vaginal epithelium when removing the speculum.

Table 1.1 Bishop score

	Score			
	0	1	2	3
Dilation of cervix (cm)	0	1 or 2	3 or 4	5 or more
Consistency of cervix	Firm	Medium	Soft	
Length of cervical canal	>2	2–1	1–0.5	<0.5
Position	Posterior	Central	Anterior	
Station of presenting part (cm above ischial spine)	3	2	1 or 0	Below

A digital examination may be performed when an assessment of the cervix is required. This can provide information about the consistency and effacement of the cervix that is not obtainable from a speculum examination.

The patient should be positioned as before. Examining from the patient's right, two fingers of the gloved right hand are gently introduced into the vagina and advanced until the cervix is palpated. Prior to induction of labour, a full assessment of the Bishop score can be made (Table 1.1).

Other aspects of the examination

In the presence of hypertension and in women with headache, fundoscopy should be performed. Signs of chronic hypertension include silver-wiring and arteriovenous nipping. In severe pre-eclampsia and some intracranial conditions (space-occupying lesions, benign intracranial hypertension), papilloedema may be present.

Oedema of the extremities affects 80 per cent of term pregnancies. Its presence should be noted, but it is not a good indicator for pre-eclampsia as it is so common. To assess pre-tibial oedema, press reasonably firmly over the pre-tibial surface for 20 seconds. This can be very painful if there is excessive oedema, and when there is it is so obvious that testing for pitting is not necessary. More importantly, facial oedema should be commented upon.

When pre-eclampsia is suspected, the reflexes should be assessed. These are most easily checked at the ankle. The presence of more than three beats of clonus is pathological (see Chapter 10, Pre-eclampsia and other disorders of placentation).

Presentation skills

Part of the art of taking a history and performing an examination is to be able to pass this information on to others in a clear and concise format. It is not necessary to give a full list of negative findings; it is enough to summarize negatives such as: there is no important medical, surgical or family history of note. Adapt your style of presentation to meet the situation. A very concise presentation is needed for a busy ward round. In an examination, a full and thorough presentation may be required. Be very aware of giving sensitive information in a ward setting where other patients may be within hearing distance.

Key points

- Always introduce yourself and say who you are.
- Make sure you are wearing your identity badge.
- Wash your hands or use alcohol gel.
- Be courteous and gentle.
- Always ensure the patient is comfortable and warm.
- Always have a chaperone present when you examine patients.
- Tailor your history and examination to find the key information you need.
- Adapt to new findings as you go along.
- Present in a clear way.
- Be aware of giving sensitive information in a public setting.

History template

Demographic details

- Name
- Age
- Occupation
- Make a note of ethnic background
- Presenting complaint or reason for attending

This pregnancy

- Gestation, LMP or EDD
- Dates as calculated from ultrasound
- Single/multiple (chorionicity)
- Details of the presenting problem (if any) or reason for attendance (such as problems in a previous pregnancy)
- What action has been taken?
- Is there a plan for the rest of the pregnancy?
- What are the patient's main concerns?
- Have there been any other problems in this pregnancy?
- Has there been any bleeding, contractions or loss of fluid vaginally?

Ultrasound

- What scans have been performed?
- Why?
- Were any problems identified?

Past obstetric history

- List the previous pregnancies and their outcomes in order

Gynaecological history

- Periods: regularity
- Contraceptive history
- Previous infections and their treatment
- When was the last cervical smear? Was it normal? Have there ever been any that were abnormal? If yes, what treatment has been undertaken?
- Previous gynaecological surgery

Past medical and surgical history

- Relevant medical problems
- Any previous operations; type of anaesthetic used, any complications

Psychiatric history

- Postpartum blues or depression
- Depression unrelated to pregnancy
- Major psychiatric illness

Family history

- Diabetes, hypertension, genetic problems, psychiatric problems, etc.

Social history

- Smoking/alcohol/drugs
- Marital status
- Occupation, partner's occupation
- Who is available to help at home?
- Are there any housing problems?

Drugs

- All medication including over-the-counter medication
- Folate supplementation

Allergies

- To what?
- What problems do they cause?

MODERN MATERNITY CARE

Lucy Kean

OVERVIEW

Modern maternity care has evolved over more than 100 years. Many of the changes have been driven by political and consumer pressure. Only recently has any good quality research been conducted into which aspects of care actually make a difference to women and their babies. In the United Kingdom, we are in the enviable position of being able to receive quality maternity care, free at the point of need. This is not so for the majority of women across the world. Despite signing up to ambitious targets for the reduction of maternal mortality, the global community is failing to achieve reductions in mortality, making pregnancy and childbirth a life-threatening challenge for millions of women.

History of maternity care in the UK

The original impetus to address the health of mothers and children was driven by a lack of healthy recruits to fight in the Boer War. Up until this point, successive governments had paid little attention to maternal or child health. In 1929 the first government document stated a minimum standard for antenatal care that was so prescriptive in its recommendations that until very recently it was practised in many regions, despite the lack of research to demonstrate effectiveness.

The National Health Service Act 1946 came into effect on 5 July 1948 and created the National Health Service (NHS) in England and Wales. The introduction of the NHS provided for maternity services to be available to all without cost. As part of these arrangements, a specified fee was paid to the general practitioner (GP) depending on whether he or she was on the obstetric list. This encouraged a large number of GPs to take an interest in maternity care, reversing the previous trend to leave this work to the midwives.

Antenatal care became perceived as beneficial, acceptable and available for all. This was reinforced by the finding that the perinatal death rate seemed to be inversely proportional to the number of antenatal visits. In 1963, the first perinatal mortality study showed that the perinatal mortality rate was lowest for those women attending between 10 and 24 times in pregnancy. This failed to take into account prematurity and poor education as reasons for decreased visits and increased mortality. However, antenatal care became established, and with increased professional contact came the drive to continue to improve outcomes with an emphasis on mortality (maternal and perinatal), without always establishing the need for or safety of all procedures or interventions for all women.

The ability to see into the pregnant uterus in 1958 with ultrasound brought with it a revolution in antenatal care. This new intervention became quickly established and is now so much part of current antenatal care that the fact that its use in improving the outcome for low-risk women was never proven has been little questioned. Attending for the 'scan' has become such a social part of antenatal care that many surmise that it is, for many women, the sole reason for attending the hospital antenatal clinic.

The move towards hospital confinement began in the early 1950s. At this time, there were simply not the facilities to allow hospital confinement for all women, and one in three were planned home deliveries. The Cranbrook Report in 1959 recommended sufficient hospital maternity beds for 70 per cent of all confinements to take place in hospital, and the subsequent Peel Report (1970) recommended a bed available for every woman to deliver in hospital if she so wished.

The trend towards hospital confinement was not only led by obstetricians. Women themselves were pushing to at least be allowed the choice to deliver in hospital. By 1972, only one in ten deliveries were planned for home, and the publication of the Social Services Committee report in The Short Report (1980) led to further centralization of hospital confinement. It made a number of recommendations. Among these were:

An increasing number of patients should be delivered in large units; selection of patients should be improved for smaller consultant units and isolated GP units; home deliveries should be phased out further.

It should be mandatory that all pregnant women should be seen at least twice by a consultant obstetrician – preferably as soon as possible after the first visit to the GP in early pregnancy and again in late pregnancy.

This report and the subsequent reports Maternity Care in Action, Antenatal and Intrapartum Care, and Postnatal and Neonatal Care led to a policy of increasing centralization of units for delivery and consequently care. Thus home deliveries are now very infrequent events, with most regions reporting less than 2 per cent of births in the community, the majority of these being unplanned.

The gradual decline in maternal and perinatal mortality was thought to be due in greater part to this move, although proof for this was lacking. Indeed, the decline in perinatal mortality was least in those years when hospitalization increased the most. As other new technologies became available, such as continuous fetal monitoring and the ability to induce labour, a change in practice began to establish these as the norm for most women. In England and Wales between 1966 and 1974, the induction rate rose from 12.7 to 38.9 per cent.

The fact that these new technologies had not undergone thorough trials of benefit prior to introduction meant that benefit to the whole population of women was never established.

During the 1980s, with increasing consumer awareness, the unquestioning acceptance of unproven technologies was challenged. Women, led by the more vociferous groups such as the National Childbirth Trust (NCT), began to question not only the need for any intervention but also the need to come to the hospital at all. The professional bodies also began to question the effectiveness of antenatal care.

The government set up an expert committee to review policy on maternity care and to make recommendations. This committee produced the document Changing Childbirth (Department of Health, Report of the Expert Maternity Group, 1993), which essentially provided purchasers and providers with a number of action points aiming to improve choice, information and continuity for all women. It outlined a number of indicators of success to be achieved within five years:

- the carriage of hand-held notes by women;
- midwifery-led care in 30 per cent of pregnancies;
- a known midwife at delivery in 75 per cent of cases;
- a reduction in the number of antenatal visits for low-risk mothers.

Unfortunately, those targets which required significant financial input, such as the presence of a known midwife at 75 per cent of deliveries, have not been met. Nevertheless, this landmark report did provide a new impetus to examine the provision of maternity care in the UK and enshrine choice as a concept in maternity care.

The most recent government document on maternity care, Maternity Matters, aims to address inequalities in maternity care provision and uptake and is essentially a document for commissioners to assess maternity care in their area and to ensure that safe and effective care is available to all women.

The pendulum has swung back, with the government now moving towards increased choices for women including birth at home or in a stand-alone midwifery unit.

Coordination of research: the Cochrane Library

The study of the effectiveness of pregnancy care has been revolutionized by the establishment of the Cochrane Library. This has led to the evaluation of each aspect of antenatal, intrapartum and post-natal care, and allowed each to be meticulously examined on the basis of the available trials. Concentrating particularly on the randomized controlled trial design, and using meta-analysis, obstetric practice has been scrutinized to an extent unique in medicine.

The database originally grew from the publication of Archie Cochrane's *Effectiveness and efficiency: random reflections on health services in 1972*. The identification of controlled trials in perinatal medicine began in Cardiff in 1974. In 1978, the World Health Organization and English Department of Health funded work at the National Perinatal Epidemiology Unit, Oxford, UK, to assemble a register of controlled trials in perinatal medicine. Now the collaboration covers all branches of medicine. The findings are published in the Cochrane Library, which is free to access for all UK healthcare workers via the National Library for Health at www. library.nhs.uk. It is serially updated to keep up with published work and represents an enormous body of information available to the clinician.

Involvement of professional bodies and consumer groups in maternity care

Maternity care is considered so important that many clinical, political and consumer bodies are now involved in how it is provided.

National Institute for Health and Clinical Excellence

As can be seen from the above, maternity care has been the subject of political debate for the last 100 years. More recently, attention has been paid to differences in standards of health care across the UK. The National Institute for Health and Clinical Excellence (NICE) has evaluated maternity care in great detail and has published a number of important guidelines, covering antenatal, intrapartum and post-natal care. Trusts are judged by their ability to provide care to the standards set out in these guidelines. The process of guideline development is rigorous and stakeholders are consulted at each stage of development. The guidelines are available through the NICE website (www.nice.org.uk) and provide the framework for standards of care within England and Wales.

National Screening Committee

Screening has formed a part of antenatal care since its inception. Antenatal care is essentially screening in its widest form. The National Screening Committee is responsible for developing standards and strategies for the implementation of these. The National Screening Committee has unified and progressed standards for all aspects of antenatal screening across the United Kingdom.

The provision of national standards means that new tests are critically evaluated before being offered to populations. Screening for additional diseases/conditions to those given below is only considered if the test is good enough and the disease/condition meets the very stringent criteria for justification of screening. Conditions for which screening is currently not recommended, such as group B streptococcus carriage, are regularly reviewed against current evidence.

Antenatal screening is now offered for:

- Down's syndrome;
- fetal anomaly (by ultrasound);
- haemoglobinopathies;
- rubella status;
- HIV/hepatitis B status;
- Tay–Sachs disease in high-risk populations.

Newborn screening includes:

- hearing;
- phenylketonuria;
- congenital hypothyroidism;
- cystic fibrosis;
- medium chain acyl co-A dehydrogenase deficiency.

Royal College of Obstetricians and Gynaecologists

The Royal College of Obstetricians and Gynaecologists (RCOG) has many roles. These include developing guidelines, setting standards for the provision of care, training and revalidation, audit and research.

Guidelines and standards

The RCOG publishes a large number of guidelines pertinent to pregnancy with patient information leaflets to accompany many of these. They are reviewed three-yearly and are accessible to all on the college website (www.rcog.org.uk).

The RCOG works in partnership with other colleges such as the Royal College of Midwives to set standards for maternity care. These standards provide important drivers to organizations such as the Clinical Negligence Scheme for Trusts in setting standards for levels of care and performance by hospitals.

Revalidation and continuing professional development

Revalidation of professionals is increasingly important. In order to be maintained on the General Medical Council Register, all doctors will need to produce evidence that they are keeping up to date within their chosen specialty. In the near future, failure to provide evidence of revalidation will lead to the removal of a doctor's licence to practise medicine. Part of the revalidation process involves the coordination and documentation of education and professional developmental activity. The RCOG plays the major role in this important task. All practising obstetricians will need to complete a five-year cycle of education in order to be registered.

Training

The college also has an important role in ensuring quality of training of doctors wishing to become consultants. It is recognized that with the limitations on working time that have come into force as a result of the European Working Time Directive, and a government initiative to limit total time in training, junior doctors now work many fewer hours than previously. Training has changed from an apprenticeship to a much more structured programme. The need to identify specific training areas has led to the development of special skills modules in obstetrics, which include labour ward management, maternal medicine and fetal medicine. Additionally there is a longer, two to three years, training scheme in maternal and fetal medicine, aimed at those who wish to train to become sub-specialists in this area.

Confidential enquiries and audit

Another important role of the college is to coordinate national audit in conjunction with other bodies such as the Royal Colleges of Midwives, Paediatricians and Anaesthetists and NCT. The Clinical Effectiveness Support Unit produced The National Sentinel Caesarean Section Audit Report, examining Caesarean sections across the UK. The audit came about as a result of concern regarding the increasing Caesarean section rate. It has provided interesting data for the trends in Caesarean section across the UK.

The confidential enquiries are a vital source of information to clinicians and service providers. These are produced under the umbrella of the Centre for Maternal and Child Enquiries (CMACE), previously known as the Confidential Enquiries into Maternal and Child Health (CEMACH).

CMACE produce national and local audits and reports into a wide range of maternal and child health issues. From an obstetric perspective, the most important is the triennial report on maternal mortality. This report has led to important improvements in maternity care, with significant reductions in deaths from thromboembolism, hypertension and anaesthesia being seen after national recommendations made through this channel (Figure 2.1).

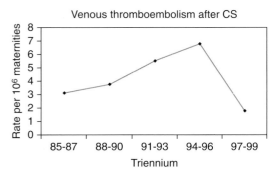

Figure 2.1 Death rates from venous thromboembolism in the triennia following new recommendations on thromboprophylaxis

Clinical Negligence Scheme for Trusts

Obstetrics is the highest litigation risk area in the NHS. It is estimated that the outstanding potential obstetric litigation bill is of the order of £200 million. As individual hospitals cannot hope to meet the cost of huge settlements, sometimes running into millions of pounds, an insurance scheme has been established. The Clinical Negligence Scheme for Trusts (CNST) was established by the NHS Executive in 1994 'to provide a means for Trusts to fund the costs of clinical negligence litigation and to encourage and support effective management of claims and risk'. The amount any individual hospital has to pay to the scheme is graded from level 0 to 3. The insurance premium is discounted by 10 per cent for a level 1 trust, 20 per cent for level 2 and 30 per cent for level 3. In 2003, it was decided to assess obstetrics separately, as many trusts were failing on the obstetric standards only. The standards set by CNST are stringent. They cover:

- organization;
- clinical care;
- high-risk conditions;
- communication;
- post-natal and newborn care.

Within each standard is a wide range of organizational and clinical standards.

Trusts are assessed at least every two years. They can bring forward an assessment if they believe they have improved, as the financial implications of improved grading are great. Improvements in maternity care are therefore linked to financial incentive, and measurable improvements in many units have been brought about as managers realize the importance of improving standards of care.

Consumer groups

There are now more consumer and support groups in existence than ever before. As well as providing support and advice for women, often at times of great need, they also allow women to have a louder voice in the planning and provision of maternity care. National consumer groups such as the NCT have representatives on many influential panels, such as the National Screening Committee and RCOG working groups. At a local level, each hospital should have a Maternity Services Liaison Committee (MSLC). When these committees work well, they can provide essential consumer input into service delivery at a local level. Consumers should make up at least one-third of the membership of the MSLCs. The influence of consumer groups can be huge: the recommendation that all women should have the right to deliver in hospital was essentially consumer led. Interestingly, it was this drive that led to the demise of many local units, the centralization of obstetric services and a huge reduction in the numbers of home deliveries, something that consumer groups are now trying to reverse. Many groups have been criticized as being unrepresentative of the whole population. This will continue to be so, as disenfranchised groups are less

able to coordinate themselves to be heard. However, many groups are making efforts to canvass the opinions of those rarely heard, such as teenagers and women who speak little or no English.

Choice is now being sought by consumers in a way never experienced before. The National Sentinel Caesarean Section Audit Report showed that maternal choice as a reason for Caesarean section is becoming increasingly common, a move driven, at least in part, by high-profile women choosing not to undergo labour with their first baby. Consumer groups will need to lead the way in deciding how far choice should be balanced against the financial constraints of a free-at-the-point-of-care health service. The guidelines on Caesarean section produced by NICE promote the ideal of Caesarean section for obstetric indications only, although they do not go as far as recommending that women's preferences be completely ignored.

Maternity care: the global challenge

In 2005, at the last survey conducted by the World Health Organization, 536 000 mothers died worldwide. In the worst areas (sub-Saharan Africa) there were 450 deaths per 10 000 live births, giving women in these areas a one in 26 risk of not surviving childbirth. At the Millennium Summit in 2000, the international community set improving maternal health as one of the eight Millennium Development Goals. The aim was to reduce the maternal mortality ratio (MMR) by three-quarters by 2015. To achieve this, a 5.5 per cent reduction in yearly maternal mortality was needed. The 2005 survey has shown that maternal mortality has fallen at less than 1 per cent per year.

Defining maternal death has been a challenge. Countries where data are easy to collect are able to collate data related to deaths in pregnancy and up to a year afterwards for all causes of death, but where data collection is more difficult a stricter definition is used. The International Statistical Classification of Diseases and Related Health Problems, Tenth Revision, 1992 (ICD-10) (WHO) defines maternal death as:

the death of a woman while pregnant or within 42 days of termination of pregnancy, irrespective of the duration and site of the pregnancy, from any cause related to or aggravated by the pregnancy or its management but not from accidental or incidental causes.

Measuring maternal deaths

In the UK, we tend to take for granted our ability to collect accurate data. However, for the international community this is a major issue. The MMR is defined as the number of maternal deaths in a population divided by the number of live births; thus, it depicts the risk of maternal death relative to the number of live births. By contrast, the maternal mortality rate (MMRate) is defined as the number of maternal deaths in a population divided by the number of women of reproductive age, reflecting not only the risk of maternal death per pregnancy or per birth (live birth or stillbirth), but also the level of fertility in the population. In addition to the MMR and the MMRate, it is possible to calculate the adult lifetime risk of maternal mortality for women in the population (Table 2.1).

Table 2.1 Statistical measures of maternal deaths (from Estimates of Maternal Mortality 2005)

Maternal mortality ratio: Number of maternal deaths during a given time period per 100 000 livebirths during the same time period

Maternal mortality rate: Number of maternal deaths in a given period per 100 000 women of reproductive age during the same time period

Adult lifetime risk of maternal death: The probability of dying from a maternal cause during a woman's reproductive period

These definitions provide the framework for reporting and collating data. However, the practicalities of data collection mean that many civil data sets are incomplete. In countries where the cause of death may not be accurately defined, it may be unusual to note or even know that a woman was or had been pregnant at the time of her death. Therefore, civil registration systems (official records of births and deaths) are augmented in many countries such as the UK by independent Confidential Enquiries. Where civil data collection is not available, household surveys are often used. These can only provide estimates, as only a proportion of the population will be surveyed and in order to collect data on uncommon

outcomes, large surveys are required, which can be expensive.

Sisterhood methods have been employed, whereby cohorts of women are questioned about the survival of their adult sisters. This method has an advantage of reducing the sample size. It is less useful in areas of lower fertility (where women have fewer than four pregnancies) and where there is substantial migration of populations.

Other types of data collection include reproductive age mortality surveys and census data. Surveys tend to be more accurate, but are very time-consuming and expensive. Census data tend to be of lesser quality, but can capture data from larger populations.

It is recognized, therefore, that data collected for analysis of worldwide maternal mortality are estimates based on the best available sources. Figure 2.2 shows the Estimates of MMR, by United Nations Population Division regions, 2005.

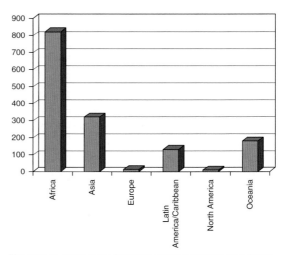

Figure 2.2 Estimates of MMR by United Nations Population Division regions, 2005

Much effort has been directed at defining why women die. Three-quarters of maternal deaths are due to a complication directly attributable to the pregnancy, such as haemorrhage or hypertension. The remaining quarter of deaths are due to conditions that may be worsened by the pregnancy, such as heart disease. Figure 2.3 shows the proportion of deaths worldwide by the individual causes.

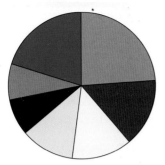

- ▨ Haemorrhage
- ■ Infection
- ☐ Unsafe abortion
- ☐ Hypertension
- ■ Obstructed labour
- ▨ Other direct causes
- ■ Other indirect causes

Figure 2.3 Causes of maternal mortality. Other direct causes include ectopic pregnancy, embolism, anaesthesia-related causes. Indirect causes include anaemia, malaria, heart disease.

Most of the common complications of childbirth do not cause death within a short time. If facilities for transfer of women are available, there can be a dramatic effect on maternal mortality. The most life-threatening complication at delivery is haemorrhage. In 2004 the WHO advocated the presence of a skilled attendant at every delivery. Despite this goal the most recent WHO figures show that a trained person attends only 46.5 per cent of women giving birth in Africa. Reaching the Millennium Goal will not be achieved at the present slow rate of change. Political pressure on governments to improve health care for women will continue to need to be high on the worldwide agenda.

Key points

- Maternity care will continue to be a political arena, as it has been for nearly 100 years.
- There is increasing public interest in the results of national audits such as the Confidential Enquiries.
- Antenatal care is subject to national standards in a way never seen before.
- The need for trusts to reduce insurance costs is leading to improved standards of care across the UK.
- National guidelines now cover almost all aspects of maternity care and should lead to standardization of care across the UK.
- The global challenge of reducing the risks of pregnancy and childbirth is not yet being met.

Additional reading

Audit Commission for Local Health Authorities and the National Health Service in England and Wales. First class delivery: improving maternity services in England and Wales. London: HSMO, 1997.

CNST standards for maternity services: available online at www.nhsla.com.

Cochrane Library: available online at www.library.nhs.uk.

Department of Health. Changing childbirth. Report of the Expert Maternity Group. London: HMSO, 1993.

Maternity Matters: choice, access and continuity of care in a safe service. London: DOH, 2007.

CHAPTER 3

PHYSIOLOGICAL CHANGES IN PREGNANCY

Keelin O'Donoghue

OVERVIEW

Every maternal organ adapts to pregnancy, each at a different time and in a different way. Maternal systems adapt as pregnancy progresses to accommodate the increasing demands of fetal growth and development. Management of both healthy and diseased pregnancy necessitates knowledge of the physiology of normal pregnancy. Understanding these adaptations enable clinicians to identify abnormal changes that lead to complications, as well as recognize changes that mimic disease, and understand altered responses to stress. This chapter outlines maternal physiological adaptations to pregnancy, indicating the potential for misinterpretation of clinical signs and providing explanations for the changes that occur.

Early pregnancy

In early pregnancy, the developing fetus, corpus luteum and placenta produce and release increasing quantities of hormones, growth factors and other substances into the maternal circulation. This triggers a cascade of events that transform the mother's cardiovascular, respiratory and renal systems. The first trimester of pregnancy is therefore a transition period between the pregnant and non-pregnant state, during which changes in all these systems take place to prepare the mother to support fetal growth. Most pregnant women report symptoms of pregnancy by the end of the sixth week after the last menstrual period. It is assumed that most physiological adaptations are completed during the first trimester, although studies examining early pregnancy physiological changes are limited, with few longitudinal measurements prior to conception and throughout the first trimester.

Following implantation, the maternal adaptation to pregnancy can be categorized based on the following functions:

1. increased availability of precursors for hormone production and fetal–placental metabolism;

2. improved transport capacity;

3. maternal–fetal exchange; and

4. removal of additional waste products.

Increased availability of metabolic substrates and hormones is achieved by increases in dietary intake, as well as endocrine changes that increase the availability of substrates like glucose. Transport capacity is enhanced by increases in cardiac output, facilitating both the transport of substrates to the placenta, and fetal waste products to maternal organs for disposal. The placenta regulates maternal–fetal exchange by 10–12 weeks gestation, but transfer occurs through other mechanisms before this. Disposal of waste products (heat, carbon dioxide and metabolic byproducts) occurs through peripheral vasodilatation and by increases in ventilation and renal filtration.

Volume homeostasis

Maternal blood volume expands during pregnancy to allow adequate perfusion of vital organs, including the placenta and fetus, and to anticipate blood loss associated with delivery. The rapid expansion of blood volume begins at 6–8 weeks gestation and plateaus at 32–34 weeks gestation. While there is some increase in intracellular water, the most marked expansion occurs in extracellular fluid volume, especially circulating plasma volume. This expanded extracellular fluid volume accounts for between 8 and 10 kg of the average maternal weight gain during pregnancy. Overall, total body water increases from 6.5 to 8.5 L by the end of pregnancy. Changes in blood volume are key to other physiological adaptations; predominantly increases in cardiac output and in renal blood flow. The interpretation of haematological indices in normal pregnancy is also affected, for example the larger increase of plasma volume relative to erythrocyte volume results in haemodilution and a physiologic anaemia (Figure 3.1).

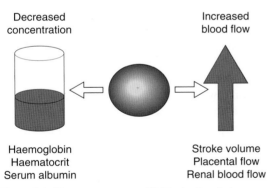

Decreased concentration

Increased blood flow

Haemoglobin
Haematocrit
Serum albumin

Stroke volume
Placental flow
Renal blood flow

Figure 3.1 The consequences of fluid retention during pregnancy. The concentrations of certain substances in the circulation decrease, whereas there are marked increases in haemodynamics

The mechanisms responsible for fluid retention and changes in blood volume are unclear. Outside of pregnancy, sodium is the most important determinant of extracellular fluid volume. In pregnancy, changes in osmoregulation and the renin-angiotensin system result in active sodium reabsorption in renal tubules and water retention. However, while there is a net retention of sodium during normal pregnancy (3–4 mmol per day) and concentrations of anti-natriuretic hormones increase, opposing natriuretic factors, such as atrial natriuretic peptide and progesterone, also increase during pregnancy. A large proportion of the retained sodium must be sequestered within fetal tissues (including placenta, membranes and amniotic fluid). As maternal plasma sodium concentration decreases slightly during pregnancy it is possible that other factors, such as changes in intracellular metabolism, may contribute to fluid retention.

Another feature of this change in fluid balance is that plasma osmolality decreases by about 10 mOsmol/kg. Whereas in the non-pregnant state such a decrease would be associated with a rapid diuresis in order to maintain volume homeostasis, the pregnant woman appears to tolerate this level of osmolality. There is also a decrease in the thirst threshold so that pregnant women feel the urge to drink at a lower level of plasma osmolality than non-pregnant women. Further, plasma osmotic pressure decreases during pregnancy, while oncotic pressure (colloid osmotic pressure) is reduced. Plasma oncotic pressure is mainly determined by albumin concentration, and this decreases by about 20 per cent during normal pregnancy to levels (23–33 g/L) that are considered abnormal outside pregnancy. As plasma oncotic pressure partly determines the degree to which fluid passes into and out of capillaries, its decrease is one of the factors responsible for the increase in glomerular filtration rate (GFR) during pregnancy and probably contributes to the development of peripheral oedema, a feature of normal pregnancy.

Key points

Factors contributing to fluid retention
- Sodium retention.
- Resetting of osmostat.
- ↓ Thirst threshold.
- ↓ Plasma oncotic pressure.

Consequences of fluid retention
- ↓ Haemoglobin concentration.
- ↓ Haematocrit.
- ↓ Serum albumin concentration.
- ↑ Stroke volume.
- ↑ Renal blood flow.

Blood

Haematology

Maternal haemoglobin levels are decreased because of the discrepancy between the 1000 to 1500 mL increases in plasma volume and the increase in erythrocyte mass, which is around 280 mL. Transfer of iron stores to the fetus contributes further to this physiological anaemia. The mean haemoglobin concentration falls from 13.3 g/dL in the non-pregnant state to 10.9 g/dL at the 36th week of normal pregnancy. A normal pregnancy haematocrit is approximately 32–34 per cent, also lower than non-pregnant values. These physiological changes may be mistaken for the development of pathological anaemia, most commonly due to iron deficiency. Pregnant women require increased amounts of iron, and absorption of dietary iron from the gut is increased as a result. Despite this adaptation, women who do not take supplementary iron during pregnancy show a reduction in iron in the bone marrow as well as a progressive reduction in mean red cell volume and serum ferritin levels. The latter are still lower at six months after delivery than in early pregnancy, suggesting that pregnancy without iron supplementation leads to depletion of iron stores.

Renal clearance of folic acid increases substantially during normal pregnancy and plasma folate concentrations fall. However, red cell folate concentrations do not decrease to the same extent. Folate supplementation for haematinic purposes in women eating an adequate diet and carrying a single fetus is therefore not routinely indicated. Finally, the maternal platelet count usually remains stable throughout pregnancy, although may be lower than in the non-pregnant state due to increased aggregation. Increases in the platelet count have been reported in the first week postpartum and this may contribute to the increased risk of thromboembolic complications in this period.

Haemostasis and coagulation

Pregnancy is a hypercoagulable state, which returns to normal around 4 weeks after delivery. Changes in the haemostatic system are presumed to occur in preparation for delivery. Almost all procoagulant factors, including factors VII, VIII, IX, X and XII and fibrinogen, are increased during pregnancy. Fibrinogen is increased by 50 per cent, from a mean of 300 mg/dL in the non-pregnant state to a mean of 450 mg/dL in pregnancy. Levels of von Willebrand factor, which serves as a carrier for factor VIII and plays a role in platelet adhesion, also increase in pregnancy. Antithrombin III levels remain unchanged, whereas protein S activity decreases, and there is an increase in activated protein C resistance. Plasma homocysteine concentrations are lower in normal pregnancy when compared with the non-pregnant state, with concentrations lowest in the second trimester before returning to non-pregnant levels postpartum. Maternal plasma D-dimer concentration increases progressively from conception until delivery, which limits the use of D-dimer testing to rule out suspected venous thromboembolism in symptomatic pregnant women. At the beginning of the second trimester, more than 50 per cent of pregnant women have a D-dimer concentration that exceeds 0.50 mg/L and by the third trimester, more than 90 per cent of women have a D-dimer concentration >0.50 mg/L.

tPA (tissue plasminogen activator) converts plasminogen into plasmin, which cleaves fibrin and fibrinogen, yielding fibrin degradation products. α2-antiplasmin, a plasmin inhibitor, and PAI-1 and PAI-2 (plasminogen activator inhibitor type 1 and type 2), prevent excess fibrin degradation by plasmin. Endothelial-derived PAI-1 increases in late pregnancy, whereas placental-derived PAI-2, detectable in the plasma during the first trimester, increases throughout pregnancy. Plasminogen levels are also increased during pregnancy, whereas levels of α2-antiplasmin are decreased. These changes, together with increases in D-dimers and fibrin degradation products, are indicative of a substantial increase in fibrinolytic system activation, possibly to counterbalance increased coagulation factors.

The increase in procoagulants, potential for vascular damage and increased venous stasis particularly in the lower extremities, explains why the incidence of venous thromboembolic complications is five times greater during pregnancy. However, this relative hypercoagulability is particularly relevant at delivery, with placental separation. At term, around 500 mL of blood flows through the placental bed every minute. Without effective and rapid haemostasis, a woman could rapidly die from blood loss. Myometrial contractions first compress the blood vessels supplying the placental bed, followed by fibrin deposition over the placental site, with up to 10 per cent of circulating fibrinogen used up for this purpose. Factors that impede this haemostatic process, such as inadequate uterine contraction or incomplete placental separation, can therefore rapidly lead to depletion of fibrinogen.

Biochemistry

Plasma protein concentrations, particularly albumin, are decreased during normal pregnancy, which not only affects the plasma oncotic pressure (as already discussed), but also affects the peak plasma concentrations of drugs that are highly protein bound. Serum creatinine, uric acid and urea concentrations are reduced during normal pregnancy, although the renal handling of uric acid changes in late gestation, resulting in increased re-absorption. Alkaline phosphatase levels increase throughout pregnancy, due to production of placental alkaline phosphatase. In contrast, levels of alanine transaminase and aspartate transaminase have been shown to be lower in uncomplicated pregnancy when compared to non-pregnant levels. Liver enzymes also change rapidly postpartum and are affected by many common obstetric events, such as delivery by Caesarean section. The lactate dehydrogenase (LDH) concentration in serum either remains unaltered or increases a small amount during normal pregnancy. The observed rise in serum LDH 1 week after delivery might originate from the involuting uterus and from damaged erythrocytes involved in the haemostatic process in the placental bed.

Normal parameters

Most laboratory parameters change during normal pregnancy (Table 3.1). However, little attention is usually paid to these gestational changes in electrolytes, or other biochemical components of the serum and haematological parameters of the blood. While all laboratories have reference intervals for healthy men and women, many lack ranges for pregnant women. It is now known that the reference values of most routine laboratory parameters change during pregnancy and the puerperium. Therefore, clinicians treating pregnant women must be aware of the physiological changes that occur during pregnancy to avoid misinterpretation of laboratory results, which could lead to erroneous diagnoses or incorrect treatment.

Table 3.1 Changes in reference values in normal pregnancy. Values vary slightly with different laboratory methods

	Non-pregnant	Pregnant (term)
Haemoglobin (g/dL)	13.3	11.0
Haematocrit (%)	38–45	32–34
White cell count ($\times 10^9$/L)	4–11	6–14
Fibrinogen (mg/dL)	300	450
Platelets ($\times 10^9$/L)	140–440	150–400
Ferritin (μg/L)	17–320	4.8–43.5
Sodium (mmol/L)	132–144	127–140
Potassium (mmol/L)	3.5–5.0	3.3–5.4
Urea (mmol/L)	4.3	3.1
Creatinine (μmol/L)	73	64
Uric acid (μmol/L)	246	269 (186–401)
Albumin (g/L)	37–48	23–38
Alanine aminotransferase (IU/L)	4–40	6–28
Alkaline phosphatase (IU/L)	30–130	133–418
Bilirubin (μmol/L)	2–20	<3.0–19.4
Triglycerides (mmol/L)	0.3–1.7	1.6–5.8
TSH (mU/L)	0.4–3.8	0.4–5.3

The immune response

Historically, pregnancy was considered an immunosuppressive state, which allowed the fetal allograft to implant and develop. It is now accepted that the placental barrier is imperfect, with bidirectional traffic of all types of maternal and fetal cells across it, and is thus an important interface of maternal–fetal immunological interaction. Approximately 30 per cent of women develop IgG antibodies against the inherited paternal human leukocyte antigen of the fetus, but the role of these antibodies is unclear and there is no evidence of attack on the fetus. This lack of maternal immune reactivity to the fetus is most likely due to reduced numbers of cytotoxic (CD8$^+$) T cells during pregnancy, with potentially harmful T cell-mediated immune responses downregulated and components of the innate immune system activated instead. Cytokine synthesis is controlled and production of pro-inflammatory cytokines tightly regulated. The antigen presenting functions and immunomodulatory abilities of monocytes means they are thought to be key in the regulation between innate and adaptive arms of the maternal immune system. However, the mechanisms by which tolerance to fetal antigens is maintained are still poorly understood.

White blood cells do not show a dilutional decrease during normal pregnancy, unlike red cells. In contrast, the total white cell count increases up to values of 14×10^9/L in the third trimester (Table 3.1). This is mainly because of increases in the numbers of polymorphonuclear leukocytes, observed as early as 3 weeks gestation and especially marked postpartum. Counts of B cells appear to be unaltered throughout pregnancy, while absolute numbers of natural killer (NK) cells increase in early pregnancy and decrease in late gestation.

The maternal brain

Women frequently report problems with attention, concentration and memory during pregnancy and in the early postpartum period. While these associations are well established, particularly the decline in memory in the third trimester, the underlying mechanisms are less clear. Proposed causes include lack of oestrogen or elevated levels of oxytocin, which has an amnesic effect, while elevated progesterone levels do not seem to be involved. However, progesterone has a sedative effect and with the increased metabolic demands of pregnancy, is likely to be responsible for some of the difficulties staying alert.

Pregnant women require less local anaesthetic in both their epidural and intrathecal spaces to produce the same dermatome level of anaesthesia compared to non-pregnant women. It has been suggested that nerves may be more sensitive to local anaesthetic agents as a result of hormonally mediated changes in diffusion barriers and concurrent activation of central endogenous analgesic systems, but the anatomical spaces also decrease in size during normal pregnancy. Finally, pregnant women appear to have greater tolerance for pain, which is biochemically mediated by increased serum levels of β-endorphins and activated spinal cord κ-opiate receptors.

The senses

Changes in the perception of odours during pregnancy are reported by a majority of pregnant women and are explained by changes in both cognitive and hormonal factors. Recent studies have shown that while pregnancy is associated with changes in olfactory performance, olfactory sensitivity actually decreases in the third trimester, and the decrease persists after delivery. Odour thresholds, but not odour discrimination or identification, are also significantly decreased during the third trimester. Aversion to some odours is a common complaint of pregnancy, but seems specific to early gestation, and is more likely to occur with potentially harmful substances, which is a suggested embryo-protective adaptation.

Corneal sensitivity decreases in most pregnant women and usually returns to normal by 8 weeks postpartum. This can be related to an increase in corneal thickness caused by oedema, and a decrease in tear production occurs during the third trimester of pregnancy in around 80 per cent of pregnant women. These changes in the cornea and tear film lead many women to become intolerant of contact lenses. The curvature of the crystalline lens can also increase, causing a myopic shift in refraction, and a transient loss of accommodation has been seen during and after pregnancy. The retinal arterioles, venules and capillaries seem unchanged in normal pregnancy, while a decrease in intraocular pressure has been reported. However, there are conflicting reports on changes in the visual fields, with defects including concentric constriction, bi-temporal constriction, homonymous hemianopia and central scotoma reported. The proposed mechanism is an increase in size of the pituitary gland affecting the optic chiasm.

Respiratory tract

Airway

The neck, oropharyngeal tissues, breasts and chest wall are all affected by weight gain during pregnancy. This, as well as breast engorgement and airway oedema, can compromise the airway leading to difficulty with visualization of the larynx during tracheal intubation. The vascularity of the respiratory tract mucosa increases and the nasal mucosa can be both oedematous and prone to bleeding. During pregnancy this is often perceived as congestion and rhinitis.

Ventilation

Ventilation begins to increase significantly at around 8 weeks of gestation, most likely in response to progesterone-related sensitization of the respiratory centre to carbon dioxide and the increased metabolic rate. As pregnancy progresses, the diaphragm is elevated 4 cm by the enlarging uterus, and the lower ribcage circumference expands by 5 cm. The increased relaxin levels of pregnancy allow the ligamentous attachments of the ribcage to relax, increasing the ribcage subcostal angle. Respiratory muscle function remains unaffected

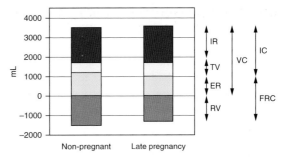

Figure 3.2 Lung volume and changes in pregnancy. ER, expiratory reserve; FRC, functional residual capacity; IC, inspiratory capacity; IR, inspiratory reserve; RV, residual volume; TV, tidal volume; VC, vital capacity. After de Swiet, *Medical disorders in obstetric practice*, 2002

in pregnancy, as do the maximum inspiratory and expiratory pressures. However, lung volumes change slightly as a result of the reconfiguration of the chest wall and the elevation of the diaphragm. There are also increases in pulmonary blood flow in pregnancy.

Significant alterations occur in the mechanical aspects of ventilation during pregnancy (Figure 3.2). Minute ventilation (or the amount of air moved in and out of the lungs in 1 minute) is the product of tidal volume and respiratory rate and increases by approximately 30–50 per cent with pregnancy. The increase is primarily a result of tidal volume, which increases by 40 per cent (from 500 to 700 mL), because the respiratory rate remains unchanged. The increase in minute ventilation is perceived by the pregnant woman as shortness of breath, which affects 60–70 per cent of women. This physiological dyspnoea is usually mild and affects 50 per cent of women before 20 weeks gestation, but resolves immediately postpartum. The incidence is highest at 28–31 weeks. There is also a 10–25 per cent decrease in functional residual capacity (FRC), which is the sum of expiratory reserve and residual volumes, both of which are decreased. FRC is further reduced in the supine position. These physiological changes do not affect the interpretation of tests of ventilation such as forced expiratory volume in 1 second (FEV_1) and peak expiratory flow rate, so non-pregnant reference values may be used to evaluate lung function in pregnant women.

Oxygenation

During pregnancy there is an increase in 2,3-diphosphoglycerate (2,3-DPG) concentration within maternal erythrocytes. 2,3-DPG preferentially binds to deoxygenated haemoglobin and promotes the release of oxygen from red cells at relatively lower levels of haemoglobin saturation (i.e. shifts the oxygen–haemoglobin dissociation curve to the right). This increases the availability of oxygen within the tissues. The fetus is also adapted to take advantage of this alteration in maternal physiology. Fetal haemoglobin differs from adult haemoglobin in that the two beta-chains are replaced by gamma-chains. Binding of 2,3-DPG to haemoglobin occurs preferentially to beta-chains, with the result that in the fetus the oxygen–haemoglobin dissociation curve is shifted to the left relative to the maternal state. In this way oxygen transfer from mother to fetus is facilitated.

Oxygen consumption increases by about 45 mL/min during the course of pregnancy, which represents an increase of about 20 per cent from oxygen consumption at rest (300 mL/min). Around one-third of the increase is necessary for the metabolic demands of placenta and fetus, and the remainder is needed for the extra metabolic work of the maternal organs. The increased oxygen consumption coupled with the decreased FRC decreases maternal oxygen reserve and predisposes the pregnant woman to hypoxaemia and hypocapnia during periods of respiratory depression or apnoea.

Arterial gases

Progesterone has respiratory stimulant properties and the greatly increased levels in pregnancy are thought to be responsible for increasing alveolar ventilation through increasing tidal volume. In consequence, there is a marked decrease (15–20 per cent) in the partial pressure of carbon dioxide (pCO_2). There is usually a slight increase in the partial pressure of oxygen (pO_2). These changes facilitate gas transfer to and from the fetus. Arterial blood gas values differ in pregnant compared to non-pregnant women, but normal ranges of arterial gases at term are not well established, and measured arterial pO_2 has been reported to be normal, low and high. Normal oxygen saturation measured non-invasively should be in excess of 95 per cent during pregnancy.

The reduction in pCO_2 has implications for acid–base balance, as carbon dioxide forms carbonic acid in the presence of water. Reductions in pCO_2 activate compensatory buffering mechanisms so that potentially hazardous alkalosis is prevented. This involves the activity of the enzyme carbonic anhydrase, which converts carbonic acid to bicarbonate, thus releasing hydrogen ions to restore pH. The kidney

then excretes the bicarbonate formed. In pregnancy, renal excretion of bicarbonate increases significantly and maternal arterial pH changes very little, being maintained at 7.40 to 7.45. An increase in the concentration of carbonic anhydrase within maternal erythrocytes has been reported, but whether this is a primary event or a secondary adaptation is uncertain.

Key points

Ventilatory changes
- Thoracic anatomy changes.
- ↑ Minute ventilation.
- ↑ Tidal volume.
- ↓ Residual volume.
- ↓ Functional residual capacity.
- Vital capacity unchanged or slightly increased.

Blood gas and acid–base changes
- ↓ pCO_2.
- ↑ pO_2.
- pH alters little.
- ↑ Bicarbonate excretion.
- ↑ Oxygen availability to tissues and placenta.

Cardiovascular system

Signs and symptoms of pregnancy mimic those of heart disease. Elevation of the diaphragm, adjustments of lung volumes and increases in minute ventilation give rise to breathlessness. Oedema in the extremities is a common finding, and results from an increase in total body sodium and water, as well as venous compression by the gravid uterus. The latter can also cause decreased venous return to the heart, leading to light-headedness and syncope. Palpitations are common and usually represent sinus tachycardia, which is normal in pregnancy. They may also occur as increased awareness of the heart beating either regularly or in association with extrasystoles, presumably related to changes in cardiac output. Premature atrial and ventricular ectopic beats are common in pregnancy and the peripheral pulse is increased in volume. Increases in plasma volume cause the jugular veins to fill and pulsate dynamically in pregnancy, but the mean right atrial pressure is unchanged and the height of the jugular venous pressure is also unchanged. Changes in the left ventricular size and volume mean the apex beat is more forceful.

In normal pregnancy, cardiac output increases as early as 5 weeks gestation (3 weeks after conception) and rises to around 40 per cent above the pre-pregnancy baseline by 24 weeks, i.e. from about 5.0 to 7.0 L/min when at rest (Table 3.2). The increase in cardiac output is caused partly by an increase in heart rate, which is detected first as early as 5 weeks, and partly by an increase in stroke volume. A progressive increase in heart rate continues until the third trimester of pregnancy, when rates are typically 10–15 beats per minute greater than those found in the non-pregnant state. There is also a progressive amplification of stroke volume (10–20 mL) during the first half of pregnancy, probably related to the changes in plasma volume at this time (Figure 3.3).

Table 3.2 Changes in cardiac output during pregnancy

	Cardiac output
Non pregnant adult female	4.5 L/min
Pregnancy (20 weeks)	↑ by 40 per cent to 6.3 L/min
Early labour	↑ by 17 per cent to 7.3 L/min
Active labour	↑ by 23 per cent to 7.7 L/min
2nd stage of labour	↓ by 34 per cent to 8.4 L/min

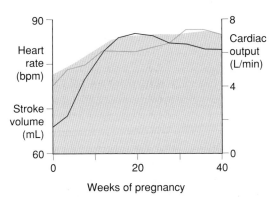

Figure 3.3 There is a marked increase in maternal cardiac output during pregnancy. Increases in both heart rate and stroke volume contribute, but changes in these components are not synchronous

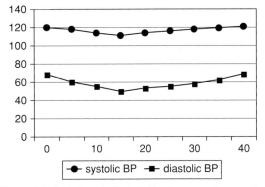

Figure 3.4 Systolic and diastolic blood pressure in normal pregnancy. After Chamberlain and Broughton Pipkin, *Clinical physiology in obstetrics*, 1998

Decreases in diastolic blood pressure (10–15 mmHg) are more marked during the antenatal period than the decrease in systolic pressure (5–10 mmHg). Thus, early pregnancy is associated with a relative increase in pulse pressure. An 11 per cent fall in mean arterial blood pressure at rest has been shown by 15 weeks gestation. Later, diastolic blood pressure increases to levels that are at least equivalent to those found in the non-pregnant state (Figure 3.4). A mean diastolic blood pressure of 66.6 mmHg has been reported in the first trimester, falling to 66.3 mmHg in the second and rising to 68.4 mmHg by 40 weeks. Accurate determination of diastolic pressure is therefore very important, and the best measurements are obtained when the fifth Korotkoff sound (disappearance of sounds) is used. As blood pressure does not rise in pregnancy, and usually falls, the increase in cardiac output is also associated with a fall in peripheral vascular resistance. A 70 per cent reduction in peripheral resistance has been demonstrated by 8 weeks gestation. The mechanisms responsible are uncertain, but alterations have been reported in production of vasoconstrictor and vasodilator agents that control peripheral arterial tone.

The cardiac output is elevated at the onset of labour to over 7.0 L/min, rising further within labour, with a 30 per cent increase in demand in the final stages (Table 3.2). This increase is due to the uterine contractions each of which squeezes 300–500 mL of blood into the maternal circulation. At delivery, a shift of blood from the empty uterus into the maternal circulation – called autotransfusion – causes an increase of 10–20 per cent in the cardiac output. Stroke volume, heart rate and cardiac output remain elevated for the first 2 days postpartum. Within the first 2 weeks after delivery the cardiac output falls rapidly, at 6 weeks postpartum it is halfway between pregnant and non-pregnant values and at 24 weeks after delivery the cardiac output falls to below 5.0 L/min.

Ausculatory changes in pregnancy are well documented. The first heart sound is loud and sometimes split, while a third heart sound is audible in 84 per cent of pregnant women by 20 weeks gestation. An ejection systolic murmur can be heard in 96 per cent of apparently normal pregnant women; this murmur is widely conducted and it disappears after delivery. The third heart sound is frequently misinterpreted as a diastolic murmur, but a true diastolic murmur occurs transiently in only 20 per cent of pregnant women, whereas 10 per cent develop continuous or systolic murmurs due to increased mammary blood flow.

Key points 🔑

Cardiovascular changes

- ↑ Heart rate (10–20 per cent).
- ↑ Stroke volume (10 per cent).
- ↑ Cardiac output (30–50 per cent).
- ↓ Mean arterial pressure (10 per cent).
- ↓ Pulse pressure.
- ↓ Peripheral resistance (35 per cent).

Gastrointestinal changes

Oral

The physiological changes of pregnancy include effects on mucous membranes, pigmentation and glandular function. Pregnancy gingivitis is the term used for inflammation and hyperplasia of the gingival mucosa occurring during gestation and from 30 to 75 per cent of pregnant women develop erythema, oedema, hyperplasia and increased bleeding of the gingival tissue. Elevated circulating oestrogen and progesterone levels are implicated in increasing vascular permeability and decreasing immune resistance, thereby increasing susceptibility to gingivitis. The hormone levels of pregnancy also affect the response of the periodontal tissues to bacterial

colonization, creating a more favourable environment for anaerobic infection. The main salivary changes in pregnancy include variations in pH and composition, with a reduction of sodium concentration that leads to a decrease in pH and increased concentration of protein. Salivary oestrogen levels are increased, resulting in an increased proliferation and desquamation of the oral mucosa. While teeth usually retain their structure, salivary changes late in pregnancy, as well as oestrogen-enhanced changes in the mucosa, predispose to dental caries. Increased tooth mobility, especially of the upper incisors, has been detected in pregnant women, even those with normal periodontal tissues.

Gut

As gestation advances, the uterus displaces the stomach and intestines upwards, which can hinder diagnosis of intra-abdominal surgical events as well as confound the routine abdominal examination. Elevated progesterone levels reduce lower oesophageal sphincter tone and increase the placental production of gastrin, increasing gastric acidity. These changes combine to increase the incidence of reflux oesophagitis and heartburn, which affect up to 80 per cent of pregnant women. Mechanical factors, the enlarging uterus and progesterone levels all contribute to delayed gastric emptying and increased stomach volume. Gastric motility decreases further during labour and emptying remains delayed during the puerperium. As a result of all of these changes, the pregnant woman is at increased risk of aspiration of gastric contents when sedated or anaesthetized after 16 weeks gestation. Delayed gastric motility and prolonged gastrointestinal transit time may also lead to constipation and alter the bioavailability of medications.

Liver

The liver, normally palpated 2 cm below the right costal margin, may become more difficult to examine because of the expanding uterus within the abdominal cavity. Physical findings such as telangiectasia and palmar erythema, otherwise suggestive of liver disease in non-pregnant women, appear in up to 60 per cent of normal pregnancies because of the hyperoestrogenic state of pregnancy, as the liver cannot easily metabolize the large quantity of placental oestrogen and progesterone. During pregnancy, absolute hepatic blood flow remains largely unaltered and hepatic function remains normal. Portal vein pressure is increased in late pregnancy, and venous pressure increases in the oesophagus. Although hepatic protein production increases, serum albumin levels decline in pregnancy due to the increase in maternal plasma volume. In contrast, an increase in serum alkaline phosphatase secondary to fetal and placental production is observed in pregnancy and persists postpartum, rendering it unhelpful diagnosing cholestasis during the third trimester (Table 3.1). Probably the most important hepatic changes in pregnancy are the increased production and plasma levels of fibrinogen and the clotting factors VII, VIII, X and XII. Finally, hypercholesterolaemia is well described in pregnancy – plasma cholesterol levels rise by around 50 per cent in the third trimester and triglycerides may rise to two or three times normal levels. Levels fall after delivery, returning to normal faster in lactating women.

The kidneys and urinary tract

Anatomic changes

The kidneys increase in size in normal pregnancy, with a 1–2 cm change in length. The calyces, renal pelvis and ureters dilate, giving the usually incorrect impression of obstruction. By the third trimester, over 80 per cent of women have some evidence of stasis or hydronephrosis, which is more marked on the right side due to uterine dextrorotation. This physical change, together with alterations in the composition of the urine itself, predisposes pregnant women to ascending urinary tract infection, a common complication of pregnancy (1–2 per cent of all pregnancies). Renal parenchymal volumes also increase during pregnancy, most likely due to increases in intrarenal fluid. By 6 weeks postpartum, renal dimensions return to pre-pregnancy values.

Functional changes

Glomerular filtration rate (GFR) rises immediately after conception and increases by about 50 per cent overall, reaching its maximum at the end of the first trimester. GFR then falls by about 20 per cent in the third trimester, returning to pre-pregnancy levels within 12 weeks of delivery (Table 3.3). Renal blood flow increases by up to 80 per cent in the second trimester, due to the combination of increased cardiac output and increased renal vasodilatation, but this is followed by a 25 per cent fall towards term (Figure 3.5). Despite chronic vasodilatation,

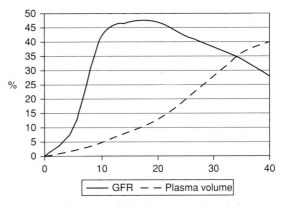

Figure 3.5 Changes in GFR and plasma volume during normal pregnancy

Table 3.3 Changes in indices of renal function during pregnancy (mean values); data from de Swiet, *Medical disorders in obstetric practice*, 2002

	Non-pregnant	1st Trimester	2nd Trimester	3rd Trimester
RPF mL/min	480	841	891	771
GFR mL/min	105	162	174	165
24 h creatinine clearance	98	151	154	129
Plasma creatinine μmol/L	73	60	54	64
Plasma urea mmol/L	4.3	3.5	3.3	3.1
Plasma urate μmol/L	246	189	214	269

the kidney is still able to autoregulate blood flow and GFR over a range of blood pressure, mainly through variations in arteriolar tone. Creatinine clearance increases by 25 per cent at 4 weeks gestation and by 45 per cent at 9 weeks, but over the course of the pregnancy a decrease back to non-pregnant values occurs. The renin-angiotensin system is also modified in normal pregnancy, with increases in plasma renin activity and plasma angiotensin-II.

As GFR increases without alterations in the production of creatinine and urea, plasma levels of these substances decrease. Creatinine levels change from a non-pregnant value of 73 mmol/L to 60, 54 and 64 mmol/L in successive trimesters. The average plasma urea level of 3.1 mmol/L in the third trimester also contrasts with the non-pregnant value of 4.3 mmol/L. Plasma urate concentrations decrease by over 25 per cent from 8 weeks gestation, but due to changes in renal absorption and excretion increase again in the third trimester to levels close to non-pregnant values (Table 3.3). There is also increased renal excretion of various nutrients, calcium and protein, mainly due to changes in renal tubular function. Sodium balance is maintained, despite the GFR increase and increases in filtration, by increasing sodium reabsorption both in proximal tubules (under the influence of oncotic pressure in the renal interstitial space) and in distal portions (under the influence of hormonal factors). Potassium metabolism remains unchanged, despite cumulative retention of potassium, necessary for fetal-placental development and expansion of maternal red blood cell mass, and increased aldosterone levels. Early morning urine is more alkaline than in non-pregnant women, but acid excretion ability of the kidney is unchanged (Table 3.1).

Glycosuria, which is rare in the absence of diabetes in the non-pregnant state, is very common during pregnancy and does not relate reliably to disorders of carbohydrate metabolism. The increase in GFR may be partially responsible, and a reabsorptive mechanism in the proximal renal tubule may become saturated so that the 'renal threshold' is exceeded, explaining the increased amount of glucose in the urine. Glucose reabsorption occurs secondarily to the absorption of sodium and therefore other factors contributing to volume homeostasis and sodium retention may also be involved in the physiological glycosuria of pregnancy.

Key points

Renal changes

- ↑ Kidney size (1 cm).
- Dilatation of renal pelvis and ureters.
- ↑ Blood flow (60–75 per cent).
- ↑ Glomerular filtration (50 per cent).
- ↑ Renal plasma flow (50–80 per cent).
- ↑ Clearance of most substances.
- ↓ Plasma creatinine, urea and urate.
- Glycosuria is normal.

Reproductive organs

Uterus

Uterine blood flow increases 40-fold to approximately 700 mL/min at term, with 80 per cent of the blood distributed to the intervillous spaces of the placentae, and 20 per cent to the uterine myometrium. Oestrogen mediates the adaptation of the uterine smooth muscle to pregnancy. High levels of maternal oestradiol and progesterone induce both hyperplasia and hypertrophy of the myometrium, increasing the weight of the uterus from 50–60 g prior to pregnancy to 1000 g by term. The growing size of the uterine contents is an important stimulus, with individual muscle fibres increasing in length by up to 15-fold. The uterine arteries also undergo hypertrophy in the first half of pregnancy, although in the second half increasing uterine distension is matched by arterial stretching. Progesterone helps maintain lower myogenic tone in the uterine vessels despite the increased blood flow. Maternal cortisol also regulates local uterine blood flow, through effects on vascular endothelium and smooth muscle. By the third trimester, the uterus is described in lower and upper segments. The lower segment is the part of the uterus and upper cervix which lies between the attachment of the peritoneum of the uterovesical pouch superiorly and the level of the internal cervical os inferiorly. It is thinner, contains less muscle and fewer blood vessels and is the site of incision for the majority of Caesarean sections (Figure 3.6).

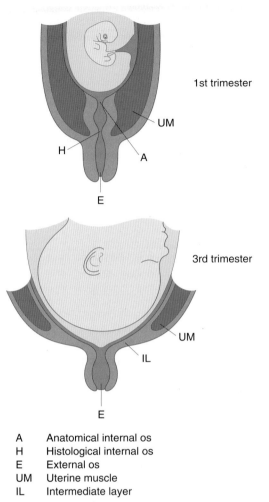

A   Anatomical internal os
H   Histological internal os
E   External os
UM   Uterine muscle
IL   Intermediate layer

Figure 3.6 Formation of the lower uterine segment. With increasing gestation, uterine stretch occurs. This has the effect of drawing the anatomical internal cervical os (A) further from the histological internal cervical os (H). The retraction of the thick intermediate layer (IL) of muscle with increasing gestation thins the lower segment

As well as changes in the size and number of myometrial cells, specialized cellular connections also develop with increasing gestation. These intercellular gap junctions allow changes in membrane potential to spread rapidly from one cell to another, facilitating the spread of membrane depolarization, and subsequent myometrial contraction. Steroid hormones also have an effect on signalling pathways. As these junctions mature, uterine contractions become more frequent. These are apparent initially as Braxton Hicks, painless contractions that are noticed in the second half of pregnancy. Subsequently, these allow the pacemaker activity of the uterine fundus to promote the co-ordinated, fundal-dominant contractions necessary for labour.

Cervix

The cervix is described as looking bluer during pregnancy, which is due to its increased vascularity. It becomes swollen and softer during pregnancy under the influence of progesterone and oestradiol; the latter also stimulates growth of the columnar epithelium of the cervical canal. This becomes visible on the ectocervix and is called an ectropion, which is prone to contact bleeding. In addition, the mucous glands of the cervix become distended and increase in complexity. Prostaglandins induce a remodelling of cervical collagen in late gestation, while collagenase released from leukocytes locally also aids in softening the cervix. Under the influence of oestrogens, the vaginal epithelium becomes more vascular during pregnancy, and there is increased desquamation resulting in increased vaginal discharge. This discharge has a more acid pH than non-pregnant vaginal secretions (4.5–5.0) and may protect against ascending infection.

Breasts and lactation

The cyclical changes seen in breast tissue with the menstrual cycle are accentuated during pregnancy. Deposition of fat around glandular tissue occurs, and the number of glandular ducts is increased by oestrogen, while progesterone and human placental lactogen (hPL) increase the number of gland alveoli. Prolactin is essential for the stimulation of milk secretion and during pregnancy prepares the alveoli for milk production. Although prolactin concentration increases throughout pregnancy, it does not then result in lactation since it is antagonized at an alveolar receptor level by oestrogen. The rapid fall in oestrogen concentration over the first 48 hours after delivery removes this inhibition and allows lactation to begin. Towards the end of pregnancy, and in the early puerperium, the breasts produce colostrum, a thick yellow secretion rich in immunoglobulins. Lactation is initiated by early suckling, which stimulates the anterior and posterior pituitary to release prolactin and oxytocin, respectively. During the first 2–3 days

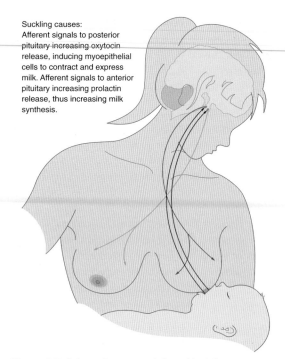

Suckling causes:
Afferent signals to posterior pituitary increasing oxytocin release, inducing myoepithelial cells to contract and express milk. Afferent signals to anterior pituitary increasing prolactin release, thus increasing milk synthesis.

Figure 3.7 Schematic representation of lactation. Suckling induces afferent signals to the anterior and posterior pituitary. This results in the release of prolactin and oxytocin. Prolactin induces milk production by the glandular tissue of the breast. Oxytocin causes contraction of the myoepithelial cells surrounding the glandular ducts, squeezing milk towards the nipple

Table 3.4 Hormones produced within the pregnant uterus

Type	Name
Pregnancy specific	Human chorionic gonadotrophin (hCG) Human placental lactogen (hPL)
Hypothalamus	Gonadotrophin-releasing hormone (GnRH) Corticotrophin-releasing hormone (CRH)
Pituitary	Prolactin Human growth hormone (hGH) Adrenocorticotrophic hormone (ACTH)
Steroids	Oestradiol Progesterone
Other peptides	Insulin-like growth factor-I and II 1,25 Dihydroxycholecalciferol Parathyroid hormone-related peptide Renin Angiotensin-II

of the puerperium, prolactin promotes breast engorgement and the alveoli become distended with milk. Oxytocin released from the posterior pituitary causes contraction in myoepithelial cells surrounding the alveoli and small ducts, squeezing milk towards the nipple. Released during labour as well, oxytocin facilitates the rapid onset of maternal–infant bonding as well as an altered emotional state (Figure 3.7).

Endocrinology

Complex endocrinological changes occur in pregnancy. Many physiological adaptations to pregnancy are organized by the maternal brain, predominantly through changes in neuroendocrine systems, and the hormones of pregnancy primarily drive these changes. Other hormones exert their actions indirectly, by interacting with cytokines and

chemokines. The production and activity of these substances are also significantly altered in pregnancy. Finally, during pregnancy, both the placenta and the fetus produce some hormones otherwise produced by the endocrine glands in the non-pregnant state (Table 3.4).

Pituitary gland

The pituitary gland enlarges during normal pregnancy and concentrations of prolactin reach levels during pregnancy that are 15-fold higher than in the non-pregnant state. Oestrogen has a stimulatory role in this process and hPL is inhibitory. The endocrinological mechanisms that regulate prolactin production in the non-pregnant state, such as sleep, which increases and dopamine agonists, which reduce prolactin concentration, remain effective during pregnancy. Therefore prolactin production by the anterior pituitary gland continues despite intrauterine production from cells within the decidua. Receptors for prolactin are also present on trophoblast cells and within the amniotic fluid. Increased prolactin production is essential for lactation (as already discussed) but also acts in the brain to reduce responses to stress. Further, prolactin may play a role in the regulation of insulin secretion and glucose homeostasis in the post-natal period. In contrast to prolactin, there is evidence that human growth hormone (hGH) production by the anterior pituitary gland is suppressed during pregnancy, and circulating concentrations are also reduced. It is likely that hPL is also involved in suppressing hGH release.

Thyroid function

Human chorionic gonadotrophin (hCG) has thyrotrophic activity owing to subunit homology with thyroid-stimulating hormone (TSH) and maternal TSH production is suppressed during the first trimester of pregnancy, when hCG levels are highest. The TSH response to thyrotrophin-releasing hormone (TRH) is reduced during the first trimester but returns to normal after this. Thyroid binding globulin increases in the first 2 weeks of pregnancy and reaches a plateau by 20 weeks. This leads to increased production of total T3 (tri-iodothyronine) and T4 (thyroxine). The increased GFR of pregnancy results in an increased renal loss of iodide, which is essential for thyroid hormone synthesis, so the thyroid compensates by increasing the proportion of iodide it takes up from the circulation. Where there is relative background iodide deficiency, these changes may result in enlargement of the thyroid gland during pregnancy.

The hypermetabolic state of normal pregnancy makes clinical assessment of thyroid function more difficult and therefore thyroid function often needs to be checked biochemically. However the physiological changes of pregnancy, including the 50 per cent plasma volume expansion, increased thyroid binding globulin production and relative iodine deficiency, mean that thyroid hormone reference ranges for non-pregnant women are not appropriate in pregnancy. Free T4 (fT4), free T3 and TSH should be analysed when assessing thyroid function in pregnancy, and total T3 and T4 not used. There is a fall in TSH and a rise in fT4 concentrations in the first trimester of normal pregnancy. This is followed by a fall in fT4 concentration with advancing gestation, with the most marked effect in the third trimester (Table 3.1).

Uterus and placenta

Many pregnancy-specific peptides are produced within the uterus, but not all have been shown to have definite endocrine roles. The best known is hCG, produced by trophoblast cells. The β-subunit is pregnancy specific and used as a sensitive pregnancy test, being detectable within the maternal circulation in small quantities within days of implantation. Production of hCG is influenced both by the cytokine leukaemia inhibitory factor (LIF) and by an isoform of gonadotrophin-releasing hormone (GnRH), which is also produced within the placenta. Human chorionic gonadotrophin has a major role during early pregnancy in maintaining the function of the corpus luteum, which produces progesterone, but circulating hCG values fall off after 12 weeks, as the placental production of progesterone becomes dominant. During normal pregnancy, hCG also suppresses the secretion of FSH and LH by the anterior pituitary gland, perhaps by interaction at the hypothalamic level.

Sex steroid hormones are produced in large quantities by the placenta and fetus. Concentrations of oestrogens and progesterone increase substantially from early pregnancy, and then plateau for the remainder of the pregnancy. Both oestrogen and progesterone have effects on the myometrium, where oestrogen encourages cellular hypertrophy while progesterone discourages contraction and, together with prolactin, on the tissues of the breast. They also have effects on many other tissues during pregnancy, such as the smooth muscle of the vascular tree and of the urinary and gastrointestinal tracts.

Corticosteroids

Trophoblast cells produce adrenocorticotrophic hormone (ACTH), which has a role in regulating the activity of the fetal adrenal glands and the myometrium and possibly also the mother's adrenal glands. A progressive increase in maternal circulating concentrations of cortisol throughout normal pregnancy has been noticed from as early as

11 weeks. Cortisol reaches two-to three-fold higher concentrations than in the non-pregnant, despite a decrease in the concentration of ACTH in later gestation. Much of the cortisol is bound to cortisol-binding globulin (CBG), which doubles in concentration during pregnancy, but there is also a slight increase in unbound cortisol. The lack of diurnal variation of cortisol and the attenuated response to dexamethasone suppression suggest that placental ACTH may have a role in regulating maternal cortisol levels. Cortisol responses to stressors are reduced in pregnant women.

Circulating concentrations of the antinatriuretic hormones aldosterone and deoxycorticosterone increase ten-fold in pregnancy. Plasma aldosterone levels rise seven to eight-fold during the first trimester, but the diurnal rhythm of levels is preserved throughout pregnancy. Progesterone has natriuretic properties, and other factors that may influence aldosterone production, such as atrial natriuretic peptide and angiotensins, are produced in greater amounts during pregnancy. The increased production of angiotensins, including the vasoactive angiotensin-II, is the result of an augmented production of the enzyme renin and its substrate angiotensinogen.

Corticotrophin-releasing hormone (CRH) is produced by the placenta in the second half of pregnancy. One function of placental CRH expression is to stimulate the fetal adrenals to synthesize and release dihydroepiandrosterone (DHEA), which the placenta then converts to oestrogens. Another function is to stimulate the fetal adrenal gland (both directly and through stimulation of the fetal pituitary) to synthesize and release cortisol. Fetal cortisol drives the placental-fetal adrenal axis through positive feedback that results in increasing oestrogen production over gestation, and also works by maturing other fetal organs.

Plasma CRH, ACTH and cortisol concentrations increase several-fold with the onset of labour and delivery, with peak CRH levels 48 hours before delivery. Maternal plasma ACTH levels are ten-fold higher in labour than when not pregnant. Thus the progression of gestation is linked to the timing of fetal development, and infants are born with appropriately mature organs. The placental regulation of its own metabolism through effects on the fetus, with subsequent effects on maternal uterine physiology, and possibly the onset of labour, has been called the 'placental clock' theory.

Key points

Endocrine changes

- ↑ Prolactin concentration.
- Human growth hormone is suppressed.
- ↑ Corticosteroid concentrations.
- ↓ TSH in early pregnancy.
- ↓ fT4 in late pregnancy.
- hCG is produced.
- Insulin resistance develops.

Metabolism

Energy requirements and weight gain

Energy requirements during pregnancy are defined as the level of energy intake from food needed to balance energy expenditure, presuming the woman has a body size and level of physical activity consistent with good health. The energy cost of pregnancy includes energy deposited in maternal and fetal tissues, and the increase in energy expenditure attributed to maintenance and physical activity. As a result of the increased tissue mass the energy cost of maintenance, as well as physical activity, rises during pregnancy. In healthy well-nourished women, the increases in basal metabolic rate (BMR) range from 124 to 210 MJ, with an average increase of 157 MJ for the whole pregnancy (corresponding to an average gestational weight gain of 12.5 kg).

Weight gain during pregnancy consists of the products of conception (fetus, placenta, amniotic fluid), the increase of various maternal tissues (uterus, breasts, blood, extracellular fluid), and the increase in maternal fat stores. The increase in weight is largely fluid, with today body water increasing by around 8 L. Rates of weight gain vary across the trimesters of pregnancy, with estimates of 1.6 kg gained in the first trimester, 0.45 kg per week in the second and 0.4 kg per week in the third trimester reported. The appropriate gestational weight gain for optimal pregnancy outcome is the subject of much debate, and is modified by pre-pregnancy body mass index (BMI) measurements. Ranges of weight gain recommended for women with low pre-pregnancy BMI ($<$20) are 12.5–18.0 kg, compared to 11.5–16.0 kg for those with normal pre-pregnancy BMI (20–26). However, women with a lower BMI must gain more weight to produce infants with birthweights comparable to women with a normal BMI. Women with high BMI not only deliver infants with higher birthweights, but also can do so with lower gestational weight gains.

Carbohydrate metabolism

Changes in carbohydrate and lipid metabolism occur during pregnancy to ensure a continuous supply of nutrients to the growing fetus. In the first half of pregnancy, fasting plasma glucose concentrations are reduced with little change in insulin levels. An oral glucose tolerance test at this time shows an enhanced response compared to the non-pregnant state, with a normal pattern of insulin release but reduced blood glucose values. This pattern changes during the second half of pregnancy, where an increase in glucose values throughout the test despite significant increases in plasma insulin concentrations suggests relative insulin resistance. Insulin action in late normal pregnancy is 50–70 per cent lower than in non-pregnant women and insulin resistance is thought to allow shunting of nutrients to the fetus. This change may involve hPL or other growth-related hormones, such as prolactin or cortisol, which reduce peripheral insulin sensitivity. Pregnancy is also associated with alterations in insulin receptor binding, similar to those described in non-pregnant women who have non-insulin-dependent diabetes mellitus. Whether this results from increased transplacental transfer of glucose or from the growth-promoting characteristics of insulin is unclear. During lactation, glucose levels fall and insulin resistance returns to normal, as glucose homeostasis is reset.

Lipid metabolism

Changes in hepatic and adipose metabolism alter circulating concentrations of triacylglycerols, fatty acids, cholesterol and phospholipids, which all increase after the eighth week of pregnancy. Both the higher concentration of oestrogen and insulin resistance are thought to be responsible for the hypertriglyceridaemia of pregnancy. HDL-cholesterol increases by 12 weeks in response to oestrogen and remains elevated throughout pregnancy, while total and LDL-cholesterol concentrations decrease initially, but then increase in the second and third trimesters. Changes in lipid metabolism influenced by increased oestrogen, progesterone and insulin promote the accumulation of maternal fat stores in early pregnancy and inhibit lipolysis. In late pregnancy, fat mobilization is enhanced to allow pregnant women to use stored lipid for energy needs and minimize protein catabolism, preserving glucose and amino acids for the fetus.

Calcium metabolism

Around 40 per cent of circulating calcium is bound to albumin. Since plasma albumin concentrations decrease during pregnancy, total plasma calcium concentrations also decrease, which is not evidence of true hypocalcaemia. There is little change in the circulating concentration of unbound ionized calcium. In pregnancy, a number of adaptive changes must occur to facilitate positive calcium balance in favour of the developing fetus, which needs to equilibrate its own calcium level and ensure skeletal development. The fetal demand for calcium is substantial and transplacental flux rates of about 6.5 mmol per day have been estimated. There are three potential methods of maternal adaptation: increasing gut absorption, mobilizing skeletal calcium reserves or restricting renal losses. The pregnant woman usually increases the rate or efficiency of gut absorption and slightly decreases excretion, thereby coping with little overall change in transfer rates into and out of bone stores. The increase in gut calcium absorption is a result of increased production of a metabolite of vitamin D_3, 1,25-dihydroxycholecalciferol (1,25-$(OH)2D_3$). Production of 1,25-$(OH)2D_3$ is under the influence of parathyroid hormone (PTH), which increases by about one-third during pregnancy. No consistent changes have been reported in circulating concentrations of other agents involved in calcium metabolism, for example calcitonin and other metabolites of vitamin D_3. However, in situations of abundant calcium, maternal PTH levels are suppressed and renal calcium retention is overridden to allow excretion. Observational studies have shown either no change or a small decline in maternal storage forms of vitamin D during pregnancy.

Omega-3 fatty acids

Omega-3 fatty acids are essential and can only be obtained from the diet. Requirements in pregnancy have not been established but are presumed to be higher than in the non-pregnant state. It is known that these fatty acids are essential for the developing fetus. Docosahexaenoic acid (DHA), the most important omega-3 fatty acid, is an important component of neural and retinal membranes, and accumulates in the fetal brain during gestation. There is a recognized association between maternal fatty acid intake in pregnancy and fetal visual and cognitive development. In addition, observational studies show an association with prolonging gestation and reducing preterm delivery risk. Pregnant women are usually advised to eat greater quantities of sources of omega-3 fatty acids (namely vegetable oils and oily fish), but as the average western diet is deficient in omega-3 fatty acids, additional fish-oil supplements are increasingly recommended. At present, while higher levels of DHA in pregnancy and lactation are linked to better developmental outcomes, few clinical studies demonstrate evidence for routine maternal supplementation.

Skin

Hyperpigmentation can be localized or generalized and affects almost 90 per cent of pregnant women, being more obvious in women with darker skin. Pre-existing moles, freckles and recent scars also tend to become darker, as do areas of skin that are already normally pigmented – including the areolae, nipples, axillae and periumbilical skin. The linea alba darkens to a brown line along the midline of the abdomen, which reaches the symphysis pubis, and is called the linea nigra. Growth and increase in the number of naevi have also been reported, but there is no evidence of an increased risk of malignant change. All of these changes appear to regress after delivery, but may recur in subsequent pregnancies. Melasma, also called chloasma, is an acquired hypermelanosis characterized by symmetrical, irregular, macular brown-grey pigmentation of the face, reported in up to 75 per cent of pregnant women. This hyperpigmentation results from the deposition of melanin in the epidermis, dermis, or both, with epidermal deposition producing a brown coloration, whereas dermal involvement produces a grey tone. The underlying cause is uncertain, but the hormonal influences of pregnancy are involved, as well as exposure to ultraviolet radiation, and

the number of melanocytes in the skin is also increased. Pigmentation usually regresses after delivery but may persist in less than 10 per cent of those affected.

Striae gravidarum (stretch marks) occur in most pregnant women, usually by the end of the second trimester, with a reported incidence of 90 per cent in Caucasians. Linear violaceous bands develop on the abdomen and sometimes on the thighs, arms, breasts, axillae and buttocks, then slowly progress into pale, skin-coloured, atrophic bands around the time of delivery. Pruritus of the abdomen may be an accompanying feature. The cause of striae is not fully understood but is probably related to destruction of elastic fibres. Several factors affect their development, including the degree of abdominal distension and maternal weight gain, genetic predisposition and hormonal changes (oestrogen, relaxin), which influence connective tissue formation. Striae persist postpartum but become less evident.

Sebaceous gland activity is increased during the second half of pregnancy with greasy skin, especially on the face, a common complaint. Acne may also commence during pregnancy. Montgomery tubercles are small sebaceous glands on the areolae of the breasts that enlarge and hypertrophy during early pregnancy, and they present as multiple elevated brown papules, being one of the first signs of pregnancy.

Hirsuitism, defined as excessive growth of body hair, is seen in many pregnant women, especially those with dark or abundant hair. Women often notice thickening of scalp hair during pregnancy and a prolonged anagen phase has been demonstrated. However, one to four months after delivery, a large proportion of hair enters the telogen phase, resulting in increased hair shedding known as telogen effluvium. This shedding may persist for several months postpartum and is most likely precipitated by the sudden hormonal changes at delivery as well as the stress of labour.

Key points

Skin changes
- Hyperpigmentation.
- Striae gravidarum.
- Hirsuitism.
- ↑ Sebaceous gland activity.

Summary

Many physiological changes occur with normal pregnancy and these changes impact every organ system, affecting both structure and function. Most are advantageous and allow the mother to cope with the increased physical and metabolic demands of the pregnancy. Some have important clinical implications: adjusting normal measurements and values, mimicking disease or altering responses to trauma and stress.

Additional reading

Butte NF, King JC. Energy requirements during pregnancy and lactation. *Public Health Nutrition.* 2005; **8**(7A): 1010–27.

Chamberlain G, Broughton-Pipkin F. *Clinical physiology in obstetrics.* Oxford, Blackwell Science, 1998.

de Swiet M. *Medical disorders in obstetric practice.* Oxford, Blackwell Science, 2002.

Gorman SR, Rosen MA. Anesthetic implications of maternal physiological changes during pregnancy. *Seminars in Anesthesia* 2000; **19**: 1–9.

Hameed AB, Sklansky MS. Pregnancy: maternal and fetal heart disease. *Current Problems in Cardiology.* 2007; **32**: 419–94.

Hill CC, Pickinpaugh J. Physiologic changes in pregnancy. *Surgical Clinics of North America* 2008; **88**: 391–401, vii.

Holmes VA, Wallace JM. Haemostasis in normal pregnancy: a balancing act? *Biochemical Society Transactions.* 2005; **33**(Pt 2): 428–32.

Larsson A, Palm M, Hansson LO, Axelsson O. Reference values for clinical chemistry tests during normal pregnancy. *BJOG* 2008; **115**: 874–81.

Muallem MM, Rubeiz NG. Physiological and biological skin changes in pregnancy. *Clinics in Dermatology.* 2006; **24**: 80–3.

Weissgerber TL, Wolfe LA. Physiological adaptation in early human pregnancy: adaptation to balance maternal-fetal demands. *Applied Physiology, Nutrition, and Metabolism.* 2006; **31**: 1–11.

CHAPTER 4

NORMAL FETAL DEVELOPMENT AND GROWTH

Gary Mires

OVERVIEW

An understanding of normal development, growth and maturation is important for understanding the complications that may arise in pregnancy and for the neonate. For example, an understanding of the development of the lungs will explain why preterm infants are at risk of respiratory distress syndrome and term infants are not and why bowel protruding into the umbilical cord at 10 weeks gestation is normal and not diagnosed as an omphalocele.

This chapter provides an overview of the development, growth and maturation of the main body organs and systems and the implications of disordered growth.

Fetal growth

The failure of a fetus to reach its full growth potential, known as fetal growth restriction (FGR), is associated with a significant increased risk of perinatal morbidity and mortality. Growth-restricted fetuses are more likely to suffer intrauterine hypoxia/asphyxia and, as a consequence, be stillborn or demonstrate signs and symptoms of hypoxic-ischaemic encephalopathy (HIE), including seizures and multiorgan damage or failure in the neonatal period. Other complications to which these growth-restricted babies are more prone include neonatal hypothermia, hypoglycaemia, infection and necrotizing enterocolitis. In the medium term, cerebral palsy is more prevalent and it is now recognized from large epidemiological studies that low birthweight infants are more likely to develop hypertension, cardiovascular disease (ischaemic heart disease and stroke) and diabetes in adult life, indicating the impact that FGR is long lasting. It is important to note, however, that not all small for gestational age (SGA) fetuses are growth restricted; some of these babies are constitutionally small and have reached their full growth potential. In addition, not all growth-restricted fetuses are SGA in that while their birthweight is within the normal range for gestation they have failed to reach their full growth potential. One of the challenges in obstetric practice is to identify potentially growth-restricted fetuses and then, from this group, those that are 'small and healthy' and those that are 'small and unhealthy'.

Determinants of fetal birthweight?

Determinants of birth weight are multifactorial, and reflect the influence of the natural growth potential of the fetus dictated largely by the fetal genome and by the intrauterine environment. The latter is influenced by both maternal and placental factors. The ultimate birthweight is therefore the result of the interaction between the fetal genome and the maternal uterine environment. Fetal growth is dependent on adequate transfer of nutrients and oxygen across the placenta. This in itself is dependent on appropriate maternal nutrition and placental perfusion. Factors affecting these are discussed below and in Chapter 10, Pre-eclampsia and other disorders of placentation. Other factors are important in determining fetal growth and include, for example, fetal hormones. They affect the metabolic rate, growth of tissues and maturation of individual organs. In particular, insulin-like growth factors (IGFs) coordinate a precise and orderly increase in growth throughout late gestation. Insulin and thyroxine (T4) are required through late gestation to ensure appropriate growth in normal and adverse nutritional circumstances. Fetal hyperinsulinaemia, which occurs in association with maternal diabetes mellitus when maternal glycaemic control is suboptimal, results in fetal macrosomia with, in particular, excessive fat deposition.

Other factors relate to fetal, maternal and placental influences.

Fetal influences

Genetic

It is recognized that fetal genome plays a significant role in determining fetal size. Obvious and sometimes severe FGR is seen in fetuses with chromosomal defects such as the trisomies particularly of chromosomes 13 (Patau's syndrome) and 18 (Edward's syndrome). Less severe FGR is common in trisomy 21 (Down's syndrome). The other genetic influence is fetal sex with slightly greater birthweights in males.

Infection

Although relatively uncommon in the UK, infection has been implicated in FGR, particularly rubella, cytomegalovirus, toxoplasma and syphilis.

Maternal influences

Physiologic influences

In normal pregnancy, maternal physiologic influences on birthweight include maternal height and pre-pregnancy weight, age and ethnic group. Heavier and taller mothers tend to have bigger babies and certain ethnic groups lighter babies (e.g. South Asian and Afro-Caribbean). Parity is also an influence with increasing parity being associated with increased birthweight. Age influences relate to the association with age and parity, i.e. older mothers are more likely to be parous but conversely in older women the increased risk of chromosomal abnormalities and maternal disease, for example hypertension, lead to lower birthweights. Teenage pregnancy is also associated with FGR.

Behavioural

Maternal behavioural influences are also important with smoking, alcohol and drug use all associated with reduced fetal growth. Babies born to mothers who smoke during pregnancy deliver babies up to 300 g lighter than non-smoking mothers. This effect may be through toxins, for example carbon monoxide, or vascular effects on the uteroplacental circulation. Alcohol crosses the placenta and a dose-related effect has been noted with up to 500 g reduction in birthweight along with other anomalies occurring in women who drink heavily (>2 drinks per day). The use of drugs is often associated with smoking and alcohol use but there is evidence to suggest that heroin is independently associated with a reduction in birthweight.

Chronic disease

Chronic maternal disease may restrict fetal growth. Such diseases are largely those that affect placental function or result in maternal hypoxia. Conditions include hypertension (essential or secondary to renal disease) and lung or cardiac conditions (cystic fibrosis, cyanotic heart disease). Hypertension can lead to placental infarction which impairs its function. Maternal thrombophilia can also result in placental thrombosis and infarction.

Placental influences

The placenta is the only way in which the fetus can receive oxygen and nutrients from the mother from early pregnancy. Placental infarction secondary to maternal conditions such as those mentioned above or premature separation as in placental abruption can impair this transfer and hence fetal growth. These conditions are discussed further in Chapter 10, Pre-eclampsia and other disorders of placentation.

Fetal development

Cardiovascular system and the fetal circulation

The fetal circulation is quite different from that of the adult (Figure 4.1). The fetal circulation is characterized by four shunts which ensure that the best, oxygenated blood from the placenta is delivered to the fetal brain. These shunts are the:

- umbilical circulation;
- ductus venosus;
- foramen ovale;
- ductus arteriosus.

The umbilical circulation carries fetal blood to the placenta for gas and nutrient exchange. The umbilical arteries arise from the caudal end of the dorsal aorta and carry deoxygenated blood from the fetus to the placenta. Oxygenated blood is returned to the fetus via

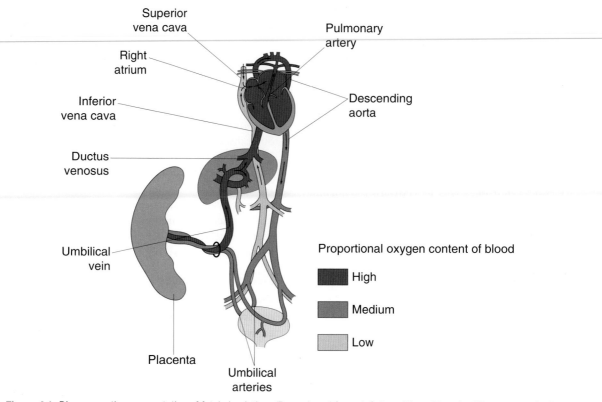

Figure 4.1 Diagrammatic representation of fetal circulation. (Reproduced from *A Colour Atlas of Doppler Ultrasonography in Obstetrics*, by K. Harrington and S. Campbell. London: Arnold, 1995.)

the umbilical vein to the liver. A small proportion of blood oxygenates the liver but the bulk passes through the ductus venosus to bypass the liver and joins the inferior vena cava (IVC) as it enters the right atrium. The ductus is a narrow vessel and high blood velocities are generated within it. This streaming of the ductus venosus blood, together with a membranous valve in the right atrium (the crista dividens), prevents mixing of the well-oxygenated blood from the ductus venosus with the desaturated blood of the inferior vena cava. The ductus venosus stream passes across the right atrium through a physiological defect in the atrial septum called the foramen ovale to the left atrium; from here, blood passes through the mitral valve to the left ventricle and hence to the aorta. About 50 per cent goes to the head and upper extremities; the remainder passes down the aorta to mix with blood of reduced oxygen saturation from the right ventricle. Deoxygenated blood returning from the head and lower body flows through the right atrium and ventricle and into the pulmonary artery after which it bypasses the lungs to enter the descending aorta via

the ductus arteriosus which connects the two vessels. Only a small portion of blood from the right ventricle passes to the lungs, as they are not functional. By this means, the desaturated blood from the right ventricle passes down the aorta to enter the umbilical arterial circulation and to return to the placenta for reoxygenation.

Prior to birth, the ductus remains patent due to the production of prostaglandin E2 and prostacyclin, which act as local vasodilators. Premature closure of the ductus has been reported with the administration of cyclooxygenase inhibitors. At birth, the cessation of umbilical blood flow causes cessation of flow in the ductus venosus, a fall in pressure in the right atrium and closure of the foramen ovale. Ventilation of the lungs opens the pulmonary circulation, with a rapid fall in pulmonary vascular resistance. The ductus arteriosus closes functionally within a few days of birth.

Occasionally, this transition from fetal to adult circulation is delayed, usually because the pulmonary vascular resistance fails to fall despite adequate breathing. This delay, termed persistent fetal circulation, results in left-to-right shunting of blood from the aorta through the ductus arteriosus to the lungs. The baby remains cyanosed and can suffer from life-threatening hypoxia. This delay in closure of the ductus arteriosus is most commonly seen in premature infants. It results in congestion in the pulmonary circulation and a reduction in blood flow to the gastrointestinal tract and brain, and is implicated in the pathogenesis of necrotizing enterocolitis and intraventricular haemorrhage.

Respiratory system

The lung first appears as an outgrowth from the primitive foregut at about 3–4 weeks post-conception and by 4–7 weeks epithelial tube branches and vascular connections are forming. By 20 weeks the conductive airway tree and parallel vascular tree is well developed. By 26 weeks, with further development of the airway and vascular tree, type I and II epithelial cells are beginning to differentiate and surfactant production from these latter cells starts from about 30 weeks. Dilatation of the gas exchanging airspaces, alveolar formation and maturation of the surfactant system continues between this time and delivery at term. The fetal lung is filled with fluid, the production of which starts in early gestation and ends in the early stages of labour. At birth, the production of this fluid ceases and the fluid present is absorbed. Adrenaline, to which the pulmonary epithelium becomes increasingly sensitive towards term, appears to play a major role in this process. With the clearance of the fluid and with the onset of breathing, the resistance in the vascular bed falls and results in an increase in pulmonary blood flow. A consequent increased pressure in the left atrium leads to closure of the foramen ovale.

Surfactant prevents the collapse of small alveoli during expiration by lowering surface tension. It is a mix of phospholipid and protein. The predominant phospholipid (80 per cent of the total) is phosphatidylcholine (lecithin). The production of lecithin is enhanced by cortisol, growth restriction and prolonged rupture of the membranes, and is delayed in diabetes. Inadequate amounts of surfactant result in poor lung expansion and poor gas exchange. In infants delivering preterm, prior to the maturation of the surfactant system, this results in a condition known as respiratory distress syndrome. It typically presents within the first few hours of life with signs of respiratory distress, including tachypnoea and cyanosis. It occurs in more than 80 per cent of infants born between 23 and 27 weeks, falling to 10 per cent of infants born between 34 and 36 weeks. Acute complications include hypoxia and asphyxia, intraventricular haemorrhage and necrotizing enterocolitis. The incidence and severity of RDS can be reduced by administering steroids antenatally to mothers at risk of preterm delivery.

Numerous, but intermittent, fetal breathing movements occur *in utero*, especially during rapid eye movement (REM) sleep, and along with an adequate amniotic fluid volume appear to be necessary for lung maturation. Oligohydramnios (reduced amniotic fluid volume), decreased intrathoracic space (e.g. diaphragmatic hernia), or chest wall deformities can result in pulmonary hypoplasia, which leads to progressive respiratory failure from birth.

Gastrointestinal system

The primitive gut is present by the end of the fourth week, having been formed by folding of the embryo in both craniocaudal and lateral directions with the resulting inclusion of the dorsal aspect of the yolk sac into the intra-embryonic coelom. The primitive gut consists of three parts, the foregut, midgut and hindgut and is suspended by a mesentery through which the blood supply, lymphatics and nerves reach the gut parenchyma. The foregut endoderm gives rise to the oesophagus, stomach, proximal half of the duodenum, liver and pancreas. The midgut endoderm gives rise to the distal half of the duodenum, jejunum, ileum, caecum, appendix, ascending colon and the transverse colon. The hindgut endoderm develops into the descending colon, sigmoid colon and the rectum.

Between 5 and 6 weeks, as a result of lack of space in the abdominal cavity as a consequence of the rapidly enlarging liver and elongation of the intestine, the midgut is extruded into the umbilical cord as a physiological hernia. While herniated, the gut undergoes rotation prior to re-entering the abdominal cavity by 12 weeks. Failure of the gut to re-enter the abdominal cavity results in the development of an omphalocele and this condition is associated with chromosomal anomaly (Figure 4.2).

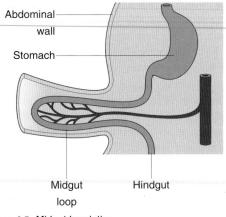

Figure 4.2 **Midgut herniation**

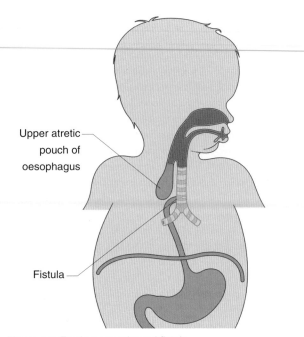

Figure 4.3 **Tracheo-oesophageal fistula**

Other malformations include those which result from failure of the normal rotation of the gut, fistulae and atresias. Malrotation anomalies can result in volvulus and bowel obstruction. Atresias exist when there is a segment of bowel in which the lumen is not patent and are most commonly seen in the upper gastrointestinal tract, i.e. the oesophagus or duodenum. As the fetus continually swallows amniotic fluid, any obstruction which prevents this will result in polyhydramnios (excess amniotic fluid). The most common fistula is the tracheo-oesophageal fistula (TOF), in which a connection exists between the bottom end of the oesophagus and the trachea (Figure 4.3). Without surgical intervention, this causes air to pass from the trachea to the oesophagus and stomach or swallowed milk and stomach acid to pass into the lungs. Some babies with TOF also have other congenital anomalies. This is known as VACTERL (vertebral, anal, cardiac, tracheal, (o)esophageal, renal and limb).

Peristalsis in the intestine occurs from the second trimester. The large bowel is filled with meconium at term. Defecation *in utero*, and hence meconium in the amniotic fluid, is associated with post-term pregnancies and fetal hypoxia. Aspiration of meconium-stained liquor by the fetus at birth can result in meconium aspiration syndrome and respiratory distress.

While body water content gradually diminishes, glycogen and fat stores increase about five-fold in the last trimester. Preterm infants have virtually no fat, and a severely reduced ability to withstand starvation. This is aggravated by an incompletely developed alimentary system, and may manifest in a poor

and unsustained suck, uncoordinated swallowing mechanism, delayed gastric emptying, and poor absorption of carbohydrates, fat and other nutrients. Growth-restricted fetuses also have reduced glycogen stores and are therefore more prone to hypoglycaemia within the early neonatal period.

Liver, pancreas and gall bladder

The pancreas, liver and epithelial lining of the biliary tree derive from the endoderm of the foregut. The liver and biliary tree appear late in the third week or early in the fourth week as the hepatic diverticulum, which is an outgrowth of the ventral wall of the distal foregut. The larger portion of this diverticulum gives rise to the parenchymal cells (hepatocytes) and the hepatic ducts, while the smaller portion gives rise to the gall bladder.

By the sixth week, the liver performs haematopoiesis. This peaks at 12–16 weeks and continues until approximately 36 weeks.

In utero, the normal metabolic functions of the liver are performed by the placenta. For example, unconjugated bilirubin from haemoglobin breakdown is actively transported from the fetus to the mother, with only a small proportion being conjugated in the liver and secreted in the bile (the mechanism after birth). The fetal liver also differs from the adult organ in many processes, for example the fetal liver has a reduced ability to conjugate bilirubin because of relative deficiencies in the necessary enzymes such as glucuronyl transferase. The loss of the placental route of excretion of unconjugated bilirubin, in the presence of reduced conjugation, particularly in the premature infant, may result in transient unconjugated hyperbilirubinaemia or physiological jaundice of the newborn.

Glycogen is stored within the liver in small quantities from the first trimester, but storage is maximal in the third trimester, with abundant stores being present at term. Growth-restricted and premature infants have deficient glycogen stores; this renders them prone to neonatal hypoglycaemia.

Kidney and urinary tract

The kidney, recognized in its permanent final form (metanephric kidney), is preceded by the development and subsequent regression of two primitive forms; the pronephros and mesonephros. The pronephros originates at about 3 weeks in a ridge which forms on either side of the midline in the embryo which is known as the nephrogenic ridge. In this region, epithelial cells arrange themselves in a series of tubules and join laterally with the pronephric duct. The pronephros is non-functional in mammals.

Each pronephric duct grows towards the tail of the embryo. As it does so it induces intermediate mesoderm in the thoracolumbar area to become epithelial tubules called mesonephric tubules. The pronephros degenerates while the mesonephric (Wolffian) duct extends towards the most caudal end of the embryo, ultimately attaching to the cloaca.

During the fifth week of gestation the ureteric bud develops as an out-pouching from the Wolffian duct. This bud grows towards the head of the embryo and into the intermediate mesoderm and as it does so it branches to form the collecting duct system (ureter, pelvis, calyces and collecting ducts) of the kidney and induces the formation of the renal secretory system (glomeruli, convoluted tubes, loops of Henle).

In humans, all of the branches of the ureteric bud and the nephronic units have been formed by 32–36 weeks of gestation. However, these structures are not yet mature, and the maturation of the excretory and concentrating ability of the fetal kidneys is gradual and continues after birth. In the preterm infant this may lead to abnormal water, glucose, sodium or acid-base homeostasis.

As fetal urine forms much of the amniotic fluid, renal agenesis will result in severe reduction or absence of amniotic fluid (oligohydramnios). Babies born with bilateral renal agenesis (Potter's syndrome), which is associated with other features such as widely spaced eyes, small jaw and low set ears, results secondary to oligohydramnios, do not pass urine and usually die either as a consequence of 'renal failure' or pulmonary hypoplasia, again secondary to severe oligohydramnios.

The most common sites of congenital urinary tract obstructive uropathies are at the pyeloureteric junction, the vesicoureteric junction or as a consequence of posterior urethral valves. Severe obstruction *in utero* can lead to hydronephrosis and renal interstitial fibrosis.

Skin and homeostasis

Fetal skin protects and facilitates homeostasis. The skin and its appendages (nails, hair) develop from the ectodermal and mesodermal germ layers. The epidermis develops from the surface ectoderm and the dermis and the hypodermis, which attaches the dermis of the skin to underlying tissues, develop from mesenchymal cells in the mesoderm.

By the fourth week following conception, a single-cell layer of ectoderm surrounds the embryo. At about 6 weeks this ectodermal layer differentiates into an outer periderm and an inner basal layer. The periderm eventually sloughs as the vernix, a creamy protective coat that covers the skin of the fetus. The basal layer produces the epidermis and the glands, nails and hair follicles.

Over the ensuing weeks, the epithelium becomes stratified and by 16–20 weeks all layers of the epidermis are developed and each layer assumes a structure characteristic of the adult. Preterm babies have no vernix and thin skin; this allows a proportionately large amount of insensible water loss. Thermal control in cool, ambient temperatures is limited by a large surface-to-body weight ratio and poor thermal insulation. Heat may be conserved by peripheral vasoconstriction and can be generated by brown fat catabolism, but this is deficient in preterm or growth-restricted babies because of the small amount of subcutaneous fat and immaturity of vascular tone regulation in the former. The response to warm ambient temperatures is also poor and can result in overheating of the infant.

Hair follicles begin to develop as hair buds between 12 and 16 weeks from the basal layer of the epidermis. By 24 weeks the hair follicles produce delicate fetal hair called lanugo, first on the head and then on other parts of the body. This lanugo is usually shed before birth.

Blood and immune system

Red blood cells and immune effector cells are derived from pluripotent haematopoietic cells first noted in the blood islands of the yolk sac. By 8 weeks the yolk sac is replaced by the liver as the source of these cells and by 20 weeks almost all of these cells are produced by the bone marrow.

Circulating monocytes are present by 16 weeks and granulocytes appear in the fetal spleen and liver by 8 weeks and in the circulation by 12–14 weeks. Complement proteins are present by the middle of the second trimester and reach 50 per cent of adult levels at term. Immunoglobulin G (IgG) originates mostly from the maternal circulation and crosses the placenta to provide passive immunity to the fetus and neonate. The fetus normally produces only small amounts of IgM and IgA, which do not cross the placenta. Detection of IgM/IgA in the newborn, without IgG, is indicative of fetal infection.

Most haemoglobin in the fetus is fetal haemoglobin (HbF), which has two gamma-chains (alpha-2, gamma-2). This differs from the adult haemoglobins HbA and HbA2, which have two beta-chains (alpha-2, beta-2) and two delta-chains (alpha-2, delta-2) respectively. Ninety per cent of fetal haemoglobin is HbF between 10 and 28 weeks gestation. From 28 to 34 weeks, a switch to HbA occurs, and at term the ratio of HbF to HbA is 80:20; by six months of age, only 1 per cent of haemoglobin is HbF. A key feature of HbF is a higher affinity for oxygen than HbA. This, in association with a higher haemoglobin concentration (at birth, the mean capillary haemoglobin is 18 g/dL), enhances transfer of oxygen across the placenta.

Abnormal haemoglobin production results in thalassaemia. The thalassaemias are a group of genetic haematological disorders characterized by reduced or absent production of one or more of the globin chains of haemoglobin. Beta-thalassaemia results from reduced or absent production of the beta-globin chains. As the switch from HbF to HbA described above occurs, the absent or insufficient beta-globin chains shorten red cell survival, with destruction of these cells within the bone marrow and spleen. Beta-thalassaemia major results from the inheritance of two abnormal beta genes; without treatment, this leads to severe anaemia, fetal growth restriction, poor musculoskeletal development and skin pigmentation due to increased iron absorption. In the severest form of alpha-thalassaemia, in which no alpha-globulin chains are produced, severe fetal anaemia occurs with cardiac failure, hepatosplenomegaly and generalized oedema. The infants are stillborn or die shortly after birth.

Endocrine system

Major components of the hypothalamic–pituitary axis are in place by 12 weeks gestation. Thyrotropin releasing hormone (TRH) and gonadotrophin releasing hormone (GnRH) have been identified in the fetal hypothalamus by the end of the first trimester. Testosterone produced by the interstitial cells of the testis is also synthesized in the first trimester of pregnancy and increases to 17–21 weeks, which mirrors the differentiation of the male urogenital tract. Growth hormone is similarly present from the early pregnancy and detectable in the circulation from 12 weeks. The thyroid gland produces thyroxine from 10 to 12 weeks. Growth-restricted fetuses exist in a state of relative hypothyroidism which may be a compensatory measure to decrease metabolic rate and oxygen consumption.

Behavioural states

From conception, the fetus follows a developmental path with milestones which continue into childhood. The first activity is the beating of the fetal heart followed by fetal movements at 7–8 weeks. These start as just discernable movements and graduate through startles to movements of arms and legs, breathing movements and by 12 weeks yawning, sucking and swallowing. This means that in the first trimester of pregnancy the fetus exhibits movements which are observed after birth. Further maturation does not add new movements but a change in respect of combinations of movements and activity which reflect fetal behavioural states. In the second trimester, for example, cycles of absence or presence of movements change, meaning that periods over which body movements are absent increase.

Four fetal behavioural states have been described annotated 1F to 4F. 1F is quiescence, 2F is characterized by frequent and periodic gross body movements with eye movements, 3F no gross body movements but eye movements and 4F vigorous continual activity again with eye movements. 1F is similar to quiet or non-REM sleep in the neonate, 2F to REM sleep, 3F to quiet wakefulness and 4F active wakefulness. An understanding of fetal behaviour can assist in assessing fetal condition and well-being.

Amniotic fluid

By 12 weeks gestation, the amnion comes into contact with the inner surface of the chorion and the two membranes become adherent, but never intimately fuse. Neither the amnion nor the chorion contains vessels or nerves, but both do contain a significant quantity of phospholipids as well as enzymes involved in phospholipid hydrolysis. Choriodecidual function is thought to play a pivotal role in the initiation of labour through the production of prostaglandins E2 and F2a.

The amniotic fluid is initially secreted by the amnion, but by the 10th week it is mainly a transudate of the fetal serum via the skin and umbilical cord. From 16 weeks gestation, the fetal skin becomes impermeable to water and the net increase in amniotic fluid is through a small imbalance between the contributions of fluid through the kidneys and lung fluids and removal by fetal swallowing. Amniotic fluid volume increases progressively (10 weeks: 30 mL; 20 weeks: 300 mL; 30 weeks: 600 mL; 38 weeks: 1000 mL), but from term there is a rapid fall in volume (40 weeks: 800 mL; 42 weeks: 350 mL). The reason for the late reduction has not been explained.

The function of the amniotic fluid is to:

- protect the fetus from mechanical injury;
- permit movement of the fetus while preventing limb contracture;
- prevent adhesions between fetus and amnion;
- permit fetal lung development in which there is two-way movement of fluid into the fetal bronchioles; absence of amniotic fluid in the second trimester is associated with pulmonary hypoplasia.

Major alterations in amniotic fluid volume occur when there is reduced contribution of fluid into the amniotic sac in conditions such as renal agenesis, cystic kidneys or fetal growth restriction; oligohydramnios results. Reduced removal of fluid in conditions such as anencephaly and oesophageal/duodenal atresia is associated with polyhydramnios.

CASE HISTORY

A 26-year-old is admitted to the labour ward at 32 weeks gestation. She gives a history suggestive of preterm rupture of membranes and is experiencing uterine contractions. On vaginal examination, the cervix is found to be 8 cm dilated and she rapidly goes on to deliver a male infant weighing 1650 g. At birth he is intubated because of poor respiratory effort and transferred to the neonatal intensive care unit.

As a premature infant, from which complications is he particularly at risk?

Fetal growth
Deficient glycogen stores in the liver increase the risk of hypoglycaemia. This is compounded by the increased glucose requirements of premature infants.

Cardiovascular system
Patent ductus arteriosus may result in pulmonary congestion, worsening lung disease and decreased blood flow to the gastrointestinal tract and brain. The duct can be closed by administering prostaglandin synthetase inhibitors, for example indomethacin, or by surgical ligation.

Respiratory system
Respiratory distress syndrome and apnoea of prematurity may lead to hypoxia. The administration of antenatal steroids to the mother reduces the risk and severity of respiratory distress syndrome. For benefit to be gained, steroids need to be administered at least 24 hours before delivery. In this case, delivery occurred too rapidly for steroids to be administered. The severity of respiratory distress syndrome can also be reduced by giving surfactant via the endotracheal tube used to ventilate the baby.

Fetal blood
Anaemia of prematurity is common because of low iron stores and red cell mass at birth, reduced erythropoiesis and decreased survival of red blood cells. Treatment is by blood

continued ➤

transfusion, iron supplementation or, in some cases, the use of erythropoietin.

Immune system

Preterm babies have an increased susceptibility to infection due to impaired cell-mediated immunity and reduced levels of immunoglobulin. Suspected infection should be treated early with antibiotics because deterioration in these premature small infants can be rapid.

Skin and homeostasis

Hypothermia is common in preterm infants secondary to a relatively large body surface area, thin skin, lack of subcutaneous fat and lack of a keratinized epidermal layer of skin. High insensible water losses due to skin immaturity may aggravate dehydration and electrolyte problems secondary to immaturity in renal function (see below). The environment can be controlled by nursing this type of infant in an incubator.

Alimentary system

Necrotizing enterocolitis is an inflammatory condition of the bowel leading to necrosis, and is thought to be secondary to alterations in gut blood flow, hypotension, hypoxia, infection and feeding practices. Feeding problems are common in preterm infants because they have immature suck and swallowing reflexes and

gut motility. Parenteral nutrition is usually required in these very premature infants, with gradually increasing volumes of milk given by nasogastric tube.

Liver and gall bladder

Jaundice (hyperbilirubinaemia) secondary to liver immaturity and a shorter half-life of red blood cells is common in premature infants. Treatment with phototherapy is required because premature infants are at greater risk of bilirubin encephalopathy.

Kidney and urinary tract

Immaturity of the kidneys can lead to a poor ability to concentrate or dilute urine. This can result in dehydration and electrolyte disturbances: hypernatraemia and hyponatraemia, hyperkalaemia and metabolic acidosis.

Neurological

Periventricular and intraventricular haemorrhages result from bleeding from the immature rich capillary bed of the germinal matrix lining the ventricles. Such haemorrhages are more likely in the presence of hypoxia. Major degrees of haemorrhage can result in hydrocephalus and neurological abnormalities such as cerebral palsy. Periventricular leukomalacia is ischaemic necrosis in the white matter surrounding the lateral ventricles, and commonly leads to cerebral palsy.

A 16-year-old is admitted to the labour ward at 38 weeks gestation. She gives a history suggestive of rupture of membranes and is experiencing uterine contractions. She was seen at 10 weeks gestation for consideration of termination of pregnancy and had a scan at that time which confirmed her gestational age. She opted to continue with the pregnancy but did not attend for antenatal care. She admitted to smoking 20 cigarettes per day. Vaginal examination confirms that the cervix is 8 cm dilated. A CTG demonstrates a baseline fetal heart rate of 165 bpm with variable decelerations, and fetal scalp pH is 7.14 with a base deficit of 12 mmol/L. A Caesarean section is performed and a male infant weighing 1900 g is delivered. Apgar scores are 3 at 1 minute and 8 at 5 minutes.

From which complications are such severely growth-restricted infants particularly at risk?

Reduced oxygen supply *in utero* can result in the fetus being stillborn or suffering damage from acute asphyxia. In the latter case, the neonate may demonstrate features of hypoxic ischaemic

encephalopathy (HIE), which may lead to death from multiorgan failure. If the infant survives, neurological damage and cerebral palsy may result. Chronic hypoxia *in utero* can also result in neurological damage without the acute manifestations of HIE. Other consequences of reduced oxygen supply *in utero* include increased haemopoiesis and cardiac failure. Increased haemopoiesis can in turn result in coagulopathy, polycythaemia and jaundice in the newborn.

Neonatal hypothermia and hypoglycaemia are also more common in this type of infant and result from reduced body fat and glycogen stores. Both of these conditions, if untreated, can lead to increased mortality and neurological damage.

Reduced supply of amino acids *in utero* can impair immune function, increasing the risk of infection in the newborn.

Growth-restricted babies are also at increased risk of chronic diseases such as coronary heart disease, stroke, hypertension and non-insulin-dependent diabetes in adulthood. This is thought to be because the fetal adaptation to undernutrition *in utero* results in the permanent resetting of homeostatic mechanisms, and this leads to later disease.

Key points

- Determinants of birth weight are multifactorial, and reflect the influence of the natural growth potential of the fetus and the intrauterine environment.

- The fetal circulation is quite different from that of the adult. Its distinctive features are:
  - oxygenation occurs in the placenta, not the lungs;
  - the right and left ventricles work in parallel rather than in series;
  - the heart, brain and upper body receive blood from the left ventricle, while the placenta and lower body receive blood from both right and left ventricles.

- Surfactant prevents collapse of small alveoli in the lung during expiration by lowering surface tension. Its production is maximal after 28 weeks.

- Respiratory distress syndrome is specific to babies born prematurely and is associated with surfactant deficiency.

- The fetus requires an effective immune system to resist intrauterine and perinatal infections. Lymphocytes appear from 8 weeks and, by the middle of the second trimester, all phagocytic cells, T and B cells and complement are available to mount a response.

- Fetal skin protects and facilitates homeostasis.

- *In utero*, the normal metabolic functions of the liver are performed by the placenta. The loss of the placental route of excretion of unconjugated bilirubin, in the face of conjugating enzyme deficiencies, particularly in the premature infant, may result in transient unconjugated hyperbilirubinaemia or physiological jaundice of the newborn.

- Growth-restricted and premature infants have deficient glycogen stores; this renders them prone to neonatal hypoglycaemia.

- The function of the amniotic fluid is to:
  - protect the fetus from mechanical injury;
  - permit movement of the fetus while preventing limb contracture;
  - prevent adhesions between fetus and amnion;
  - permit fetal lung development in which there is two-way movement of fluid into the fetal bronchioles; absence of amniotic fluid in the second trimester is associated with pulmonary hypoplasia.

CHAPTER 5

ANTENATAL CARE

Alec McEwan

OVERVIEW

The overall purpose of antenatal care is to optimize the outcome of pregnancy for the mother, her child and the rest of her family.

History taking, examination and the use of investigations are tailored to each individual pregnancy to assess risk and to screen for potential physical, psychological and social problems.

If a potential problem is identified, appropriate action can be taken to minimize the impact it has on the pregnancy. This may involve recruiting help from other professionals.

Models of antenatal care vary throughout the world. Although this chapter discusses the UK model, the principles of high calibre care targeted at the woman's needs are applicable throughout all health care settings.

Aims of antenatal care

The aims of antenatal care are:

- to prevent, detect and manage those factors that adversely affect the health of mother and baby;
- to provide advice, reassurance, education and support for the woman and her family;
- to deal with the 'minor ailments' of pregnancy;
- to provide general health screening.

The original model of antenatal care established in the 1930s involved as many as 15 visits to a doctor or a midwife. This scheme was not evidence based but persisted for many years because of fears that reducing the number of visits would lead to an increase in maternal and perinatal morbidity and mortality. Newer models of antenatal care have questioned the need for so many reviews and in problem-free pregnancies without additional risk factors there is no evidence that fewer visits compromise outcomes. However, the identification of factors which may increase the risks of complications is critical if extra care is to be appropriately targeted. Risk assessment should be viewed as an ongoing exercise throughout the pregnancy so that the type of care offered to a woman can change as new issues and concerns come to light. The community midwife should be seen as the overall coordinator of care, assisting the woman to access specialist services as and when they become necessary. Even if no adverse factors are identified, a minimum standard of care is still to be expected. This chapter focuses on this basic plan for antenatal care and describes how the process of risk assessment is carried out.

The newest models of antenatal care aim to make the woman the focus. Women should be treated with kindness and dignity at all times, and due respect given to personal, cultural and religious beliefs. Services should be readily accessible and there should be continuity of care. There is a need for high quality, culturally appropriate, verbal and written information on which women can base their choices, through a truly informed decision-making process which is led by them. This may seem obvious, however, it remains the case that many pregnant women struggle to engage with what they currently see as a rigid non-individualized system of antenatal care which they feel does not serve their best interests.

Classification of antenatal care

In the UK, maternity care for an individual woman is provided by a community-based team of midwives and GPs, a hospital consultant team, or a combination of the two. A small number of women have such complex pregnancies that the vast majority of their antenatal care is provided by a hospital-based obstetric team and they are said to have 'consultant care'. Many more women have pregnancies where there are no overtly complicating factors and these women usually have community-based care and are said to be 'booked under the midwife'. A further group have factors identified at booking, for example previous Caesarean section, which mandate involvement by obstetricians but where the majority of routine care can still be provided by the community team. Some call this 'shared care'.

In reality, these distinctions are blurred. Women with highly complex pregnancies may nevertheless find helpful the different kind of support and information provided by their community midwife, while women booked under midwifery care will frequently attend hospital day assessment units, and sometimes consultant clinics, when concerns arise. They need not necessarily be reclassified as consultant care if no problem is identified. It remains important though that the woman herself knows who is primarily responsible for the provision of her antenatal care.

Ultrasound scanning is usually performed in a maternity unit, whatever kind of care is accessed. Dating and detailed scans will be organized for a woman whether she is community or consultant booked. There is, however, a movement towards also offering these specialist scanning services in the community and, where this is already happening, there is no need for a woman with a straightforward pregnancy to have any antenatal care or investigation in hospital. Antenatal appointments in the community may be provided in GP surgeries, community hospitals, polyclinics and children's centres. Women should be able to access maternity care easily and should be seen in an environment that allows the

confidential and safe discussion of difficult issues such as domestic violence, sexual abuse, psychiatric illness and substance misuse.

Most women booked under a hospital consultant will have risk factors which recommend delivery of the baby within the obstetric maternity unit, but not all. It may be entirely reasonable for a consultant-booked patient to later choose a home birth, for example. This will depend on the original reason for referral to the consultant. Community-booked women may have a choice between home birth, delivery in a midwife run unit, or delivery in a consultant unit. In some areas, women who are booked with a community midwife, but who choose delivery in hospital, may be looked after in labour by a member of the community team who attends hospital for the birth. This continuity of care can be difficult to achieve.

Whichever form of care is chosen, a pregnant woman will receive a set of client-held records in which all healthcare professionals will write each time she is seen. The booking proforma (Figure 5.1) is found within these notes, as are the results of investigations and plans for the delivery. This improves communication and allows access for all healthcare staff to the same information.

Most maternity units now also provide day-care facilities. Hospital-booked or community-booked patients can be referred to these units for assessment or review of a wide variety of antenatal problems, including hypertension in pregnancy and reduced fetal movements. The units are staffed by experienced midwives, many of whom are trained in ultrasonography. Day-care units help to reduce admissions to antenatal wards which can cause enormous social and domestic disruption.

Advice, reassurance and education

Pregnancy is a time of great uncertainty, and the physical changes experienced by the woman during her pregnancy add to this. She may need explanation and reassurance to help her cope with a wide variety of symptoms, including nausea, heartburn, constipation, shortness of breath, dizziness, swelling, backache, abdominal discomfort and headaches. Mostly, these represent the physiological adaptation of her body to the pregnancy and are often called the 'minor complaints' of pregnancy. Although usually

NAME/ADDRESS/POSTCODE: Parvinder Singh 7, Birchwood Avenue Newtown	AFFIX PATIENT IDENTIFICATION LABEL HERE IF AVAILABLE ALTERNATIVELY WRITE INFORMATION IN BOX PROVIDED	D.O.B: 31-01-63	DATE OF BOOKING	05-02-02	
		Religion:	Marital Status:	Married	
			Previous Name/s:	/	
			Country of Origin:	Pakistan	
			ETHNIC GROUP	Patient	Partner
			White		
Telephone Home:	Telephone Work:		Black Caribbean		
HOSPITAL No.	OCCUPATION: Housewife		Black African		
CONSULTANT: Mr. Jackson	PARTNER'S OCCUPATION: Plumber		Black Other		
PLACE OF DELIVERY: Newtown maternity unit	NHS No:		Indian		
LMP: 12/11/01 EDD: 19/08/02	Silver Stat Card Y/N		Pakistani	✓	✓
FAMILY DOCTOR: Address: Telephone No:			Bangladeshi		
Name: Dr. P. Smith Newtown M/C			Chinese		
HUSBAND/~~PARTNER~~ Address: Telephone No:			Any other group		
Name: Davinder Singh – as above			Not Given		
NEXT OF KIN: Address: Telephone No:					
Relationship: Husband – as above					
Computer information explained Y/N	Signature of Midwife		Printed Name:		
Social Worker	Telephone:		Referral Date:		

MEDICAL AND SURGICAL HISTORY

	YES	NO		YES	NO
1. Cardiac/Hypertension	✓		14. Special Diet		✓
2. Thromboembolism	✓		15. Vegetarian		✓
3. Respiratory		✓	16. Drug Misuse*		✓
4. Renal		✓	17. Bacterial Infections		✓
5. Alimentary		✓	18. Viral Infections		✓
6. Liver		✓	19. Chickenpox		✓
7. Endocrinological	✓		20. Genetic		✓
8. Neurological		✓	21. Previous Surgery	✓	
9. Haematological	✓		22. Previous Infertility		✓
10. Blood Transfusion	✓		23. Other		✓
11. Contraception		✓	24. Mental Health		✓
12. Drugs in Pregnancy		✓	25. Alcohol (units per week)		✓
13. Allergies		✓	26. Smoking		✓

COMMENTS:

1. Previous pre-eclampsia
   Essential hypertension also
2. Previous deep vein thrombosis (left)
7. Hypothyroidism: on thyroxine
9. Anaemia in previous pregnancy
10. and 21. Previous transfusion after C/S.

ANTENATAL INVESTIGATION

BOOKING		DATE	RESULT
B.T.S. Number			
ABO Group			B Pos
Antibodies			Neg
H.I.V.			Neg
VDRL			Neg
Hepatitis	A		Neg
	B		Neg
	C		
Electrophoresis			
Rubella Titre			Immune
AFP			
MSU			
Cytology			
Amniocentesis			
CVS			
Down's Screening			
Other			
PREVIOUS ANTI-D GIVEN YES/NO			
DATES GIVEN			

Figure 5.1   A typical booking proforma contained in patient-held records

Name: Parvinder Singh   Hospital No. ....

PREVIOUS ANAESTHETIC PROBLEMS
(see anaesthetic referral guide lines)

Booking:- Weight

            Height

            BM Index 42

	YES	NO
REFERRAL		

FAMILY HISTORY

	YES	NO		YES	NO		YES	NO
1. Multiple Birth		✓	4. Diabetes	✓		6. Congenital Abnormalities		✓
2. Hypertension	✓		5. Tuberculosis		✓	7. Deafness (Congenital)		✓
3. Thromboembolism	✓		Other					

Comments:

2. Essential hypertension – both Parvinder's parents.
3. Parvinder's mother and sister have both had pulmonary emboli
4. Parvinder's mother has non–insulin dependent diabetes mellitus

OBSTETRIC HISTORY

Menstrual Cycle:	$\frac{5}{28}$				GRAVIDA: 6		PARITY: 4 + 1		

LMP: 12/11/01	EDD: 19/08/02	NORMAL YES/NO		BLEEDING SINCE LMP YES/NO					
DATE	PLACE	DURATION OF PREGNANCY	METHOD OF DELIVERY	SEX	WT.	CONDITION AT BIRTH	NAME OF CHILD
1985	NMU	38 wks	NVD	♂	2.7 kg	A + W	
			(Induced for PET)				
1987	NMU	39 wks	NVD	♀	2.65 kg	A + W	
1990	NMU	39 wks	NVD	♀	2.8 kg	A + W	
1992	NMU	8/40	Miscarriage				
1993	NMU	40 wks	Elective Caesarean	♂	3.0 kg	A + W	
			section. Transverse				
			lie. PPH. Transfusion				

INFORMATION GIVEN

HEA. Pregnancy Booklet   Yes/No   Screening Tests   Yes/No   FW8 Form   Yes/No

Figure 5.1 (*continued*)

of minimal harm, they can be extremely distressing and cause significant anxiety. Occasionally they will be the first presentation of a more serious problem. A skilled community midwife will differentiate those women who need referral to hospital from those who can be reassured and managed with simple advice.

Information regarding smoking, alcohol consumption and the use of drugs during pregnancy (both legal and illegal) is extremely important. In some populations almost a third of women smoke during pregnancy despite its association with fetal growth restriction, preterm labour, abruption and intrauterine fetal death. A major role of antenatal care is to help women limit these harmful behaviours during pregnancy, for example by inclusion in smoking cessation programmes. Alcohol or illegal substance misuse may require more specialized skills from a psychiatric service. Women also need advice on a whole variety of other issues (see below). The information given should be of high quality, and evidence-based. It should be provided in a manner appropriate to the woman, and in written format where possible.

Parentcraft is the term used to describe formal group education of issues relating to pregnancy, labour and delivery and care of the newborn. These sessions offer an opportunity for couples to meet others in the same situation and help to establish a network of social contacts that may be useful after the delivery. They usually include a tour of the maternity department, the aim of which is to lessen anxiety and increase the sense of maternal control surrounding delivery.

Common issues requiring advice and education during pregnancy

- Food hygiene, dietary advice, vitamin supplementation.
- The risks of smoking during pregnancy, smoking cessation, nicotine replacement therapy.
- Alcohol consumption.
- Use of medications.
- Recreational drug misuse.
- Exercise and sexual intercourse.
- Mental health issues.
- Foreign travel, DVT prophylaxis and correct use of seatbelts.

- Maternity rights and benefits.
- Female genital mutilation and domestic violence.
- Screening for fetal problems (Down's syndrome, anomalies, haemoglobinopathies).
- Screening for maternal conditions (diabetes, hypertensive disorders, UTI, anaemia).
- Management of prolonged pregnancy.
- Place of birth and labour.
- Pain relief in labour.
- Breastfeeding and vitamin K prophylaxis.
- Care of the new baby and newborn screening.

Accessing antenatal care: the 'booking visit'

When a woman believes herself to be pregnant she is encouraged to make contact with a community midwife, or less commonly her GP, who will confirm the pregnancy with a urine and/or serum pregnancy test. This initial contact with a health care professional should be an easy process which can occur in a variety of settings. At this point, or shortly afterwards, the community midwife will take a detailed history, examine the woman and perform a series of routine investigations (with the woman's consent) in order that appropriate care can be offered. This is known as 'the booking visit'. If risk factors are identified which may negatively impact on the pregnancy outcome, the midwife will access specialized services on behalf of the woman. This may mean referral to a hospital consultant obstetric clinic, or specialist substance misuse or perinatal mental health teams. Issues raised at the booking visit may need to be explored in some depth.

Confirmation of the pregnancy

The symptoms of pregnancy (breast tenderness, nausea, amenorrhoea, urinary frequency) combined with a positive urinary or serum pregnancy test are usually sufficient confirmation of a pregnancy, and an internal examination to assess uterine size is usually not necessary. All pregnant women should be offered a 'dating scan' (see below), which both confirms the pregnancy and accurately dates it. It may be possible to hear the fetal heart with the Doppler ultrasound from approximately 12 weeks onwards.

Dating the pregnancy

Setting a reliable 'expected date of delivery' (EDD) is an important function of antenatal care. Precise dating of a pregnancy becomes extremely important both at preterm gestations, when it may influence the timing of the delivery if there are fetal or maternal problems, and when the pregnancy is prolonged. A number of different screening tests also rely on an accurate gestation if their interpretation is to be meaningful (see Serum screening for neural tube defects and Down's syndrome in Chapter 7, Prenatal diagnosis). A pregnancy can be dated either by using the date of the first day of the last menstrual period (LMP) or, more accurately, by ultrasound scan.

Menstrual EDD

Chapter 1, Obstetric history taking and examination, explains how the EDD can be calculated from the first day of the last menstrual period. However, this method assumes a 28-day menstrual cycle, ovulation on day 14 of this cycle, and an accurate recollection by the woman of her LMP. In reality, the timing of ovulation is variable within a cycle and most women do not have a period every 28 days. Furthermore, many studies have shown poor recollection of the LMP.

Dating by ultrasound

For these reasons, dating by an ultrasound scan in the first or early second trimester is generally considered to be more accurate, especially if there is menstrual irregularity or uncertainty regarding the LMP. National recommendations state that all women should be offered a dating scan, ideally between 10 and 14 weeks, and that the EDD predicted by this scan should be used in preference to the menstrual EDD.

Benefits of a dating scan

- Accurate dating in women with irregular menstrual cycles or poor recollection of LMP.
- Reduced incidence of induction of labour for 'prolonged pregnancy' (see Chapter 8, Antenatal obstetric complications).
- Maximizing the potential for serum screening to detect fetal abnormalities (see Chapter 7, Prenatal diagnosis).
- Early detection of multiple pregnancies.
- Detection of otherwise asymptomatic failed intrauterine pregnancies.

Before 20 weeks gestation there is minimal variation in fetal size between individual pregnancies, so measurements can be plotted on standard fetal biometry charts and the gestation calculated (Figure 5.2). The crown–rump length (CRL) is used up until 13 weeks + 6 days, and the head circumference (HC) from 14 to 20 weeks. Beyond 20 weeks gestation, the effects of genes and environmental factors will cause significant variability in fetal size. Dating a pregnancy by ultrasound scan therefore becomes progressively less accurate as the gestation advances. This is just one of the potential problems of 'late booking'.

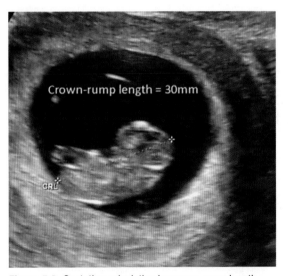

Figure 5.2 Gestation calculation by crown–rump length

CASE HISTORY

Mrs A attends an antenatal booking clinic on 26th June 2009. She has an irregular menstrual cycle and has a poor memory regarding her LMP; she thinks it was 3rd April 2009. From this LMP, her EDD should be 10th January 2010 and at this booking visit she should be 12 weeks gestation. An ultrasound is requested to date the pregnancy and the result is shown in Figure 5.2. The CRL of the fetus is 30 mm. This is plotted to the 50th centile on the CRL chart and found to correspond to 9 weeks and 4 days. The new EDD, based on the scan, is the 25th January 2010.

The booking history

A detailed history is of vital importance if the right kind of care is to be made available from the outset. Past medical, obstetric and gynaecological histories are explored in depth, as these may have a major impact on the pregnancy risk assessment. Family history and social factors may have an even greater impact on the pregnancy than clinical factors. Age and racial origin must be noted at booking. Women at the extremes of reproductive ages are at greater risk of certain pregnancy complications (e.g. fetal chromosomal abnormalities in older women) and specific racial groups carry higher risks of medical conditions, both genetic (e.g. sickle-cell disease and thalassaemias) and otherwise (vitamin D deficiency, diabetes and fibroids, for example). Women from ethnic minorities, or those with sensory impairments, may find it more difficult to access medical care and good quality information. Interpreters are frequently required to overcome language barriers.

CASE HISTORY

Mrs Singh is approximately 8 weeks gestation and attends a booking visit with her community midwife, who fills out her client-held records. The history page is shown in Figure 5.1. A number of issues have been raised which must be addressed when planning her antenatal care.

Mrs Singh is originally from Pakistan, although she has been a UK citizen for many years. This makes a language problem less likely. However, there is no record that a thalassaemia screen has ever been performed. This is important because thalassaemia trait (carrier status) might contribute to maternal anaemia. Furthermore, if the father of this baby is also a carrier, the child will have a one in four chance of having thalassaemia proper. It is reassuring that all the children are fit and well, but this does not exclude the possibility that they are both carriers.

Mrs Singh is 39 years old. This slightly increases the risks of dysfunctional labour and pre-eclampsia, but more significantly is associated with an increase in the risk of certain fetal chromosomal abnormalities, principally Down's syndrome. The decision to undergo screening and invasive testing is a personal one, often influenced by cultural and religious beliefs, but an offer of screening should be made to all women. Mrs Singh has essential hypertension (possibly related to her body weight) but is not currently requiring medication. This, her previous history of pre-eclampsia (in her first pregnancy), and her age all increase the risk of pre-eclampsia occurring in this pregnancy. Regular antenatal checks will be needed to detect a recurrence. There is a worrying personal history of deep vein thrombosis and a family history of pulmonary emboli. It is possible that this family has an inherited thrombophilia (increased blood-clotting tendency) such as protein C or S deficiency. Confirming or excluding this possibility is important because thrombophilias are associated with a high thrombotic risk in pregnancy and an increase in the risk of fetal growth restriction, placental abruption and pre-eclampsia. Many of these complications can be prevented by the use of antenatal and post-natal low-dose aspirin and heparin injections.

Mrs Singh's children have all been of low birthweight. It is difficult to determine whether they were constitutionally (genetically) small, but healthy, or whether they were pathologically small (i.e. growth restricted). It would be important to organize serial growth scans during this pregnancy as surveillance for fetal growth restriction.

Hypothyroidism corrected by thyroxine supplements rarely causes complications during pregnancy. Anaemia is common and usually responds to oral iron supplements. Dietary advice may be necessary and other causes of anaemia must always be considered. Mrs Singh is at risk of Vitamin D deficiency, and should be offered supplements. The blood transfusion after her last delivery has been noted. No red cell antibodies have arisen as a result, but these will need to be checked for again later in the pregnancy.

Mrs Singh has a raised body mass index (BMI) and this increases her risks of anaesthetic complications (such as failure to intubate or successfully site a spinal anaesthetic) and also her risks of developing gestational diabetes. An oral glucose tolerance test will be recommended at 28 weeks gestation to screen for this.

Finally, the previous Caesarean section is an issue which will require discussion. The transverse lie was probably secondary to uterine laxity, but this would need to be confirmed by reading the old notes. Malpresentation at term may occur again, but even if it does not the options for mode of delivery (vaginal birth after Caesarean 'VBAC' versus elective repeat Caesarean section 'ERCS') will need to be discussed.

In conclusion, Mrs Singh has a number of factors that increase the risks of complications in this pregnancy. Shared care under a hospital consultant would be the appropriate form of antenatal care.

The community midwife subsequently refers Mrs Singh to an obstetric consultant clinic where she is seen at 12 weeks gestation, with a dating scan. She opts not to have an NT scan, but is keen to have a detailed scan at 20 weeks. She is seen in the consultant clinic, with fetal growth scans, on three further occasions. The community midwife also meets with Mrs Singh regularly, in between these appointments. Her oral glucose tolerance test is normal, and her blood pressure does not rise significantly. At the final hospital visit at 36 weeks gestation she expresses her desire for a vaginal birth. The fetus remains in a cephalic presentation and she labours spontaneously at 39 weeks gestation, giving birth normally to a healthy male infant weighing 2.5 kg.

A detailed guide to obstetric history taking is given in Chapter 1, Obstetric history taking and examination. It is helpful to remember the following areas which must be covered; past medical and surgical history, past obstetric and gynaecological history, family history and social history. A set of client-held records should be completed by the midwife during this booking visit. Although these vary from region to region, they are similar and a simplified example is shown in Figure 5.1. An example case history is provided which demonstrates why this history taking is so important.

The booking examination

Historically a full physical examination was carried out at the booking visit. This included the cardiovascular and respiratory systems as well as an abdominal, full pelvic and breast examination, as detailed in Chapter 1, Obstetric history taking and examination. The value of this has been questioned as the detection of significant pathology in the absence of specific symptoms is uncommon. Loud heart sounds and flow murmurs can be heard in most pregnant women and usually result from the hyperdynamic circulation characteristic of pregnancy, rather than from pathology. Speculum examination in the absence of bleeding or discharge is likely to be unhelpful, uncomfortable and embarrassing for the woman, and routine breast examination has a higher false-positive rate due to pregnancy-related physiological changes in breast tissue. Furthermore, excessive anxiety can be caused by the subsequent referrals that are made to other specialists when spurious 'signs' are found.

Most of these 'rituals' have been dispensed with in low-risk women, but thorough examination must be carried out if there are symptoms or risk factors of concern. Recent immigrants, for example, should have a full chest and cardiac examination. Subclinical rheumatic heart disease and congenital cardiac anomalies may have gone previously unrecognized and will usually become clinically significant during pregnancy.

For most healthy women, without complicating medical problems, the booking examination will include the following:

- Accurate measurement of blood pressure.
- Abdominal examination to record the size of the uterus.
- Recognition of any abdominal scars indicative of previous surgery.
- Measurement of height and weight for calculation of the BMI. Women with a low BMI are at greater risk of fetal growth restriction and obese women are at significantly greater risk of most obstetric complications, including gestational diabetes, pre-eclampsia, need for emergency Caesarean section and anaesthetic difficulties.
- Urine dip testing for protein, glucose, leukocytes, nitrates and blood.

Booking investigations

Full blood count

A full blood count is a screen for anaemia and thrombocytopenia, both of which may require further investigation. Anaemia in pregnancy is most frequently caused by iron deficiency; however, a wide variety of other causes must be considered, especially if the haemoglobin value is below 9.0 g/dL. A haemoglobin level of 11 g/dL or more is considered normal early in pregnancy, with the upper limit of the 'normal range' dropping to 10.5 g/dL by 28 weeks gestation. Routine iron supplements are not recommended unless the Hb falls below these values and tests suggest iron deficiency. A full blood count is normally repeated at 28 weeks gestation.

Blood group and red cell antibodies

Recording the blood group at this point will help with cross-matching blood at a later date if an emergency arises. Women found to be rhesus D negative will be offered prophylactic anti-D administration to prevent rhesus D iso-immunization and haemolytic disease of the fetus and newborn in future pregnancies (see Chapter 8, Antenatal obstetric complications). Prophylactic anti-D is either given as a single dose at 28 weeks gestation, or in divided doses at 28 and 34 weeks. Other possible isoimmunizing events, such as threatened miscarriage after 12 weeks gestation, antepartum haemorrhage and delivery of the baby, will require additional anti-D prophylaxis in rhesus D-negative women. Other red cell antibodies may also cause fetal and neonatal haemolysis, and problems with blood cross-matching in the event of maternal haemorrhage. These atypical red cell antibodies most commonly arise from previous blood transfusions and screening tests for these antibodies are performed for a second time in all women at 28 weeks gestation.

Urinalysis

A midstream urine sample should be sent early in pregnancy to detect asymptomatic bacteriuria, which is common in pregnancy. Treating otherwise unidentified urinary infections reduces the chances of developing pyelonephritis.

Rubella

Vertical transmission of rubella from a mother to her fetus carries a high risk of causing serious congenital abnormalities, especially in the first trimester. Women who are found to be rubella non-immune should be strongly advised to avoid infectious contacts and should undergo rubella immunization after the current pregnancy to protect their future pregnancies. The theoretical risk of viral reactivation from the vaccine means it should not be given during pregnancy, and pregnancy should be avoided for the three months following immunization. A history of previous immunization is not a guarantee of permanent immunity.

Hepatitis B

The presence of antibodies to the hepatitis B surface antigen represents immunity resulting either from previous infection or from immunization and should not cause concern. The presence of the surface antigen itself, or the 'e' antigen, represents either a recent infection or carrier status. Vertical transmission to the fetus may occur, mostly during labour, and horizontal transmission to maternity staff or the newborn infant can follow contact with bodily fluids. Immunization of the baby after birth minimizes the transmission risk. All babies born to hepatitis B carriers should be actively immunized (vaccination) and those born to women who are highly infective should also receive passive immunization with hepatitis B immunoglobulin (HBIG).

Human immunodeficiency virus

Without screening, less than half of all pregnant women infected with human immunodeficiency virus (HIV) are aware of their status. In known HIV-positive mothers, the use of antiretroviral agents, elective Caesarean section and avoidance of breastfeeding may reduce the vertical transmission rate from approximately 30 per cent to less than 1 per cent. Knowledge of HIV infection is therefore vital if the offspring are to be protected. Screening only those women at high risk of HIV infection (e.g. intravenous drug abusers, recent immigrants from central Africa) misses a significant number of cases. The Department of Health guidelines now recommend that all pregnant women should be offered an HIV test at booking.

Syphilis

The incidence of syphilis has been rising over the last ten years. It can be vertically transmitted to the fetus, with serious consequences. This transmission can be prevented simply by treatment of the mother with antibiotics, and screening in pregnancy can be justified. Serological screening tests for syphilis are notorious for giving false positive results. Other treponemal infections (endemic in some countries) and a variety of other medical conditions may give positive results in the absence of syphilis. Women who have been successfully treated in the past may still have positive serology. Interpretation of positive screening results requires specialist skills, and genitourinary medicine teams are usually consulted.

Haemoglobin studies

All women should be offered screening for haemoglobinopathies. The thalassaemias and sickle-cell diseases are carried in an autosomal recessive fashion and the partner of a carrier, or fully affected woman, should also be offered carrier testing. If both the woman and the father of the baby are found to be carriers there is a one in four risk that the pregnancy will be affected by the full condition. Prenatal genetic tests following chorionic villus sampling (CVS) or amniocentesis can usually definitively diagnose or exclude the condition in the fetus. In areas where the prevalence of these conditions is low, screening is performed using the Family Origin Questionnaire and a routine full blood count. Women from the Eastern Mediterranean, India, West Indies, South-East Asia and the Middle East are at greatest risk. If the questionnaire indicates a high risk of thalassaemia or sickle-cell disease, or if the mean corpuscular haemoglobin is low, then formal laboratory screening with liquid chromatography should be carried out. Where disease prevalence is high, all pregnant women should be offered laboratory screening with high performance liquid chromatography.

Other routine booking investigations

At the current time, the evidence base does not support routine screening for bacterial vaginosis, cytomegalovirus, toxoplasmosis, hepatitis C or group B streptococcus colonization. Routine screening for chlamydia is not recommended by NICE, however women under the age of 25 should be informed of their local National Chlamydia Screening Programme. Cervical smears and vaginal swabs are not routinely taken at the booking visit. However, smears should be performed during pregnancy on women with an abnormal cervix on examination or those who are overdue for a smear and are likely to default in the post-natal period. The request form should state clearly that the woman is pregnant, as this will affect interpretation of the cytology.

Screening for fetal abnormalities

This is a routine aspect of antenatal care, offered to all women in some form or another. Initial discussion of these screening tests usually occurs at the booking visit to establish the wishes of the couple. Provision of high-quality unbiased information is critical at this point so that women and their partners can make an informed choice. These tests are not mandatory, and many choose not to have them.

The tests themselves are carried out between 11 and 22 weeks gestation and include:

- screening for Down's syndrome. A wide variety of methods exist and these are discussed in detail in Chapter 7, Prenatal diagnosis. Essentially they include a nuchal translucency scan at 11–14 weeks gestation, with or without biochemical tests, or biochemical blood tests in isolation at 15–20 weeks;
- screening for neural tube defects (e.g. spina bifida, anencephaly) with maternal serum alpha-fetoprotein levels at 15–20 weeks gestation. This blood test has been mostly superseded by routine detailed structural scanning at 18–20 weeks and is likely to become obsolete in the near future;
- screening for structural congenital abnormalities by ultrasound examination at 18 to 20 + 6 weeks

gestation (details in Chapter 6, Antenatal imaging and assessment of fetal well-being).

Screening for clinical conditions later in pregnancy

Gestational diabetes

Policies for screening for gestational diabetes mellitus (GDM) have previously varied widely within regions and across the country. The NICE clinical guideline on 'Diabetes in pregnancy' (number 63), issued in July 2008, has introduced a degree of uniformity. All women should be assessed at booking for risk factors for gestational diabetes (see box below). If risk factors are present, the woman should be offered a 2-hour 75 g oral glucose tolerance test (OGTT) at 24–28 weeks gestation. It is imperative that the woman is informed why these tests have been recommended, and what the implications of a positive screening result would be. A previous history of gestational diabetes should prompt glucose monitoring, or an OGTT, at 16–18 weeks. If these results are normal, the test should be repeated at 24–28 weeks. Further details are given in Chapter 12, Medical diseases complicating pregnancy.

> **Risk factors for screening for gestational diabetes**
>
> - BMI above 30 kg/m².
> - Previous baby weighing 4.5 kg, or above.
> - Previous gestational diabetes.
> - First-degree relative with diabetes.
> - Family origin from high prevalence area (South Asian, black Caribbean and Middle Eastern).

Pre-eclampsia and preterm birth

All women should be screened at every antenatal visit for pre-eclampsia by measurement of blood pressure and urinalysis for protein. Extra antenatal visits, above the minimum schedule, will be indicated for women with risk factors for pre-eclampsia elicited by the booking history and examination, or for women who have a rise in blood pressure above certain limits, or those who develop proteinuria or symptoms suggestive of pre-eclampsia. Other screening tests for pre-eclampsia, based on blood tests or ultrasound scanning, are not recommended for routine antenatal care. Women without a history of preterm birth should not be routinely offered screening tests for preterm labour, such as bacterial swabs, or cervical length scans.

Fetal growth and well-being

Symphysis-fundal height measurements should be performed with a tape-measure at every antenatal appointment from 25 weeks gestation and the values plotted on a centile chart, ideally customized to the woman herself. Concerns that fetal growth may be slow, or has stopped altogether, should be addressed by ultrasound scanning. However, routine growth scans are not recommended in the absence of specific risk factors, and the evidence base does not support their use if the uterus is felt to be large-for-dates, unless there are concerns about polyhydramnios. Women should not be advised to routinely count fetal movements in normal pregnancies, however, further fetal assessment is indicated if the woman perceives a reduction in movements. It is still common practice to listen to the fetal heart at each antenatal visit in the second and third trimester, either with a Pinnard stethoscope or Doppler ultrasound. This is no longer supported by NICE if the fetus is active, but it is recognized as reasonable if the woman requires reassurance.

Follow-up visits

NICE has published a clinical guideline (Number 62) which details a recommended schedule of antenatal appointments for women who are healthy and whose pregnancies remain uncomplicated. This is summarized in Table 5.1. Primiparous women are scheduled to have two more routine checks than multiparous women. Pre-eclampsia is a common complication of first pregnancies, particularly in the late third trimester. It can develop very rapidly and the two additional visits for primiparous women are designed to maximize detection at an early stage. Additional appointments may need to be scheduled if there are factors which are recognized to increase the risks of problems developing. It is clear from the schedule that maternal blood pressure and urine

should be examined at each and every visit, and that the symphysiofundal height should be measured from 25 weeks gestation. Fetal presentation and degree of engagement should be assessed from 36 weeks. Maternal weight is no longer recorded routinely after the initial booking examination. Rhesus D-negative women should be offered routine antenatal prophylaxis, either as a single large dose at 28 weeks gestation, or in smaller divided doses at 28 and 34 weeks gestation.

Common problems detected in routine antenatal care are hypertensive disorders of pregnancy, anaemia, abnormalities of uterine size ('small-for-dates' and 'large-for-dates') and abnormal fetal presentations. Further investigation in hospital will usually be necessary.

Each follow-up visit should be seen as an opportunity for women to express their anxieties and to educate them in the details of delivery, infant feeding and parenting skills. A recommended schedule of information giving and education is also suggested in the NICE guideline (Table 5.1).

Customized antenatal care

Through the process of booking and routine antenatal follow up, it may become apparent that a woman and her pregnancy have risk factors or special needs not met by standard care. Referrals to other hospital consultants, psychiatric services, social services and physiotherapists are common in pregnancy. Indeed, 'high-risk' antenatal clinics staffed by specially skilled obstetricians and doctors from other disciplines can usually be found in tertiary centres.

Antenatal complications dealt with in customized antenatal clinics

- Endocrine (diabetes, thyroid, prolactin and other endocrinopathies).
- Miscellaneous medical disorders (e.g. secondary hypertension and renal disease, autoimmune disease).
- Haematological (thrombophilias, bleeding disorders).
- Substance misuse.
- Preterm labour.
- Multiple gestation.
- Teenage pregnancies.

Table 5.1 Recommended schedule of antenatal visits (NICE Clinical Guideline 62)

Visit	Purpose	Primips	Multips
Initial contact	Information giving, including folic acid supplementation, food hygiene Lifestyle issues and screening tests offered	•	•
Booking (by 10w)	Extensive information giving Identification of women needing additional care Offer screening tests Offer dating scan, Down's syndrome (DS) screening and detailed scan Calculate BMI, measure BP, test urine	•	•
Dating scan (10–14w)	To accurately determine gestational age, finalize EDD and to detect multiple pregnancies	•	•
16w	Review test results. Offer quadruple test if not yet screened for DS Provide information with focus on the detailed scan BP/urine dip	•	•
18–20w	Ultrasound for structural anomalies	•	•
25w	Information giving, BP/urine dip/symphysiofundal height measurement (SFH)	•	
28w	Information giving, BP/urine dip/SFH Second screen for anaemia and red cell antibodies Anti-D prophylaxis for RhD-negative women	•	•
31w	Information giving, BP/urine dip/SFH	•	
34w	Provide information with a focus on labour and birth BP/urine dip/SFH 2nd dose of prophylactic anti-D (depending on local dosage schedule)	•	•
36w	Provide information with a focus on breastfeeding, Vitamin K for the newborn, care of the baby, post-natal issues Palpation for fetal presentation BP/urine dip/SFH	•	•
38w	Provide information with a focus on prolonged pregnancy Palpation for fetal presentation BP/urine dip/SFH	•	•
40w	Provide further information with a focus on prolonged pregnancy Palpation for fetal presentation BP/urine dip/SFH	•	
41w	Offer membrane sweep and formal induction of labour Palpation for fetal presentation BP/urine dip/SFH	•	•

Furthermore, a number of regions are fortunate in having dedicated perinatal mental health teams to care for pregnant women with psychiatric problems. Included in the team are psychiatrists, counsellors, community psychiatric nurses and social workers who have a special interest in pregnancy and its interaction with psychiatric and psychological problems (see Chapter 18, Psychiatric disorders and the puerperium).

New developments

- The community midwife should be viewed as the lead professional, helping the woman access specialist services, as and when required.

- Vitamin D deficiency is common in pregnant women from certain high risk groups. Vitamin D supplements are found in multivitamin preparations designed for pregnancy, and women should be encouraged to take these, particularly if they have risk factors for deficiency.

- Down's syndrome screening should be offered to all women, and the test offered should have a high sensitivity and a low false positive rate. Consent for all forms of fetal anomaly screening should be documented.

Key points

- Antenatal care improves pregnancy outcomes and a variety of models exist.

- There are key visits during the pregnancy when essential investigations or decisions are taken regarding antenatal care and delivery.

- Antenatal care should be seen as an opportunity for education, reassurance and screening for potential problems.

- Continued efforts should be made to improve the access to antenatal care for disadvantaged and minority groups.

CHAPTER 6

ANTENATAL IMAGING AND ASSESSMENT OF FETAL WELL-BEING

Gary Mires

OVERVIEW

Ultrasound is the principal imaging modality used in obstetrics. Indeed, diagnostic ultrasound is used to screen all pregnancies in most developed countries. Ultrasound is used to date pregnancies and chart antenatal growth of the fetus and to identify congenital abnormalities. Colour and spectral Doppler can identify placental and fetal blood vessels and provide information on placental function and the fetal circulatory response to hypoxia.

Antenatal tests of fetal well-being are now principally based on ultrasound techniques and are designed to identify the fetuses that are in the early or late stages of fetal hypoxia. Continuous wave Doppler ultrasound is employed to provide continuous tracings of the fetal heart rate, the patterns of which alter when the fetus is hypoxic.

Three-dimensional ultrasound and increasingly magnetic resonance imaging (MRI) are used to provide further information when a fetal abnormality is suspected.

Diagnostic ultrasound in obstetric practice

In 1959, Professor Ian Donald, the Regius Chair of Midwifery at Glasgow University, noted that clear echoes could be obtained from the fetal head using ultrasound. Since the reporting of this initial discovery, the technique of ultrasound has developed into one which now plays an essential role in the care of nearly every pregnant woman in the developed world.

The ultrasound technique uses very high frequency sound waves of between 3.5 and 7.0 mega hertz emitted from a transducer. Transducers can be placed and moved across the maternal abdomen (transabdominal, Figure 6.1) or mounted on a probe which can be inserted into the vagina (transvaginal, Figure 6.2)

Transvaginal ultrasonography is useful in early pregnancy, for examining the cervix later in pregnancy and for identifying the lower edge of the placenta. It is also useful in early pregnancy in women with significant amounts of abdominal adipose tissue through which abdominal ultrasound waves would need to travel and

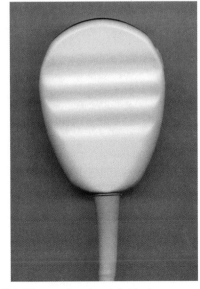

Figure 6.1 Ultrasound probe; abdominal

hence be attenuated prior to reaching the uterus and its contents, making visualization difficult. In general, however, after 12 weeks gestation, an abdominal transducer, which is a flat or curvilinear probe with a

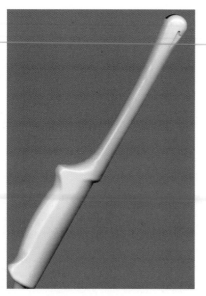

Figure 6.2 Ultrasound probe; trans vaginal

much wider array, is used. Crystals within the transducer emit a focused ultrasound beam in a series of pulses and then receive the reflected signals from within the uterus between the pulses. The strength of the reflected sound wave depends on the difference in 'acoustic impedance' between adjacent structures. The acoustic impedance of a tissue is related to its density; the greater the difference in acoustic impedance between two adjacent tissues the more reflective will be their boundary. The returning signals are transformed into visual signals and generate a continuous picture of the moving fetus. Movements such as fetal heart beat and malformations in the fetus can be assessed and measurements can be made accurately on the images displayed on the screen. Such measurements enable the assessment of gestational age, size and growth in the fetus. Ultrasound images obtained can also be processed with computer software to produce three-dimensional (3D) images and even four-dimensional (moving 3D images) which provide more detail on fetal anatomical structure and the identification of anomalies.

The use of Doppler ultrasound allows the assessment of the velocity of blood within fetal and placental vessels and provides indirect assessment of fetal and placental condition. Doppler ultrasound makes use of the phenomenon of the Doppler frequency shift, where the reflected wave will be at a different frequency from the transmitted one if it interacts with moving structures, such as red blood cells flowing along a blood vessel with the change in

frequency being proportional to the velocity of the blood cells. If the red blood cells are moving towards the beam, the reflected signal will be at a higher frequency than the transmitted one and conversely the reflected beam will be at a lower signal if the flow is away from the beam. In this modality, signals from a particular vessel can be isolated and displayed in graphic form, with the velocity plotted against time. The significance of changes observed in waveform patterns obtained from placental and fetal vessels and how these observations can be used in clinical practice will be discussed later in the chapter.

Ultrasound scanning is currently considered to be a safe, non-invasive, accurate and cost-effective investigation in the fetus. This chapter will consider the diagnostic use of these techniques in more detail.

Clinical applications of ultrasound

The main uses of ultrasonography in pregnancy are in the areas discussed below.

Diagnosis and confirmation of viability in early pregnancy

The gestational sac can be visualized from as early as 4–5 weeks of gestation and the yolk sac at about 5 weeks (Figure 6.3). The embryo can be observed and measured at 5–6 weeks gestation. A visible heartbeat can be visualized by about 6 weeks.

Transvaginal ultrasound plays a key role in the diagnosis of disorders of early pregnancy, such as incomplete or missed miscarriage, blighted ovum where no fetus is present (Figure 6.4) and ectopic

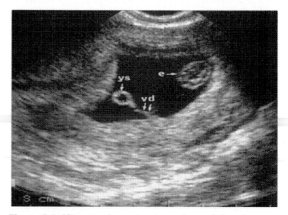

Figure 6.3 Ultrasound sac showing yolk sac (ys) and embryo (e) with the vitelline duct (vd)

pregnancy. In a missed miscarriage, for example, the fetus can be identified, but with an absent fetal heart and in a blighted ovum, the absence of fetal development results in the presence of a gestational sac which is empty. An ectopic pregnancy is suspected if, in the presence of a positive pregnancy test, an ultrasound scan does not identify a gestation sac within the uterus, there is an adnexal mass with or without a fetal pole, or there is fluid in the pouch of Douglas.

Determination of gestational age and assessment of fetal size and growth

Up to approximately 20 weeks gestation the range of values around the mean for measurements of fetal length, head size and long bone length is narrow and hence assessment of gestation based on these measures is accurate. The crown–rump length (CRL) is used up to 13 weeks + 6 days, and the head circumference (HC) from 14 to 20 weeks gestation. The biparietal diameter (BPD) (Figure 6.5) and femur length (FL) (Figure 6.6) can also be used to determine gestational age. Essentially, the earlier the measurement is made, the more accurate the prediction, and measurements made from an early CRL (accuracy of prediction ± 5 days) will be preferred to a biparietal diameter at 20 weeks (accuracy of prediction ± 7 days).

In the latter part of pregnancy, measuring fetal abdominal circumference (AC) (Figure 6.7) and HC will allow assessment of the size and growth of the fetus and will assist in the diagnosis and management

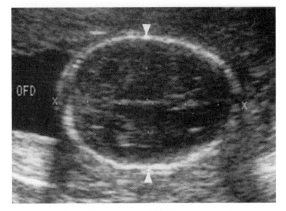

Figure 6.5 Biparietal diameter (BPD)

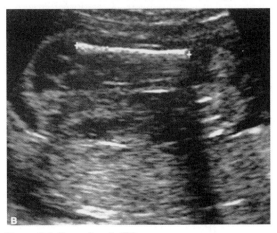

Figure 6.6 Femur length (FL)

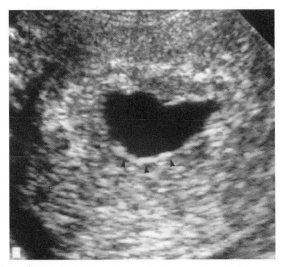

Figure 6.4 Ultrasound image showing empty gestation sac in a case of blighted ovum

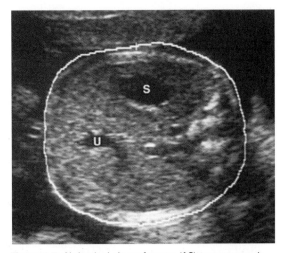

Figure 6.7 Abdominal circumference (AC) measurement demonstrating the correct section showing the stomach (S) and the umbilical vein (U)

of fetal growth restriction. In addition to AC and HC, BPD and FL, when combined in an equation, provide a more accurate estimate of fetal weight (EFW) than any of the parameters taken singly.

In pregnancies at high risk of fetal growth restriction (FGR), serial measurements are plotted on the normal reference range. Growth patterns are helpful in distinguishing between different types of growth restriction (symmetrical and asymmetrical). Asymmetry between head measures (BPD, HC) and AC can be identified in FGR, where a brain-sparing effect will result in a relatively large HC compared with the AC (Figure 6.8). The opposite would occur in a diabetic pregnancy, where the abdomen is disproportionately large due to the effects of insulin on the fetal liver and fat stores. Cessation of growth is an ominous sign of placental failure.

Gestational age cannot be accurately calculated by ultrasound after 20 weeks gestation because of the wider range of normal values of AC and HC around the mean.

Multiple pregnancy

Ultrasound is now the most common way in which multiple pregnancies are identified (Figure 6.9). In addition to identifying the presence of more than one fetus, it can also be used to determine the chorionicity of the pregnancy.

Monochorionic twin pregnancies (i.e. those who 'share' a placenta) are associated with an increased risk of pregnancy complications and a higher perinatal mortality rate than dichorionic twin pregnancies. It is therefore clinically useful to be able to determine chorionicity early in pregnancy (see Chapter 9, Twins and higher multiple gestations).

The dividing membrane in monochorionic twins is formed by two layers of amnion and in dichorionic twins by two layers of chorion and two of amnion. Dichorionic twins therefore have thicker membranes than monochorionic twins and this can be perceived qualitatively on ultrasound. Ultrasonically, dichorionic twin pregnancies in the first trimester of pregnancy have a thick inter-twin separating membrane (septum), flanked on either side by a very thin amnion. This is in contrast to a monochorionic twin pregnancy, which on two-dimensional ultrasound has a very thin inter-twin septum.

Another method of determining chorionicity in the first trimester uses the appearance of the septum at its origin from the placenta. On ultrasound, a

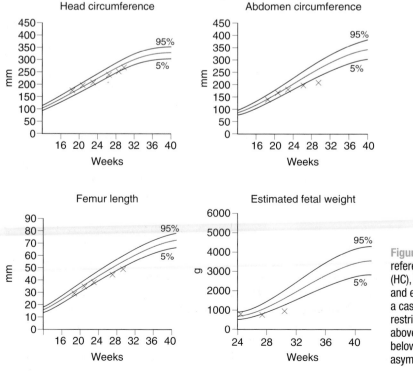

Figure 6.8 Ultrasound plots on reference range for head circumference (HC), abdominal circumference (AC) and estimated fetal weight (EFW) in a case of early onset fetal growth restriction (FGR). Note that HC remains above 5th centile while the AC falls below 5th centile. This is a case of asymmetric FGR with head sparing

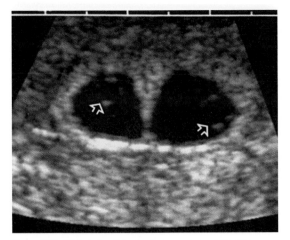

Figure 6.9 Early twin dichorionic pregnancy; note the 'peaked' inter twin membrane

tongue of placental tissue is seen within the base of dichorionic membranes and has been termed the 'twin peak' or 'lambda' sign. The optimal gestation at which to perform such ultrasonic chorionicity determination is 9–10 weeks. Dichorionicity will also be confirmed by the identification of two placental masses and later in pregnancy by the presence of different-sex fetuses.

Ultrasound is also invaluable in the management of twin pregnancy in terms of confirming fetal presentations, which may be difficult on abdominal palpation, evidence of growth restriction, fetal anomaly and the presence of placenta praevia, all of which are more common in this type of pregnancy, and any suggestion of twin-to-twin transfusion syndrome.

Diagnosis of fetal abnormality

Major structural abnormalities occur in 2–3 per cent of pregnancies and many can be diagnosed by an ultrasound scan at around or before 20 weeks gestation. Common examples include spina bifida and hydrocephalus, skeletal abnormalities such as achondroplasia, abdominal wall defects such as exomphalos and gastroschisis, cleft lip/palate and congenital cardiac abnormalities.

Detection rates of between 40 and 90 per cent have been reported. This means that a 'normal scan' is not a guarantee of a normal baby. A number of factors can influence the success of detecting an abnormality. Some are very difficult to visualize or to be absolutely certain about. Some conditions, for

example hydrocephalus, may not have been obvious at the time of early scans. The position of the baby in the uterus will influence visualization of organs such as the heart, face and spine. Repeat scans are sometimes required if visualization is a problem in anticipation that the fetus will be in a more accessible position.

First trimester ultrasonic 'soft' markers for chromosomal abnormalities such as the absence of fetal nasal bone, an increased fetal nuchal translucency (the area at the back of the neck) are now in common use to enable detection of fetuses at risk of chromosomal anomalies such as Down's syndrome.

Placental localization

Placenta praevia can cause life-threatening haemorrhage in pregnancy. Ultrasonography has become indispensible in the localization of the site of the placenta and thus ultrasonographic identification of the lower edge of the placenta to exclude or confirm placenta praevia as a cause for antepartum haemorrhage is now a part of routine clinical practice. The transvaginal approach, undertaken with caution, can be helpful in clearly identifying the lower placental edge if not seen clearly with an abdominal probe.

At the 20 weeks scan, it is customary to identify women who have a low-lying placenta. At this stage, the lower uterine segment has not yet formed and most low-lying placentas will appear to 'migrate' upwards as the lower segment stretches in the late second and third trimesters. About 5 per cent of women have a low-lying placenta at 20 weeks, and only 5 per cent of this group will eventually be shown to have a placenta praevia.

Amniotic fluid volume assessment

Ultrasound can be used to identify both increased and decreased amniotic fluid volumes. The fetus has a role in the control of the volume of amniotic fluid. It swallows amniotic fluid, absorbs it in the gut and later excretes urine into the amniotic sac. Congenital abnormalities that impair the fetus's ability to swallow, for example anencephaly or oesophageal atresia, will result in an increase in amniotic fluid. Congenital abnormalities that result in a failure of urine production or passage, for example renal agenesis and posterior urethral valves, will result in reduced or absent amniotic fluid. Fetal growth restriction can be associated with reduced amniotic fluid because of reduced renal perfusion and hence urine output. Variation from the normal range of amniotic fluid volume calls for a further detailed ultrasound assessment of possible causes.

Assessment of fetal well-being

Ultrasound can be used to assess fetal well-being by evaluating fetal movements, tone and breathing in the Biophysical Profile. Doppler ultrasound can be used to assess placental function and identify evidence of blood flow redistribution in the fetus, which is a sign of hypoxia. These aspects of ultrasound use will be discussed later in the chapter.

Measurement of cervical length

Evidence suggests that approximately 50 per cent of women who deliver before 34 weeks gestation will have a short cervix. The length of the cervix can be assessed using transvaginal scanning.

Other uses

Ultrasonography is also of value in other obstetric conditions such as:

- confirmation of intrauterine death;
- confirmation of fetal presentation in uncertain cases;
- diagnosis of uterine and pelvic abnormalities during pregnancy, for example fibromyomata and ovarian cysts.

Scanning schedule in clinical practice

The National Institute for Health and Clinical Excellence (NICE) recommend that all pregnant women should be offered scans at between 10 and 14 weeks and 18 and 21 weeks gestation (Antenatal Care: Routine Care for the Healthy Pregnant Woman, 2008). The earlier scan is principally to determine gestational age, to detect multiple pregnancies and to determine nuchal translucency as part of screening for Down's syndrome. The 18–21 week scan primarily screens for structural anomalies. Scans performed after this stage in pregnancy are only performed if there is a clinical indication such as concern about fetal growth or well-being, discussed later in the chapter. Evidence suggests that routine ultrasound in early pregnancy appears to enable better gestational age assessment, earlier detection of multiple pregnancies and earlier detection of clinically unsuspected fetal malformation at a time when termination of pregnancy is possible.

Ultrasound in the assessment of fetal well-being

Amniotic fluid volume

The amount of amniotic fluid in the uterus is a guide to fetal well-being in the third trimester. The influence of congenital abnormalities on amniotic fluid volume in early pregnancy has already been described.

A reduction in amniotic fluid volume is referred to as 'oligohydramnios' and an excess is referred to as 'polyhydramnios'. Definitions of oligohydramnios and polyhydramnios are based on sonographic criteria. Two ultrasound measurement approaches give an indication of amniotic fluid volume. These are maximum vertical pool and amniotic fluid index.

The maximum vertical pool is measured after a general survey of the uterine contents. Measurements of less than 2 cm suggest oligohydramnios, and measurements of greater than 8 cm suggest polyhydramnios.

The Amniotic Fluid Index (AFI) is measured by dividing the uterus into four 'ultrasound' quadrants. A vertical measurement is taken of the deepest cord free pool in each quadrant and the results summated. The AFI alters throughout gestation, but in the third trimester it should be between 10 and 25 cm; values below 10 cm indicate a reduced volume and those below 5 cm indicate oligohydramnios, while values above 25 cm indicate polyhydramnios.

Amniotic fluid volume is decreased in fetal growth restriction as a consequence of redistribution of fetal blood away from the kidneys to vital structures such as the brain and heart with a consequent reduction in renal perfusion and urine output.

The cardiotocograph

The cardiotocograph (CTG) is a continuous tracing of the fetal heart rate used to assess fetal well-being. The Doppler effect detects fetal heart motion and allows the interval between successive beats to be measured, thereby allowing a continuous assessment of fetal heart rate. Fetal cardiac behaviour is regulated through the autonomic nervous system and by vasomotor, chemoceptor and baroreceptor mechanisms. Pathological events, such as fetal hypoxia, modify these signals and hence cardiac response including variation in heart rate patterns, which can be detected and recorded in the CTG. Features which are reported from a CTG to define normality and identify abnormality and potential concern for fetal well-being include the:

- baseline rate;
- baseline variability;
- accelerations;
- decelerations;

and each of these is discussed further below.

Interpretation of the CTG must be in the context of any risk factors, for example suspected FGR, and all features must be considered in order to make a judgement about the likelihood of fetal compromise.

The recording is obtained with the pregnant woman positioned comfortably in a left lateral or semi-recumbent position to avoid compression of the maternal vena cava. An external ultrasound transducer for monitoring the fetal heart and a tocodynometer (stretch gauge) for recording uterine activity are secured overlying the uterus. Recordings are then made for at least 30 minutes with the output from the CTG machine producing two 'lines', one a tracing of fetal heart rate and a second a tracing of uterine activity.

Baseline fetal heart rate

The normal fetal heart rate at term is 110–150 bpm. Higher rates are defined as fetal tachycardia and lower rates fetal bradycardia. The baseline fetal heart rate falls with advancing gestational age as a result of maturing fetal parasympathetic tone and prior to term 160 bpm is taken as the upper limit of normal. The baseline rate is best determined over a period of 5–10 minutes. Fetal tachycardias can be associated with maternal or fetal infection, acute fetal hypoxia, fetal anaemia and drugs such as adrenoceptor agonists, for example ritodrine.

Baseline variability

Under normal physiological conditions, the interval between successive heart beats (beat-to-beat) varies. This is called 'short-term variability' and increases with increasing gestational age. It is not visible on a standard CTG but can be measured with computer-assisted analysis. In addition to these beat-to-beat variations in heart rate, there are longer-term fluctuations in heart rate occurring between two and six times per minute. This is known as 'baseline variability'. Normal baseline variability reflects a normal fetal autonomic nervous system. Baseline variability is considered abnormal when it is less than 10 beats per minute (bpm) (Figure 6.10). As well as gestational age, baseline variability is modified by fetal sleep states and activity, and also by hypoxia, fetal infection and drugs suppressing the fetal central nervous system, such as opioids, and hypnotics (all of which reduce baseline variability). As fetuses display deep sleep cycles of 20–30 minutes at a time, baseline variability may be normally reduced for this length of time, but should be preceded and followed by a period of trace with normal baseline variability.

Fetal heart rate accelerations

These are increases in the baseline fetal heart rate of at least 15 bpm, lasting for at least 15 seconds. The presence of two or more accelerations on a 20–30-minute CTG defines a reactive trace and is indicative of a non-hypoxic fetus, i.e. they are a positive sign of fetal health.

Fetal heart rate decelerations

These are transient reductions in fetal heart rate of 15 bpm or more, lasting for more than 15 seconds. Decelerations can be indicative of fetal hypoxia or umbilical cord compression. There is a higher chance of hypoxia being present if there are additional abnormal features such as reduced variability or baseline tachycardia (Figure 6.11).

From the above descriptions, a normal antepartum fetal CTG can therefore be defined as a baseline of 110–150 bpm, with baseline variability exceeding 10 bpm, and with more than one acceleration being seen in a 20–30 minute tracing. Reduced baseline variability, absence of accelerations and the presence of decelerations are all suspicious features. A suspicious CTG must be interpreted within the clinical context. If many antenatal risk factors have already been identified, a suspicious CTG may warrant delivery of the baby, although where no risk factors exist, a repeated investigation later in the day may be more appropriate (Figure 6.12).

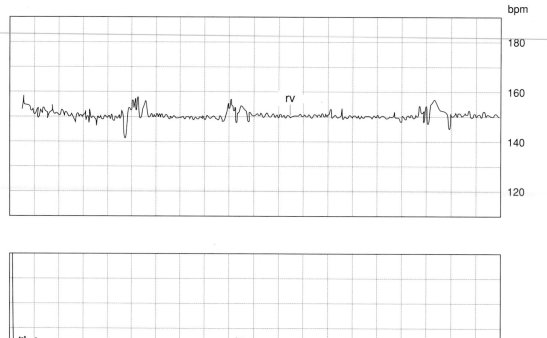

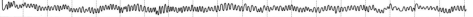

Figure 6.10 A fetal cardiotocograph showing a baseline of 150 beats per minute (bpm) but with reduced variability (rv)

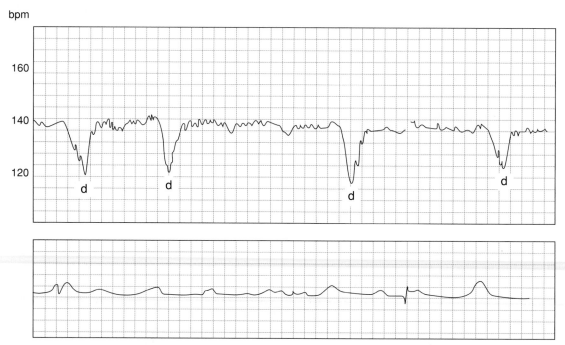

Figure 6.11 An admission cardiotocograph from a term pregnancy. Although the baseline fetal heart rate is normal, there is reduced variability, an absence of fetal heart rate accelerations, and multiple decelerations (d). The decelerations were occurring after uterine tightening and are therefore termed 'late'

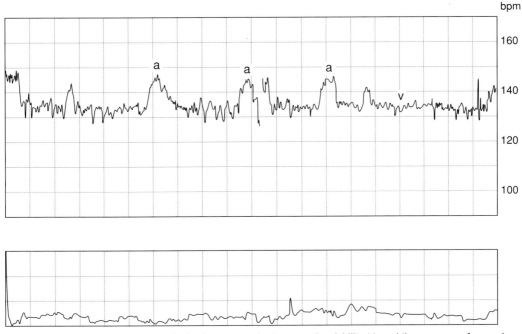

Figure 6.12 A normal fetal cardiotocograph showing a normal rate, normal variability (v), and the presence of several accelerations (a)

The computerized cardiotocograph

The basis of fetal CTG is pattern recognition, and this leads to differences in interpretation amongst different clinicians. Computerized CTG interpretation packages have been developed. These packages have been shown to be equal (or superior) to human interpretation in differentiating normal from abnormal outcome.

Biophysical profile

In an effort to refine the ability of fetal CTG to identify antenatal hypoxia, investigators have looked at additional fetal parameters such as fetal breathing movements, gross body movements, flexor tone and accelerations in fetal heart rate related to movements, all of which are abolished in the hypoxic state. A biophysical profile is a long (30 minute) ultrasound scan which observes fetal behaviour, measures amniotic fluid volume and includes a CTG. By assigning each of the active variables, and also amniotic fluid volume and the CTG scores of either 2 (normal) or 0 (suboptimal), it is possible to assign an individual fetus score of between 0 and 10. A score of 0, 2 or 4 is considered abnormal and a score of 8 or 10 normal. A score of 6 is equivocal and requires

repeat within a reasonable timescale (hours) to exclude a period of fetal sleep as a cause. This is the basis of fetal biophysical profiling (Figure 6.13).

Early observational studies suggested that delivery at a score of less than 6 was associated with a lower perinatal mortality than in similar high risk

Parameter	Score 2	Score 0
Non-stress CTG	Reactive	Fewer than two accelerations in 40 minutes
Fetal breathing movements	≥30 seconds in 30 minutes	Less than 30 seconds of fetal breathing in 30 minutes
Fetal body movements	≥3 movements in 30 minutes	Two or fewer gross body movements in 30 minutes
Fetal tone	One episode of limb flexion	No evidence of fetal movement or flexion
Amniotic fluid volume*	Largest cord-free pocket of fluid over 1 cm	Less than 1 cm pocket of fluid

Figure 6.13 Biophysical profile scoring system

pregnancies in which biophysical profiles (BPPs) were not performed. However, despite this early promise, widespread use did not occur. There appear to be several reasons for this lack of implementation. Biophysical profiles can be time consuming. Fetuses spend approximately 30 per cent of their time asleep, during which time they are not very active and do not exhibit breathing movements. It is therefore necessary to scan them for long enough to exclude this physiological cause of a poor score. Another problem with fetal BPPs is that by the time a fetus develops an abnormal score prompting delivery, it is likely to already be severely hypoxic. While delivery may reduce the perinatal death rate (death *in utero*, or within the first week of life), it may not increase long-term survival and, in particular, survival without significant mental and physical impairment.

More recent evidence in the form of a meta-analysis however, which included five trials involving 2974 women, found no significant differences between the groups in respect of perinatal deaths or poor fetal condition at birth as assessed by an Apgar score less than seven at 5 minutes. The authors concluded that there is currently insufficient evidence from randomized trials to support the use of BPP as a test of fetal well-being in high-risk pregnancies.

Doppler investigation

The principles of Doppler have already been discussed. Waveforms can be obtained from both the umbilical and fetal vessels. Data obtained from the umbilical artery provide indirect information about placenta function, whereas data from the fetal vessels provide information on the fetal response to hypoxia.

Umbilical artery

Waveforms obtained from the umbilical artery provide information on placental resistance to blood flow and hence indirectly placenta 'health' and function. An infarcted placenta secondary to maternal hypertension, for example, will have increased resistance to flow. A normal umbilical arterial waveform is shown in Figure 6.14. This is a plot obtained using Doppler ultrasound of velocity of blood flow against time and demonstrates forward flow of blood throughout the whole cardiac cycle, i.e. including diastole. A useful analogy to understand the concept of umbilical Doppler and placental resistance is to consider the umbilical artery as a hose carrying

water towards a placenta which in a healthy pregnancy will act like a sponge and in an infarcted placenta will act more like a brick wall. So, with a normal pregnancy blood will flow through the placenta without difficulty like water from a hose directed at the sponge and will pass straight through the sponge, whereas in a diseased placenta the blood will reflect back from the high resistance placenta like water from a hose being directed back from the wall at which it is directed. In the former, the normal constant forward flow in diastole will be seen and in the abnormal absent or reversed diastolic flow will be seen (Figure 6.15).

Most studies investigating the value of using this technique in clinical practice have looked at resistance to flow, which is reflected in the diastolic component. A small amount of diastolic flow implies high resistance downstream to the vessel being studied and implies low perfusion (Figure 6.16). A high diastolic component indicates low downstream resistance and

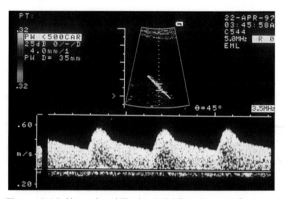

Figure 6.14 Normal umbilical arterial Doppler waveform

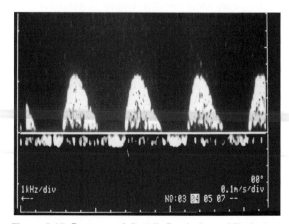

Figure 6.15 Reverse end diastolic flow in the umbilical artery

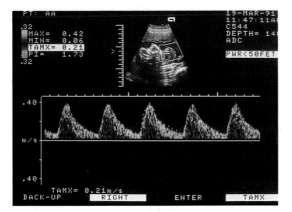

Figure 6.16 Reduced end diastolic flow in umbilical artery compared to normal in Figure 6.14

implies high perfusion. A measure of the amount of diastolic flow relative to systolic is provided by several indices, such as the pulsatility index or resistance index, which essentially compare the amount of diastolic flow to systolic flow. When these indices are high, this indicates high resistance to flow; when the indices are low, resistance to flow is low. Normally, diastolic flow in the umbilical artery increases (i.e. placental resistance falls) throughout gestation. Absent or reversed end-diastolic flow in the umbilical artery is a particularly serious development with a strong correlation with fetal distress and intrauterine death.

An analysis of randomized controlled trials of the use of umbilical Doppler in high risk pregnancy involving nearly 7000 women found that compared to no Doppler ultrasound, Doppler ultrasound in high risk pregnancy (especially those complicated by hypertension or presumed impaired fetal growth) was associated with a trend to a reduction in perinatal deaths. The use of Doppler ultrasound was also associated with fewer inductions of labour and fewer admissions to hospital without reports of adverse effects. The use of Doppler ultrasound in high-risk pregnancies appears therefore to improve a number of obstetric care outcomes and appears promising in helping to reduce perinatal deaths.

Fetal vessels

Falling oxygen levels in the fetus result in a redistribution of blood flow to protect the brain, heart and adrenal glands, and vasoconstriction in all other vessels. Several fetal vessels have been studied, and reflect this 'centralization' of flow. The middle cerebral artery will show increasing diastolic flow as hypoxia

increases (Figure 6.17), while a rising resistance in the fetal aorta reflects compensatory vasoconstriction in the fetal body. Absent diastolic flow in the fetal aorta implies fetal acidaemia. Perhaps the most sensitive index of fetal acidaemia and incipient heart failure is demonstrated by increasing pulsatility in the central veins supplying the heart, such as the ductus venosus and inferior vena cava. When late diastolic flow is absent in the ductus venosus (Figures 6.18 and 6.19), delivery should be considered as fetal death is imminent.

Measurement of velocity of blood in the middle cerebral artery also gives an indicator of the presence of fetal anaemia. The peak systolic velocity increases in this situation. This technique is particularly useful in the assessment of the severity of Rhesus disease and twin-to-twin transfusion syndrome which results in anaemia in the donor twin.

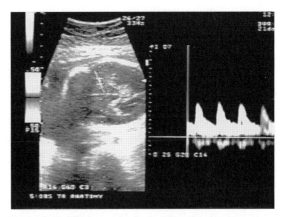

Figure 6.17 Middle cerebral artery Doppler showing increased diastolic flow with possible redistribution to brain in hypoxia

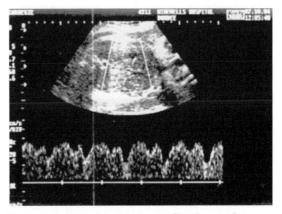

Figure 6.18 Normal ductus venosus Doppler waveform

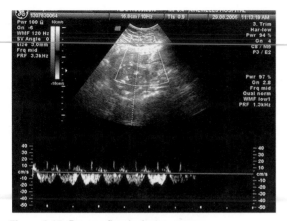

Figure 6.19 Reverse flow in ductus venosus

Doppler ultrasound and the prediction of adverse pregnancy outcome

Doppler studies of the uterine artery during the first and early second trimester have been used to predict pregnancies at risk of adverse outcome, particularly pre-eclampsia. The proposed pathogenic model of pre-eclampsia is one of incomplete physiological invasion of the spiral arteries by the trophoblast, with a resultant increase in uteroplacental vascular resistance (see Chapter 10, Pre-eclampsia and other disorders of placentation). This is reflected in the Doppler waveforms obtained from the maternal uterine circulation. Doppler ultrasound studies of the uterine arteries may demonstrate markers of increased resistance to flow including the diastolic 'notch' in the waveform (Figure 6.20) in early diastole, thought to result from increased vascular resistance in the uteroplacental bed. Studies have provided evidence of the association between high-resistance

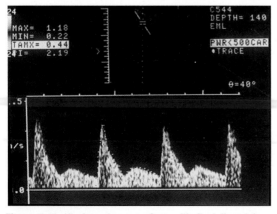

Figure 6.20 Uterine artery waveform with diastolic notch

waveform patterns and adverse outcomes, including pre-eclampsia, fetal growth restriction and placental abruption. Sixty to seventy per cent of women at 20–24 weeks gestation with bilateral uterine notches will subsequently develop one or more of these complications. Consequently, such pregnancies will require close monitoring of fetal growth rate increased surveillance for the possible development of maternal hypertension and proteinuria.

Ultrasound and invasive procedures

Ultrasound is used to guide invasive diagnostic procedures such as amniocentesis, chorion villus sampling and cordocentesis, and therapeutic procedures such as the insertion of fetal bladder shunts or chest drains. If fetoscopy is performed, the endoscope is inserted under ultrasound guidance. This use of ultrasound has greatly reduced the possibility of fetal trauma, as the needle or scope is visualized throughout the procedure and guided with precision to the appropriate place.

Summary of the aims of obstetric ultrasound

The early pregnancy scan (11–14 weeks)

The principal aims of this scan are:

- to confirm fetal viability;
- to provide an accurate estimation of gestational age;
- to diagnose multiple gestation, and in particular to determine chorionicity;
- to identify markers which would indicate an increased risk of fetal chromosome abnormality such as Down's syndrome;
- to identify fetuses with gross structural abnormalities.

The 20 week scan (18–22 weeks)

The principal aims of this scan are:

- to provide an accurate estimation of gestational age if an early scan has not been performed;
- to carry out a detailed fetal anatomical survey to detect any fetal structural abnormalities or markers for chromosome abnormality;

- to locate the placenta and identify the 5 per cent of women who have a low-lying placenta for a repeat scan at 34 weeks to exclude placenta praevia;
- to estimate the amniotic fluid volume.

Also, in some centres:

- to perform Doppler ultrasound examination of maternal uterine arteries to screen for adverse pregnancy outcome, for example pre-eclampsia;
- to measure cervical length to assess the risk of preterm delivery.

Ultrasound in the third trimester

The principal aims of ultrasound in the third trimester are:

- to assess fetal growth;
- to assess fetal well-being.

Magnetic resonance imaging

MRI utilizes the effect of powerful magnetic forces on spinning hydrogen protons, which when knocked off their axis by pulsed radio waves, produce radio frequency signals as they return to their basal state. The signals reflect the composition of tissue (i.e. the amount and distribution of hydrogen protons) and thus the images provide significant improvement over ultrasound in tissue characterization. Ultrafast MRI techniques enable images to be acquired in less than 1 second to eliminate fetal motion. Such technology has led to increased usage of fetal MRI which provides multiplanar views, better characterization of anatomic details of, for example, the fetal brain, and information for planning the mode of delivery and airway management at birth.

CASE HISTORY

An 18-year-old in her first pregnancy attends for review at the antenatal clinic at 34 weeks gestation. Her dates were confirmed by ultrasound at booking (12 weeks). She is a smoker. The midwife measures her fundal height at 30 cm. An ultrasound scan is performed because of the midwife's concern that the fetus is SGA, and the measurements are plotted in Figure 6.21.

Do the ultrasound findings support the clinical diagnosis of SGA?

Yes, because the fetal AC is below the 5th centile for gestation. This finding does not give an indication of the well-being of the fetus and is compatible with FGR secondary to placental insufficiency or a healthy, constitutionally small baby.

What additional features/measures on ultrasound assessment could give an indication of fetal well-being?

Liquor volume

Amniotic fluid volume is decreased in FGR associated with fetal hypoxia with redistribution of fetal blood flow away from the kidneys to vital structures such as the brain and heart, with a consequent reduction in renal perfusion and urine output.

Doppler ultrasound

Umbilical artery

Waveforms from the umbilical artery provide information on feto-placental blood flow and placental resistance. Diastolic flow in the umbilical artery increases (i.e. placental resistance falls)

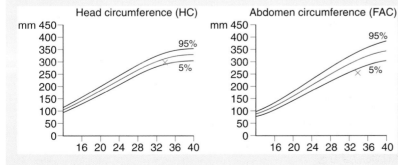

Figure 6.21 Plot of fetal head circumference and fetal abdominal circumference (FAC) for case history

continued ➤

throughout gestation. If the resistance index (RI) in the umbilical artery rises above the 95th centile of the normal graph, this implies faulty perfusion of the placenta, which may eventually result in fetal hypoxia. Absent or reversed end-diastolic flow in the umbilical artery is a particularly serious development, with a strong correlation with fetal distress and intrauterine death.

Fetal vessels

Falling oxygen levels in the fetus result in a redistribution of blood flow to protect the brain, heart, adrenals and spleen, and vasoconstriction in all other vessels. The middle cerebral artery will show increasing diastolic flow as hypoxia increases, while a rising resistance in the fetal aorta reflects compensatory vasoconstriction in the fetal body. When diastolic flow is absent in the fetal aorta, this implies fetal acidaemia. Increasing pulsatility in the central veins supplying the heart, such as the ductus venosus and inferior vena cava, is an indicator of fetal acidaemia and impending heart failure; when late diastolic flow is absent in the ductus venosus, fetal death is imminent.

Cardiotocography

Fetal tachycardia, reduced variability in heart rate, absence of accelerations and presence of decelerations identified on a CTG are associated with fetal hypoxia.

Additional reading

Alfirevic Z, Neilson JP. Doppler ultrasound for fetal assessment in high risk pregnancies. *Cochrane Database of Systematic Reviews*. 1996; (**4**): CD000073.

Lalor JG, Fawole B, Alfirevic Z, Devane D. Biophysical profile for fetal assessment in high risk pregnancies. *Cochrane Database of Systematic Reviews*. 2008; (**1**): CD000038.

CHAPTER 7

PRENATAL DIAGNOSIS

Sarah Vause

OVERVIEW

This chapter will discuss why prenatal diagnostic tests may be performed and the types of non-invasive and invasive tests available. It will discuss factors which should be taken into consideration prior to offering testing, and emphasize the importance of good communication with women and multidisciplinary working.

Definition

Prenatal diagnosis is the identification of a disease prior to birth.

Why is prenatal diagnostic testing performed?

Prenatal diagnosis is usually performed because something leads to the suspicion of disease being present. For example:

- family history – genetic disease with a known recurrence risk;
- past obstetric history – RhD alloimmunization;
- serum screening tests – trisomy 21;
- ultrasound screening – 20 week anomaly scan.

Prenatal diagnosis frequently follows a prenatal screening test, whether this is simply the history taking at the booking visit, or a more formal screening test such as those offered for Down's syndrome, haemoglobinopathies or ultrasound screening.

Attributes of a screening test:

- relevance – the condition screened for must be relevant and important;
- effect on management – alternative management options must be available, for example planning

therapy or offering termination of an affected pregnancy;

- sensitivity – the test must have a high detection rate for the condition;
- specificity – the test must exclude the vast majority who do not have the condition;
- predictive value – the test must predict accurately who does, and who does not have the condition;
- affordability – the test should be cheap enough to be cost effective;
- equity – the test should be available to all.

Classification

Prenatal diagnostic tests can be divided into non-invasive tests and invasive tests.

The main non-invasive test is the use of ultrasound scanning for structural fetal abnormalities, such as neural tube defects, gastroschisis, cystic adenomatoid malformation of lung, renal abnormalities (Table 7.1).

Maternal blood can be tested for exposure to viruses (viral serology). If a woman has no IgG or IgM for a particular virus early in pregnancy, but then develops IgM and IgG later in pregnancy, it suggests that she has had a clinical or subclinical infection with that virus during pregnancy. Maternal

Table 7.1 Examples of conditions and their method of diagnosis

Diagnostic test	Condition
Ultrasound diagnosis	Neural tube defect Gastroschisis Cystic adenomatoid malformation of lung Twin to twin transfusion syndrome
Invasive test – CVB or amniocentesis	Down's syndrome Cystic fibrosis Thalassaemia
Invasive test – cordocentesis	Alloimmune thrombocytopenia
Ultrasound then invasive test	Congenital diaphragmatic hernia Exomphalos Ventriculomegaly Duodenal atresia

blood is usually only tested if features on ultrasound are suggestive of infection having occurred, for example hydrops or ventriculomegaly or if there is a history of exposure to a particular virus.

Free fetal DNA can be extracted from maternal blood to determine fetal blood group in cases of alloimmunization, or to determine the sex of the fetus in X-linked disorders.

Much interest is being focused on developing prenatal diagnostic tests for aneuploid pregnancies by extracting fetal RNA from maternal blood.

Amniocentesis and chorion villus biopsy (CVB) are the two most common invasive tests and are commonly used for checking the karyotype of the fetus, or to look for single gene disorders. These tests carry a small risk of miscarriage, therefore the risk of being affected by the condition and the seriousness of the condition should be severe enough to warrant taking the risk. Rarely, cordocentesis is used as an invasive diagnostic test.

Frequently, non-invasive tests and invasive tests are used together. The ultrasound scan may diagnose a structural problem in the fetus such as a congenital diaphragmatic hernia, but since congenital diaphragmatic hernias are associated with underlying chromosomal abnormalities, an invasive test would then be offered.

Invasive testing

Pre-test counselling

Invasive tests are most frequently performed to diagnose aneuploidy, for example Down's syndrome or genetic conditions, such as cystic fibrosis or thalassaemia. Women choose to have, or not have, invasive testing. This is an important decision which may have lifelong consequences and therefore must be a decision which is fully informed.

For a clinician to discuss the option of invasive testing in a meaningful way with a woman, the clinician should know:

- about the condition suspected and its severity so that the woman can assess the effect that having a child with this disorder would have on her and her family;
- that the history is correct – involvement of colleagues from the Clinical Genetics Department is often invaluable;
- that a test is available – sometimes the mutation has not been found;
- what sample is needed, and how it should be processed;
- accurate assessment of risk – again colleagues from the Clinical Genetics Department may be helpful;
- acceptability – some women feel that they cannot accept the small risk of miscarriage;
- whether it is ethical – some conditions do not carry a significant risk of serious disability, and yet it is possible to offer prenatal diagnosis for them, for example sickle cell disease

Prior to the test, the clinician should also discuss with the women what options would be available to her if the test result shows that the fetus is affected with the condition. This is an important part of the decision-making process. There is no point doing an invasive test if it will not be of benefit to the woman or her baby.

The three options available are usually to:

1. Continue – the information from the test may facilitate plans for care around the time of delivery, or may help the woman prepare emotionally for the birth of a baby with a serious condition.

2. Influence the decision to terminate the pregnancy.

3. Terminate, but provide information which may prove useful when counselling about recurrence risks in future pregnancies.

Some women decline invasive testing as they feel that it would not provide them with useful information, and would put them at risk of miscarriage.

To ensure informed consent, the clinician needs to be certain that the woman understands the procedure, why it is being offered, the risks, limitations and subsequent management options. The clinician also needs to be sure that the woman in not under duress from others such as her family, community or religious groups. It is good practice to complete a consent form as a formal record that the discussion has taken place.

Chorion villus sampling (also known as chorion villus biopsy)

Fetal trophoblast cells in the mesenchyme of the villi divide rapidly in the first trimester. A CVB procedure aims to take a sample of these rapidly dividing cells from the developing placenta. This is done either by passing a needle under ultrasound guidance through the abdominal wall into the placenta, or by passing a fine catheter (or biopsy forceps) through the cervix into the placenta (Figure 7.1).

The woman is scanned initially:

• to confirm that the pregnancy is viable prior to the procedure;

• to ensure that it is a singleton pregnancy (prenatal diagnosis in multiple pregnancy is more complex);

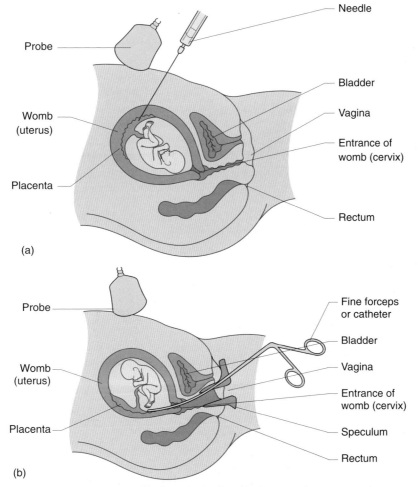

Figure 7.1 (a and b) Pictures adapted from RCOG information leaflet of both approaches

- to confirm gestational age (should not be performed before 10 weeks gestation);
- to localize the placenta and determine whether a transabdominal or transcervical approach is more appropriate. Transabdominal procedures are performed more commonly, but may not be feasible if the uterus is retroverted or the placenta is low on the posterior wall of the uterus.

The additional overall risk of miscarriage from chorion villus sampling (CVS) is approximately 2 per cent. This is in addition to the background (natural) risk of miscarriage for a first trimester pregnancy.

Many laboratories can provide a result for common aneuploidies (T21, 18 and 13) within 48 hours for a CVS sample. Full culture results take approximately 7–10 days and results for genetic disorders take varying amounts of time.

Placental mosaicism is sometimes found. This is the occurrence of two different cell types in the same sample, usually one cell line is normal and one cell line is abnormal. It occurs in approximately 1 per cent of CVS samples, and this is higher than for amniocentesis. The mosaic pattern may be present in the placenta, and not occur in the fetus (confined placental mosaicism). If a mosaic result is obtained on CVS, then another fetal tissue (e.g. amniotic fluid) should be sampled to determine whether this is the case. Mosaic results should be discussed with the Clinical Genetics Department to get accurate information on the impact this may have on the fetus.

Amniocentesis

Amniotic fluid contains amniocytes and fibroblasts shed from fetal membranes, skin and the fetal genitourinary tract. An amniocentesis procedure takes a sample (15–20 mL) of amniotic fluid which contains these cells. This is done by passing a needle under continuous direct ultrasound control through the abdominal wall into the amniotic cavity and aspirating the fluid (Figure 7.2).

An initial ultrasound is performed prior to the procedure. One in every 100 women who have amniocentesis from 15 weeks of pregnancy under ultrasound guidance miscarry as a result of the procedure.

Many laboratories can provide a result for common aneuploidies (T21, 18 and 13) within 48 hours for an amniocentesis sample. Full culture results take approximately 7–10 days and results for genetic disorders take varying amounts of time. This is similar to CVS.

Amniotic fluid may be used to check for viral infections, for example cytomegalovirus. In the past, it was also used for biochemical tests, for example alpha fetoprotein and spectrophotometric tests for haemolytic disease. These are needed less frequently now and have been superseded by other investigations.

The advantage of CVS over amniocentesis is that it can be performed earlier in pregnancy, at a stage when surgical termination is possible in the event of a 'bad

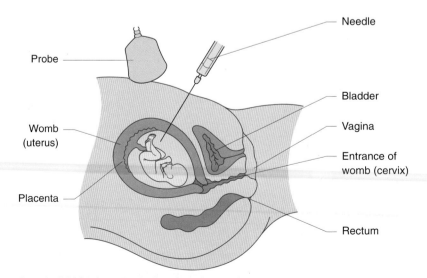

Figure 7.2 Picture from the RCOG information leaflet of amniocentesis

result', and at a stage in pregnancy before a woman has needed to disclose the pregnancy to family, friends and employers.

The disadvantage of CVS compared with amniocentesis is that it may be associated with a higher risk of miscarriage.

Cordocentesis

Cordocentesis is performed when fetal blood is needed, or when a rapid full culture for karyotype is needed. The most common reason for performing a cordocentesis as a diagnostic prenatal test is to check the fetal platelet count, when alloimmune thrombocytopenia is suspected.

A needle is passed under ultrasound guidance into the umbilical cord at the point where it inserts into the placenta. This point is chosen because the umbilical cord is fixed and does not move. Cordocentesis can be performed from about 20 weeks gestation. The risk of miscarriage varies with indication and position of the placenta (Table 7.2).

Care after any invasive test

Following any invasive procedure there should be:

- accurate labelling of the sample;
- prompt and secure transport of the sample to the appropriate laboratory;
- documentation of the procedure and any complications in the woman's notes;
- communication with the referring clinician;
- the woman should be advised to avoid strenuous exercise for the next 24 hours;
- she should be advised that while she may experience some mild abdominal pain, it should be relieved by paracetamol;
- she should be advised that if she has any bleeding, pain not relieved by paracetamol or leakage of fluid vaginally she should seek medical advice, and told how to access this;

- she should be given appropriate contact numbers;
- a process for giving results should be agreed, including who will give the results, how they will be given and when the results are likely to be available;
- if the woman is RhD negative, an appropriate dose of Anti D should be administered (with a Kleihauer test if more than 20 weeks gestation);
- a plan of ongoing care should be discussed once the results are available.

Down's syndrome

In the UK, prenatal diagnosis of Down's syndrome is the most common reason for performing invasive testing.

Most prenatal diagnostic tests arise following a 'high risk' screening test.

In the UK, NICE has recommended that all women should be offered screening for Down's syndrome as part of their routine antenatal care. It is also recommended that the screening test offered should have at least a 75 per cent detection rate for <3 per cent false-positive rate.

Several different screening tests are available but the option approved by the National Screening Committee is the combined test which is performed between 11 and 14 weeks gestation. This tests involves the combination of an ultrasound scan to measure the nuchal lucency and a blood test to measure the levels of human chorionic gonadotrophin (HCG) and pregnancy associated plasma protein-A (PAPP-A) in maternal blood.

The nuchal lucency measurement is a measurement of the thickness of a pad of skin in the nuchal (neck) region of the fetus. Fetuses with Down's syndrome tend to have a thicker nuchal lucency. If a thick nuchal lucency measurement is obtained it increases the risk of the fetus having Down's syndrome.

Table 7.2 Comparison of invasive tests

Test	CVS	Amniocentesis	Cordocentesis
Gestation from which test can be performed	11 weeks	15 weeks	Around 20 weeks
Miscarriage risk	+ 2 per cent	+ 1 per cent	+ 2–5 per cent

The risk of Down's syndrome increases with maternal age. For each woman, the individual risk can be calculated by taking her age-related risk and then adjusting this up or down based on the measurements obtained for the nuchal lucency, HCG and PAPP-A. Based on her individual result, the woman can then choose whether to have an invasive test or not.

Prior to performing the screening test, the woman should be encouraged to consider what action she would take, and how she would feel if she screened positive. It is also important to explain to women that this initial test is simply a screening test and not a diagnostic test. A low risk result does not rule out the possibility of Down's syndrome completely (even if the result shows a very low risk of 1:10 000, she could be that 1 in 10 000). With a high risk result of 1:10, 90 per cent of fetuses would be normal. The diagnostic tests available to her should be explained.

The accuracy of the screening test for Down's syndrome can be refined by adding further markers such as measuring the nasal bone, frontomaxillary nasal angle and looking for the presence of tricuspid regurgitation and at the ductus venosus wave form. These increase the sensitivity of the test and reduce the false-positive rate. However, they are resource intensive, and a prenatal diagnostic test must still be performed to reach a definitive diagnosis.

CASE HISTORIES

This section discusses the features and management of four conditions which may be diagnosed prenatally.

1. Neural tube defect – non-invasive prenatal diagnosis by ultrasound scan

N is a 22-year-old woman living in the North West of England. She found herself unexpectedly pregnant and had not been taking folic acid. When she first attended the antenatal clinic an ultrasound scan showed her to be 19 weeks pregnant. The fetus was noted to have an abnormal head shape, the cerebellum was described as banana shaped and a myelomeningocele was identified in the lumbar region. The fetus had bilateral talipes.

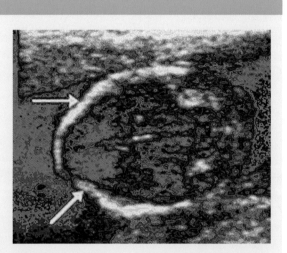

Note the scalloped head shape anteriorly (lemon shaped) marked by the white arrows and the banana shaped cerebellum (C).

How should this patient be managed?

A prenatal diagnosis of a neural tube defect has been made on ultrasound scan. Ultrasound scan will detect at least 90 per cent of all neural tube defects. Ms N should be seen by the consultant and the ultrasound findings explained to her. She should have the opportunity to discuss the prognosis with a neurosurgeon, and this may be best organized by referring her to a tertiary fetal medicine unit.

What is the outlook for the baby/child?

For women to make decisions about whether to continue with their pregnancy or not, they need an honest and realistic view of the likely outcome for their baby/child. It is always difficult to predict the outlook for the baby/child but lower lesions generally have a better prognosis.

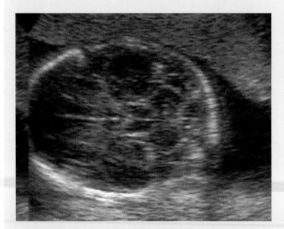

Normal intracranial anatomy imaged in the transcerebellar plane – note the ovoid head shape and the dumb bell-shaped cerebellum (C).

Similar plane in Ms N, whose fetus has a neural tube defect.

The main problems encountered are:

- problems with mobility – tend to become wheelchair bound as they get older;
- continence and voiding – both bladder and bowel;
- low IQ;
- repeated surgery – shunts, bladder and bowel, orthopaedic;
- difficulty forming normal relationships and living independently

What options does Mrs N have?

Mrs N may choose to continue with the pregnancy with support from health care professionals both before and after delivery. Parents who choose to continue with a pregnancy may benefit from contacting a parent support group such as ASBAH (Association for Spina Bifida and Hydrocephalus). Alternatively, she may opt for termination of pregnancy.

What is the risk of it happening again in a future pregnancy?

The risk of recurrence of a neural tube defect is 5 per cent after one affected pregnancy (12 per cent after two affected pregnancies and 20 per cent after three affected pregnancies).

It is more common in some geographical areas (e.g. Ireland, Scotland and North West England), if the mother has diabetes or epilepsy, if the mother is taking antiepileptic medication and in obese women.

Folic acid (400 μg) taken preconceptually and for the first trimester reduces the risk of neural tube defects.

What advice would you give about future pregnancies?

By taking folic acid for at least three months preconceptually, the risk of recurrence can be reduced. Mrs N should take a higher dose than the usual preconceptual dose (5 mg instead of the usual 400 μg). She should also ensure that she eats healthily and that her weight is normal. Any medication she is taking should be reviewed.

2. Gastroschisis – non-invasive prenatal diagnosis by ultrasound scan

Ms G is an 18-year-old woman who had her first scan at 16 weeks gestation. When the fetal abdomen was scanned, an irregular mass was seen to project from the anterior abdominal wall at the level of the umbilicus, to one side of the umbilical cord. No other fetal abnormalities were noted.

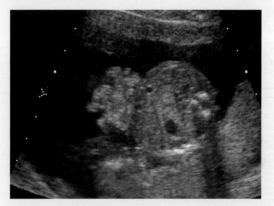

How should this patient be managed?

A prenatal diagnosis of a gastroschisis has been made on ultrasound scan. Ultrasound scan will detect at least 90 per cent of all gastroschisis defects. Ms G should be seen by the consultant and the ultrasound findings explained to her. She requires referral to a tertiary unit for ongoing management and planning of delivery. Involvement of a multidisciplinary team would be important.

What should the consultant tell her about the outlook for her baby?

The consultant should stress that the majority of babies born with gastroschisis will do well in the long term and lead normal lives.

Exomphalos	Gastroschisis
Membrane covered herniation of abdominal contents – smooth outline	Not membrane covered. Free floating bowel loops – irregular outline
Umbilical cord inserts into apex of sac	Herniation lateral (usually to the right) of the cord insertion
Very high incidence of associated abnormalities and genetic syndromes	Very low incidence of other abnormalities
High incidence of chromosomal abnormalities – karyotyping should be offered	No increase in incidence of chromosomal abnormalities
May contain stomach, liver spleen	Usually only small bowel extraabdominally
Associated with polyhydramnios	Associated with oligohydramnios

continued ≫

The consultant should stress that gastroschisis is not usually associated with any other physical problems or with learning problems (see table). It should be explained that the fetus will need to be monitored regularly during the pregnancy as fetuses with gastroschisis are often small and may have oligohydramnios. In later pregnancy, the fetal bowel may dilate and become thick walled, which can make the post natal surgery more difficult and there may be associated ischaemia and bowel atresia.

Following delivery, the baby would require an operation to repair the defect. Surgical repair ranges from reduction of bowel and suturing of defect under local anaesthetic, to the need for a silo. This is a covering placed over the abdominal organs on the outside of the baby. Gradually, the organs are squeezed by hand through the silo into the opening and returned to the body. This method can take up to a week to return the abdominal organs to the body cavity. Severe cases may require bowel resection for atresias. There is an 85 per cent survival rate with the majority of babies on full oral feeds by 4 weeks of age.

Ms G should be given the opportunity to meet the neonatal surgeons during the pregnancy and visit the neonatal surgical unit. After delivery, she should be encouraged to express breast milk to feed to her baby.

What plans would you make for delivery?

Induction around 37 weeks gestation enables delivery to be planned in a unit with appropriate neonatal surgical facilities, and may reduce the incidence of stillbirth late in pregnancy.

There does not appear to be any benefit from delivery by Caesarean section for babies with gastroschisis. If a woman has a normal delivery it makes it easier for her to visit her baby on the neonatal surgical unit in the first few days after delivery.

3. Exomphalos associated with Trisomy 18 – initial ultrasound diagnosis with subsequent CVB

Ms E is a 37-year-old woman who attended for her first scan at 13 weeks gestation.

On ultrasound scan, a smooth protrusion could be seen on the anterior abdominal wall of the fetus. It appeared to be covered by a membrane and the umbilical cord inserted into the apex of the protrusion. The sonographer described this as an exomphalos in her report.

How should this patient be managed?

A prenatal diagnosis of an exomphalos has been made on ultrasound scan. Ultrasound scan will detect at least 90 per cent of all exomphalos defects, but this diagnosis cannot be made until after 12 weeks gestation. Prior to 12 weeks, there is developmental physiological herniation of abdominal contents into the base of the umbilical cord. Ms E should be seen by the consultant and the ultrasound findings explained to her. As there is a high incidence of associated abnormalities (in 70–80 per cent of fetuses), she should be referred to a tertiary unit for detailed ultrasound. The consultant

should also explain that there is a high chance of chromosomal abnormality (approximately one-third of fetuses) and discuss the option of invasive testing (see table).

What options are available to Ms E?

- Do nothing.
- Termination of pregnancy.
- CVB now and continue if the chromosomes are normal. It is possible that other abnormalities may still be detected on ultrasound later in pregnancy. If the chromosomes are abnormal she would still have the option of a surgical termination of pregnancy up to 14 weeks gestation in some hospitals.
- Wait until after 15 weeks gestation, then have an amniocentesis with a lower risk of miscarriage. Even if the chromosomes are normal, it is still possible that other abnormalities may be detected on ultrasound later in pregnancy.

Ms E chose to have a CVB which showed that the fetus had trisomy 18. She then chose to terminate her pregnancy, as she knew that most fetuses with trisomy 18 were either stillborn or did not live beyond the first few months.

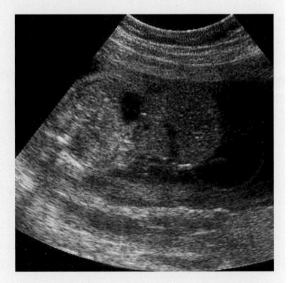

4. Duchenne muscular dystrophy – non-invasive testing for fetal sex

Mrs D has a brother with Duchenne muscular dystrophy. He has been under the care of the clinical geneticists, and Mrs D has been tested and found to be a carrier of the gene. She contacts her GP when she is 7 weeks' pregnant as she wishes to have testing to see whether the fetus is affected by Duchenne muscular dystrophy.

What are the chances of Mrs D having an affected fetus?

There is a 1:4 chance of an affected fetus.

Duchenne muscular dystrophy is an X-linked recessive condition. There is a 1:2 chance that any baby will be a girl and a 1:2 chance that it will be a boy. If the fetus is male, there is a 1:2 chance that it has inherited a normal X chromosome from Mrs D (unaffected) and a 1:2 chance that it has inherited the X chromosome carrying the abnormal gene, in which case the boy would be affected. If the fetus is female there is a 1:2 chance that it will have inherited a normal X chromosome from Mrs D and therefore not be a carrier, and a 1:2 chance that it will have inherited the X chromosome carrying the abnormal gene and therefore be a carrier. A female fetus would not be affected as this is an X-linked recessive condition, and a female fetus would have inherited a normal X chromosome from the father.

How should Mrs D be managed?

The GP should arrange an urgent referral to the antenatal clinic and also contact the Clinical Genetics Department. Mrs D requires an initial ultrasound scan to confirm that the fetus is viable, to confirm the gestation and to confirm that it is a singleton pregnancy. Testing would be much more complex if this were a twin pregnancy.

Initially, a blood test can be performed on Mrs D to ascertain the sex of the fetus. All fetuses shed small quantities of DNA into the maternal circulation. This can be amplified by a PCR technique. By testing the maternal serum for free fetal DNA from the Y chromosome the sex of the fetus can be ascertained. If Y chromosome DNA is found in the maternal serum, it must have come from a male fetus. If no Y chromosome DNA is found then it is likely that it is a female fetus. However, there is also a small possibility that the test has not worked.

Mrs D had the blood test at 8 weeks gestation which showed that she was carrying a female fetus. As this meant that she would not have an affected baby she did not need to have any further invasive testing. If the blood test had shown that she was carrying a male fetus, she would then have had a CVB to determine whether this was an affected or unaffected male. By having the blood test, she was able to avoid invasive testing.

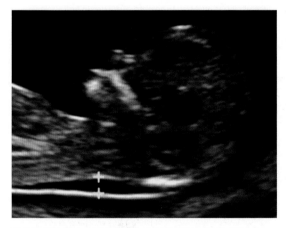

Figure 7.3 The nuchal lucency measurement is seen behind the fetal neck marked by the callipers $++$

Key points

- Detailed counselling prior to embarking on any screening or diagnostic tests is extremely important. The woman must understand the potential outcomes, the choices available to her and should be encouraged to consider how the outcome of the test would affect the decisions she made during her pregnancy.

- If a fetal abnormality is diagnosed antenatally, multidisciplinary management is important. This will help to provide the woman with the best information about the likely outcome for her baby, facilitate her decision making, and provide appropriate support from experienced professionals at a difficult time.

New developments

All fetuses release some of their DNA into the maternal circulation. By amplifying this DNA using a polymerase chain reaction (PCR), it makes it possible to check the fetal genotype. Two examples of situations where this is useful are fetal sexing and to check the fetal blood group.

Fetal sexing: If a woman carries a sex-linked condition, such as Duchenne muscular dystrophy, and wants prenatal diagnostic testing, it is important to know the sex of the fetus. If the fetus is found to be female, invasive testing can be avoided, as the fetus will not be affected. If the fetus is known to be male, there will be a 50:50 chance of it being affected and an invasive test is necessary. If the PCR test on the free fetal DNA shows that Y chromosome DNA can be amplified, then this must have come from the fetus (as the mother has no Y chromosome DNA of her own), and the test therefore shows that the fetus is male.

Fetal blood group: Similarly, if RhD-positive DNA is amplified from the blood of a RhD-negative woman, this must have come from the fetus (as the mother has no RhD-positive DNA of her own), and the test therefore shows that the fetus is RhD-positive. In RhD-negative women with Anti D antibodies, this test is used to determine the blood group of the fetus, as a RhD-positive fetus is at risk of alloimmune haemolytic disease, whereas a RhD-negative fetus is not at risk. Intensive surveillance can be instituted for the mother of the RhD-positive fetus, and the mother of the RhD-negative fetus can be reassured that problems will not occur. Fetal blood group can be determined from samples taken in the first trimester and testing for the common blood group antigens, including Rhesus and Kell, performed.

There is much promising work on a non-invasive diagnostic test for Down's syndrome which measures the ratio of alleles of a placental specific (fetal specific) messenger RNA from a gene located on chromosome 21. If these alleles are found in a ratio of 1:2 or 2:1 it suggests that the fetus has three copies of chromosome 21, i.e. Down's syndrome. This test has the potential to replace invasive prenatal diagnostic testing for Down's syndrome.

Fetal MRI has improved the diagnosis of central nervous system abnormalities in the fetus, in particular by proving a good diagnostic tool for assessing whether the corpus callosum is present in the fetus. This is a structure which is often difficult to visualize with ultrasound.

3D and 4D ultrasound are useful for surface rendering which helps in the visualization of cleft lips and palates, and for volume rendering. While this modality has aided description of anatomy to parents, it still has to find a role as a diagnostic tool.

CHAPTER 8

ANTENATAL OBSTETRIC COMPLICATIONS

Louise C Kenny

OVERVIEW

There are a variety of maternal and fetal complications which can arise during pregnancy. Some of these 'minor' conditions arise because the physiological changes of pregnancy exacerbate many irritating symptoms that in the normal non-pregnant state would not require specific treatment. While these problems are not dangerous to the mother, they can be extremely troublesome and incapacitating. Some of the more major fetal and maternal complications are discussed in detail in other chapters. Here we discuss common complications, including malpresentation, Rhesus disease and abnormalities of amniotic fluid production.

'Minor' complications of pregnancy

Musculoskeletal problems

Backache

Backache is extremely common in pregnancy and is caused by:

- hormone induced laxity of spinal ligaments;
- a shifting in the centre of gravity as the uterus grows;
- additional weight gain;

which cause an exaggerated lumbar lordosis. Pregnancy can exacerbate the symptoms of a prolapsed intervertebral disc, occasionally leading to complete immobility. Advice should include maintenance of correct posture, avoiding lifting heavy objects (including children), avoiding high heels, regular physiotherapy and simple analgesia (paracetamol or paracetamol–codeine combinations).

Symphysis pubis dysfunction

This is an excruciatingly painful condition most common in the third trimester, although it can occur at any time during pregnancy. The symphysis pubis joint becomes 'loose', causing the two halves of the pelvis to rub on one another when walking or moving. The condition improves after delivery and the management revolves around simple analgesia. Under a physiotherapist's direction, a low stability belt may be worn.

Carpal tunnel syndrome

Compression neuropathies occur in pregnancy due to increased soft-tissue swelling. The most common of these is carpal tunnel syndrome. The median nerve, where it passes through the fibrous canal at the wrist before entering the hand, is most susceptible to compression. The symptoms include numbness, tingling and weakness of the thumb and forefinger, and often quite severe pain at night. Simple analgesia and splinting of the affected hand usually help, although there is no realistic prospect of cure until after delivery. Surgical decompression is very rarely performed in pregnancy.

Gastrointestinal symptoms

Constipation

Constipation is common in pregnancy and usually results from a combination of hormonal and mechanical factors that slow gut motility. Concomitantly administered iron tablets may exacerbate the condition. Women should be given clear explanations, reassurance and advice regarding the adoption of a high-fibre diet. Medications are best avoided but if necessary, mild (non-stimulant) laxatives, such as lactulose, may be suggested.

Hyperemesis gravidarum

Nausea and vomiting in pregnancy are extremely common; 70–80 per cent of women experience these symptoms early in their pregnancy and approximately 35 per cent of all pregnant patients are absent from work on at least one occasion through nausea and vomiting. Although the symptoms are often most pronounced in the first trimester, they by no means are confined to it. Similarly, despite common usage of the term 'morning sickness', in only a minority of cases are the symptoms solely confined to the morning. Nausea and vomiting in pregnancy tends to be mild and self-limited and is not associated with adverse pregnancy outcome.

Hyperemesis gravidarum, however, is a severe, intractable form of nausea and vomiting that affects 0.3–2.0 per cent of pregnancies. It causes imbalances of fluid and electrolytes, disturbs nutritional intake and metabolism, causes physical and psychological debilitation and is associated with adverse pregnancy outcome, including an increased risk of preterm birth and low birthweight babies. The aetiology is unknown and various putative mechanisms have been proposed including an association with high levels of serum human chorionic gonadotrophin (hCG), oestrogen and thyroxine. The likely cause is multifactorial. Severe cases of hyperemesis gravidarum cause malnutrition and vitamin deficiencies, including Wernicke's encephalopathy, and intractable retching predisposes to oesophageal trauma and Mallory–Weiss tears. Treatment includes fluid replacement and thiamine supplementation. Antiemetics such as phenothiazines are safe and are commonly prescribed. Other proposed treatments including the administration of corticosteroids have not yet been adequately proven and remain empirical.

Gastroesophageal reflux

This is very common. Altered structure and function of the normal physiological barriers to reflux, namely the weight effect of the pregnant uterus and hormonally induced relaxation of the oesophageal sphincter, explain the extremely high incidence in the pregnant population. For the majority of patients, lifestyle modifications such as smoking cessation, frequent light meals and lying with the head propped up at night are helpful. When these prove insufficient to control symptoms, medications can be added in a stepwise fashion starting with simple antacids. Histamine-2 receptor antagonists and proton pump inhibitors can be used if more simple measures fail although their safety record in pregnancy is less certain. Severe, refractory dyspeptic symptoms warrant gastroenterology referral just in case a stomach ulcer or hiatus hernia is being overlooked.

Haemorrhoids

Several factors conspire to render haemorrhoids more common during pregnancy including the effects of circulating progesterone on the vasculature, pressure on the superior rectal veins by the gravid uterus and increased circulating volume. A conservative approach is usually advocated including local anaesthetic/anti-irritant creams and a high-fibre diet. Never overlook the 'warning' symptoms of tenesmus, mucus, blood mixed with stool and back passage discomfort that may suggest rectal carcinoma; a rectal digital examination should be carried out if these symptoms are suggested.

Varicose veins

Varicose veins may appear for the first time in pregnancy or pre-existing veins may become worse. They are thought to be due to the relaxant effect of progesterone on vascular smooth muscle and the dependent venous stasis caused by the weight of the pregnant uterus on the inferior vena cava.

Varicose veins of the legs may be symptomatically improved with support stockings, avoidance of standing for prolonged periods and simple analgesia. Thrombophlebitis may occur in a large varicose vein, more commonly after delivery. A large superficial varicose vein may bleed profusely if traumatized; the leg must be elevated and direct pressure applied. Vulval and vaginal varicosities are uncommon but symptomatically troublesome; trauma at the time of delivery (episiotomy, tear, instrumental delivery) may also cause considerable bleeding.

Oedema

This is common, occurring to some degree in approximately 80 per cent of all pregnancies. There is generalized soft-tissue swelling and increased capillary permeability, which allows intravascular fluid to leak into the extravascular compartment. The fingers, toes and ankles are usually worst affected and the symptoms are aggravated by hot weather. Oedema is best dealt with by frequent periods of rest with leg elevation; occasionally, support stockings are indicated. Excessively swollen fingers may necessitate removal of rings and jewellery before they get stuck. It is important to remember that generalized (rather than lower limb) oedema may be a feature of pre-eclampsia, so remember to check the woman's blood pressure and urine for protein. More rarely, severe oedema may suggest underlying cardiac impairment or nephrotic syndrome.

Other common 'minor' disorders:

- Itching
- Urinary incontinence
- Nose bleeds
- Thrush (vaginal candidiasis)
- Headache
- Fainting
- Breast soreness
- Tiredness
- Altered taste sensation
- Insomnia
- Leg cramps
- Striae gravidarum and chloasma.

Problems due to abnormalities of the pelvic organs

Fibroids (leiomyomata)

Fibroids are compact masses of smooth muscle that lie in the cavity of the uterus (submucous), within the uterine muscle (intramural) or on the outside surface of the uterus (subserous). They may enlarge in pregnancy, and in so doing present problems later on in pregnancy or at delivery (Figure 8.1). A large fibroid at the cervix or in the lower uterine segment may prevent descent of the presenting part and obstruct vaginal delivery.

Red degeneration is one of the most common complications of fibroids in pregnancy. As it grows, the fibroid may become ischaemic; this manifests clinically as acute pain, tenderness over the fibroid and frequent vomiting. If these symptoms are severe, uterine contractions may be precipitated, causing miscarriage or preterm labour. Red fibroid degeneration requires treatment in hospital, with potent analgesics (usually opiates and intravenous fluids). The symptoms usually settle within a few days. The differential diagnosis of red degeneration includes acute appendicitis, pyelonephritis/urinary tract infection, ovarian cyst accident and placental abruption.

A subserous pedunculated fibroid may tort in the same way that a large ovarian cyst can. When this happens, acute abdominal pain and tenderness may make the two difficult to distinguish from one another. In this scenario, a pertinent history followed by an ultrasound scan (transvaginal in the first trimester, transabdominal in the second and third) will aid the diagnosis.

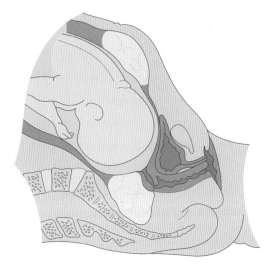

Figure 8.1 Fibroids complicating pregnancy. The tumour in the anterior wall of the uterus has been drawn up out of the pelvis as the lower segment was formed, but the fibroid arising from the cervix remains in the pelvis and will obstruct labour

Retroversion of the uterus

Fifteen per cent of women have a retroverted uterus. In pregnancy, the uterus grows and a retroverted uterus will normally 'flip' out of the pelvis and begin to fill the abdominal cavity, as an anteverted uterus would. In a small proportion of cases, the uterus remains in retroversion and eventually fills up the entire pelvic cavity; as it does so, the base of the bladder and the urethra are stretched. Retention of urine may occur, classically at 12–14 weeks, and this is not only very painful but may also cause long-term bladder damage if the bladder becomes over-distended. In this situation, catheterization is essential until the position of the uterus has changed.

Congenital uterine anomalies

The shape of the uterus is embryologically determined by the fusion of the Mullerian ducts. Abnormalities of fusion may give rise to anything from a subseptate uterus through to a bicornuate uterus and even (very rarely) to a double uterus with two cervices. These findings are often discovered incidentally at the time of a pelvic operation such as a laparoscopy, or an ultrasound scan.

The problems associated with bicornuate uterus are:

- miscarriage;
- preterm labour;
- preterm prelabour rupture of membranes (PPROM);
- abnormalities of lie and presentation;
- higher Caesarean section rate.

Ovarian cysts in pregnancy

Ovarian cysts are common in pregnant women; fortunately, the incidence of malignancy is uncommon in women of childbearing age. The most common types of pathological ovarian cyst are serous cysts and benign teratomas. Physiological cysts of the corpus luteum may grow to several centimetres but rarely require treatment, therefore asymptomatic cysts may be followed up by clinical and ultrasound examination, but large cysts (for example, dermoids) may require surgery in pregnancy.

Surgery is usually postponed until the late second or early third trimester, when there is the potential that if the baby were delivered, it would be able to survive.

The major problems are of large (>8 cm) ovarian cysts in pregnancy, which may undergo torsion, haemorrhage or rupture, causing acute abdominal pain. The resulting pain and inflammation may lead to a miscarriage or preterm labour. Symptomatic cysts, most commonly due to torsion, will require an emergency laparotomy and ovarian cystectomy or even oophorectomy if the cyst is torted. A full assessment must include a family history of ovarian or breast malignancy, tumour markers (although these are of limited value in pregnancy) and detailed ultrasound investigation of both ovaries. Surgery in the late second and third trimester of pregnancy is normally performed through a midline or paramedian incision; a low transverse suprapubic incision would not allow access to the ovary, as it is drawn upwards in later pregnancy.

Cervical cancer

Cervical abnormalities are much more difficult to deal with in pregnancy, partly because the cervix itself is more difficult to visualize at colposcopy, and also because biopsy may cause considerable bleeding. Cervical carcinoma most commonly arises in poor attenders for cervical screening. The disease is commonly asymptomatic in early stages, but later stage presentation includes vaginal bleeding (especially postcoital). Examination may reveal a friable or ulcerated lesion with bleeding and purulent discharge. The prospect of cervical carcinoma in pregnancy leads to complex ethical and moral dilemmas concerning whether the pregnancy must be terminated (depending on the stage it has reached) to facilitate either surgical treatment (radical hysterectomy) or chemotherapy. Cervical cancer is dealt with in greater detail in Chapter 14, premalignant and malignant disease of the cervix in Gynaecology by Ten Teachers, 19th edition.

Urinary tract infection

Urinary tract infections (UTIs) are common in pregnancy. Eight per cent of women have asymptomatic bacteriuria; if this is untreated, it may progress to UTI or even pyelonephritis, with the attendant associations of low birth weight and preterm delivery.

The predisposing factors are:

- history of recurrent cystitis;
- renal tract abnormalities: duplex system, scarred kidneys, ureteric damage and stones;

- diabetes;
- bladder emptying problems, for example multiple sclerosis.

The symptoms of UTI may be different in pregnancy; it occasionally presents as low back pain and general malaise with flu-like symptoms. The classic presentation of frequency, dysuria and haematuria is not often seen. On examination, tachycardia, pyrexia, dehydration and loin tenderness may be present. Investigations should include a full blood count and midstream specimen of urine (MSU) sent for urgent microscopy, culture and sensitivities. If there is a strong clinical suspicion of UTI, treatment with antibiotics should start immediately. The woman should drink plenty of clear fluids and take a simple analgesic, such as paracetamol.

The most common organism for UTI is *Escherichia coli*; less commonly implicated are streptococci, *Proteus*, *Pseudomonas* and *Klebsiella*. If more than 10^5 organisms are present at culture, this confirms a diagnosis of UTI. The commonly reported 'heavy mixed growth' is often associated with UTI symptoms and may be treated, or the MSU repeated after a week, depending on the clinical scenario. The first-line antibiotic for UTI is amoxycillin or oral cephalosporins.

Pyelonephritis is characterized by dehydration, a very high temperature (>38.5ºC), systemic disturbance and occasionally shock. This requires urgent and aggressive treatment including intravenous fluids, opiate analgesia and intravenous antibiotics (such as cephalosporins or gentamicin). In addition, renal function should be determined, with at least baseline urea and electrolytes, and the baby must be monitored with cardiotocography (CTG). Recurrent UTIs in pregnancy require MSU specimens to be sent to the microbiology laboratory at each antenatal visit, and low-dose prophylactic oral antibiotics may be prescribed. Investigation should take place after delivery, unless frank haematuria or other symptoms suggest that an urgent diagnosis is essential. Investigations might include a renal ultrasound scan, renal DMSA function scan, creatinine clearance, intravenous urogram and cystoscopy.

Abdominal pain in pregnancy

Abdominal pain is one of the most common minor disorders of pregnancy; the problem is in distinguishing pathological from 'physiological' pains. There are many possibilities to exclude. Furthermore, the anatomical and physiological changes of pregnancy may alter 'classical' presenting symptoms and signs making clinical diagnosis challenging. The causes listed in Table 8.1 are not exhaustive, but cover most possible diagnoses. The crucial point is that certain conditions are potentially

Table 8.1 Causes of abdominal pain in pregnancy

Pregnancy-caused (obstetric) conditions
Early pregnancy (<24 weeks)
Ligament stretching
Miscarriage
Ectopic pregnancy
Acute urinary retention due to retroverted gravid uterus
Later pregnancy (>24 weeks)
Labour
Placental abruption
HELLP syndrome
Uterine rupture
Chorioamnioitis

Pregnancy-unrelated conditions
Uterine/ovarian causes
Torsion or degeneration of fibroid
Ovarian cyst accident
Urinary tract disorders
Urinary tract infection (acute cystitis and acute pyelonephritis)
Renal colic
Gastrointestinal disorders
Medical gastric/duodenal ulcer
Acute appendicitis
Acute pancreatitis
Acute gastroenteritis
Intestinal obstruction or perforation
Medical causes
Sickle cell disease (abdominal crisis)
Diabetic ketoacidosis
Acute intermittent porphyria
Pneumonia (especially lower lobe)
Pulmonary embolus
Malaria

dangerous or debilitating (e.g. acute appendicitis) and may be masked by the altered anatomy and physiology of pregnancy. Obstetricians may therefore have to perform x-rays and arrange invasive assessments to make a diagnosis.

Venous thromboembolism

Venous thromboembolic disease (VTE) is the most common cause of direct maternal death in the UK. In the most recent triennium, there were 41 fatalities, giving a maternal mortality rate of 1.94 per 100 000 – more than twice that of the next most common cause (pre-eclampsia).

Pregnancy is a hypercoagulable state because of an alteration in the thrombotic and fibrinolytic systems. There is an increase in clotting factors VIII, IX, X and fibrinogen levels, and a reduction in protein S and anti-thrombin (AT) III concentrations (see Chapter 3, Physiological changes in pregnancy). The net result of these changes is thought to be an evolutionary response to reduce the likelihood of haemorrhage following delivery.

These physiological changes predispose a woman to thromboembolism and this is further exacerbated by venous stasis in the lower limbs due to the weight of the gravid uterus placing pressure on the inferior vena cava in late pregnancy and immobility, particularly in the puerperium.

Pregnancy is associated with a 6–10-fold increase in the risk of venous thromboembolic disease compared to the non-pregnant situation. Without thromboprophylaxis, the incidence of non-fatal pulmonary embolism (PE) and deep vein thrombosis (DVT) in pregnancy is about 0.1 per cent in developed countries, this increases following delivery to around 1–2 per cent and is further increased following emergency Caesarean section.

Thrombophilia

Some women are predisposed to thrombosis through changes in the coagulation/fibrinolytic system that may be inherited or acquired. There is growing evidence that both heritable and acquired thrombophilias are associated with a range of adverse pregnancy outcomes particularly recurrent fetal loss. The major hereditary forms of thrombophilia

Risk factors for thromboembolic disease
Pre-existing
• Maternal age (>35 years)
• Thrombophilia
• Obesity (>80 kg)
• Previous thromboembolism
• Severe varicose veins
• Smoking
• Malignancy
Specific to pregnancy
• Multiple gestation
• Pre-eclampsia
• Grand multiparity
• Caesarean section, especially if emergency
• Damage to the pelvic veins
• Sepsis
• Prolonged bed rest

currently recognized include: deficiencies of the endogenous anticoagulants protein C, protein S and AT III; abnormalities of procoagulant factors, factor V Leiden (caused by a mutation in the factor V gene) and the prothrombin mutation G20210A. It seems probable that there are still some thrombophilias not yet discovered or described. Heritable thrombophilias are present in at least 15 per cent of Western populations.

Acquired thrombophilia is most commonly associated with antiphospholipid syndrome (APS). APS is the combination of lupus anticoagulant with or without anti-cardiolipin antibodies, with a history of recurrent miscarriage and/or thrombosis. It may (or, more commonly, may not) be associated with other autoantibody disorders, such as systemic lupus erythematosus (SLE).

If thrombophilic disorders are taken together, more than 50 per cent of women with pregnancy-related VTE will have a thrombophilia. It is therefore vital that women with a history of thrombotic events are screened for thrombophilia. The presence of thrombophilia, with a history of thrombotic episode(s), means that prophylaxis should be considered for pregnancy.

Diagnosis of acute venous thromboembolism

Clinical diagnosis of VTE is unreliable, therefore women who are suspected of having a DVT or PE should be investigated promptly.

Deep vein thrombosis

The most common symptoms are pain in the calf with varying degrees of redness or swelling. Women's legs are often swollen during pregnancy; therefore unilateral symptoms should ring alarm bells. The signs are few, except that often the calf is tender to gentle touch. It is mandatory to ask about symptoms of PE (see next section), as a woman with PE might present initially with a DVT.

Compression ultrasound has a high sensitivity and specificity in diagnosing proximal thrombosis in the non-pregnant woman and should be the first investigation used in a suspected DVT. Calf veins are often poorly visualized, however, it is known that a thrombus confined purely to the calf veins with no extension is very unlikely to give rise to a PE.

Venography is invasive, requiring the injection of contrast medium and the use of x-rays. It does, however, allow excellent visualization of veins both below and above the knee.

Pulmonary embolus

It is crucial to recognize PE, as missing the diagnosis could have fatal implications. The most common presentation is of mild breathlessness, or inspiratory chest pain, in a woman who is not cyanosed but may be slightly tachycardic (>90 bpm) with a mild pyrexia (37.5°C). Rarely, massive PE may present with sudden cardiorespiratory collapse (see Chapter 16, Obstetric emergencies).

If PE is suspected, initial electrocardiogram (ECG), chest x-ray and arterial blood gases should be performed to exclude other respiratory diagnoses. However, these investigations are insufficient on their own to exclude or diagnose PE and it may be sensible to investigate the lower limbs for evidence of DVT by ultrasound and if positive treat with a presumptive diagnosis of PE. If all the tests are normal but a high clinical suspicion of PE remains, a ventilation perfusion (V/Q) scan or computed tomography pulmonary angiogram (CTPA) should be performed. In both cases the radiation to the fetus is below the threshold considered safe.

D-dimer is now commonly used as a screening test for thromboembolic disease in non-pregnant women, in whom it has a high negative predictive value. Outwith pregnancy, a low level of D-dimer suggests the absence of a DVT or PE, and no further objective tests are necessary, while an increased level of D-dimer suggests that thrombosis may be present and an objective diagnostic test for DVT and/or PE should be performed. In pregnancy, however, D-dimer can be elevated due to the physiological changes in the coagulation system, limiting its clinical usefulness as a screening test in this situation.

Treatment of VTE

Warfarin is given orally and prolongs the prothrombin time (PT). Warfarin is rarely recommended for use in pregnancy (exceptions include women with mechanical heart valves) as it crosses the placenta and can cause limb and facial defects in the first trimester and fetal intracerebral haemorrhage in the second and third trimesters.

Low molecular weight heparins (LMWHs) are now the treatment of choice. They do not cross the placenta and have been shown to be at least as safe and effective as unfractionated heparin (UFH) in the treatment of VTE with lower and fewer haemorrhagic complications in the initial treatment of non-pregnant subjects. In addition, LMWH is safe and easy to administer. Women are taught to inject themselves and can continue on this treatment for the duration of their pregnancy.

Following delivery, women can choose to convert to warfarin (with the need for stabilization of the doses initially and frequent checks of the international normalized ratio (INR) or remain on LMWH. Both warfarin and LMWH are safe in women who are breastfeeding.

Graduated elastic stockings should be used for the initial treatment of DVT and should be worn for two years following a DVT to prevent post phlebitic syndrome.

Prevention of VTE in pregnancy and postpartum

The Royal College of Obstetricians and Gynaecologists have recently released updated guidelines on the prevention of thrombosis and embolism in pregnancy and the puerperium (Green-top Guideline No. 37, November 2009) and these are summarized in Figure 8.2.

Antenatal thromboprophylaxis risk assessment and management

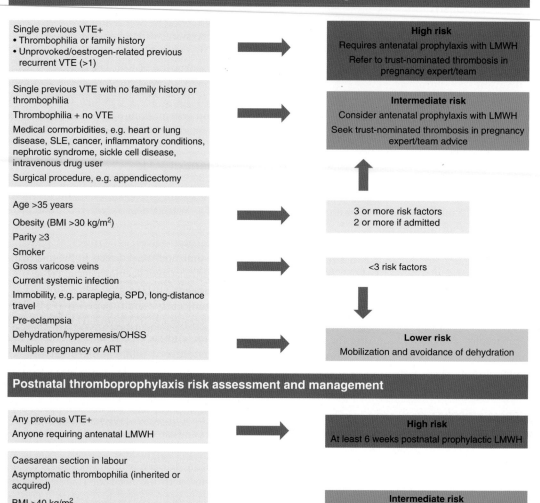

Single previous VTE+
- Thrombophilia or family history
- Unprovoked/oestrogen-related previous recurrent VTE (>1)

→ **High risk**
Requires antenatal prophylaxis with LMWH
Refer to trust-nominated thrombosis in pregnancy expert/team

Single previous VTE with no family history or thrombophilia

Thrombophilia + no VTE

Medical cormorbidities, e.g. heart or lung disease, SLE, cancer, inflammatory conditions, nephrotic syndrome, sickle cell disease, intravenous drug user

Surgical procedure, e.g. appendicectomy

→ **Intermediate risk**
Consider antenatal prophylaxis with LMWH
Seek trust-nominated thrombosis in pregnancy expert/team advice

Age >35 years

Obesity (BMI >30 kg/m^2)

Parity ≥3

Smoker

Gross varicose veins

Current systemic infection

Immobility, e.g. paraplegia, SPD, long-distance travel

Pre-eclampsia

Dehydration/hyperemesis/OHSS

Multiple pregnancy or ART

→ 3 or more risk factors
2 or more if admitted

→ <3 risk factors

→ **Lower risk**
Mobilization and avoidance of dehydration

Postnatal thromboprophylaxis risk assessment and management

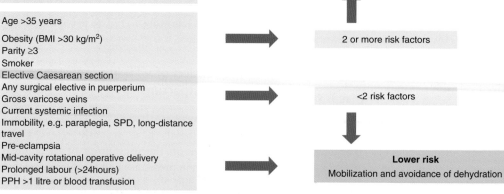

Any previous VTE+
Anyone requiring antenatal LMWH

→ **High risk**
At least 6 weeks postnatal prophylactic LMWH

Caesarean section in labour

Asymptomatic thrombophilia (inherited or acquired)

BMI >40 kg/m^2

Prolonged hospital admission

Medical cormorbidities, e.g. heart or lung disease, SLE, cancer, inflammatory conditions, nephrotic syndrome, sickle cell disease, intravenous drug user

→ **Intermediate risk**
At least 7 days postnatal prophylactic LMWH

Note: if persisting or >3 risk factors, consider extending thrombophylaxis with LMWH

Age >35 years

Obesity (BMI >30 kg/m^2)

Parity ≥3

Smoker

Elective Caesarean section

Any surgical elective in puerperium

Gross varicose veins

Current systemic infection

Immobility, e.g. paraplegia, SPD, long-distance travel

Pre-eclampsia

Mid-cavity rotational operative delivery

Prolonged labour (>24hours)

PPH >1 litre or blood transfusion

→ 2 or more risk factors

→ <2 risk factors

→ **Lower risk**
Mobilization and avoidance of dehydration

Figure 8.2 Obstetric thromboprophylaxis – risk assessment and management.

Substance abuse in pregnancy

Approximately one-third of adults who access drug services are women of reproductive age. There are approximately 6000 births to problem drug users in the UK each year (about 1 per cent of all deliveries). Multidisciplinary care is often necessary to optimize outcomes because the financial, psychological, social and domestic problems associated with drug misuse are often greater than the physical and medical concerns.

Opioids, especially heroin, remain the most commonly used drugs in the UK, although many drug users take combinations of drugs that often include cocaine or crack cocaine. Most problem drug users smoke tobacco and are heavy users of alcohol and cannabis. Taking drugs in combination greatly increases the unpredictability of their effect on the user. Intravenous injection of drugs also puts drug users at greater risk of infection with blood-borne viruses (hepatitis B and C and HIV). Many drug users live in disadvantaged communities in conditions of poverty and social exclusion. Many have had poor parenting experiences, poor education and significant mental health problems. The aims of management are to stabilize the mother's drug-taking habits and ensure contact with social/care workers and psychiatric/drug liaison services as appropriate.

It is important not to try to reduce the opiate dose too rapidly in pregnancy, as this can easily precipitate acute withdrawal in both the mother and fetus; the principle is to administer the lowest effective dose of methadone liquid in three divided doses every day.

Screening for infections such as hepatitis B and human immunodeficiency virus (HIV) is routinely offered in the UK. In many cases,

Problems frequently encountered amongst drug addicts

- Social problems: housing, crime, other children in care or abused.
- Co-existent addictions: alcohol and smoking.
- Malnutrition: especially iron, vitamins B and C.
- Risk of viral infections, e.g. human immunodeficiency virus (HIV) or hepatitis B.
- Specific fetal and neonatal risks (Table 8.2).

Table 8.2 The effects of some drugs of abuse on the fetus and neonate

Drug	Fetal and neonatal risk
Tobacco	Fetal growth restriction
Placental abruption Alcohol	Fetal growth restriction Fetal alcohol syndrome (FAS)
Opiates	Pre-term labour Neonatal withdrawal syndrome
Cocaine and derivatives	Placental abruption Fetal growth restriction Pre-term labour

multidisciplinary case conferences should be held to make arrangements and decisions for when the baby is delivered.

Alcohol

There is much debate about what is a 'safe' dose of alcohol during pregnancy. What is likely is that an intake of less than 100 g per week (approximately two drinks per day, e.g. two medium glasses of wine or one pint of beer) is not associated with any adverse effects. Doses greater than this have been related to fetal growth restriction (FGR). Massive doses, in excess of 2 g/kg of body weight (17 drinks per day), have been associated with fetal alcohol syndrome. However, the syndrome is not seen consistently in infants born to women who are heavy consumers of alcohol, and occurs only in approximately 30–33 per cent of children born to women who drink about 2 g/kg of body weight per day (equivalent to approximately 18 units of alcoholic drink per day). The differing susceptibility of fetuses to the syndrome is thought to be multifactorial and reflects the interplay of genetic factors, social deprivation, nutritional deficiencies, tobacco and other drug abuse, along with alcohol consumption.

If alcohol abuse is suspected, it may be necessary to involve social workers and arrange for formal psychiatric/addiction assessment. It is extremely difficult to 'test' for alcohol abuse, as even markers such as mean corpuscular volume and gamma GT are not reliable in pregnancy. Malnutrition is very likely in heavy alcohol abuse and requires (in addition to a change in basic diet) B vitamin supplements and iron; the problem is that the majority of such patients not only do not take their medicines but also default antenatal appointments.

Smoking and pregnancy

Smoking acutely reduces placental perfusion. Overall perinatal mortality is increased, babies are smaller at delivery and there is a higher risk of antepartum haemorrhage in smokers compared with non-smokers. It is estimated that a baby will weigh less than its target weight by a multiple of 15 g times the average number of cigarettes a woman smokes per day; smoking fewer than five cigarettes per day has a barely discernible obstetric effect and quitting by 15 weeks gestation reduces the risk as much as quitting before pregnancy. Consequently, all women should be counselled regarding smoking cessation at their booking visit.

Oligohydramnios and polyhydramnios

Amniotic fluid is produced almost exclusively from fetal urine from the second trimester onwards. It serves a vital function in protecting the developing baby from pressure or trauma, allowing limb movement, hence normal postural development, and permitting the fetal lungs to expand and develop through breathing.

Oligohydramnios

Too little amniotic fluid (oligohydramnios) is commonly defined as amniotic fluid index <5th centile for gestation. The amniotic fluid index (AFI) is an ultrasound estimation of amniotic fluid derived by adding together the deepest vertical pool in four quadrants of the abdomen. The AFI (in cm) is therefore associated with some degree of error. In general, however, it is possible to differentiate subjectively on ultrasound between 'too much', 'too little' and 'normal looking'.

Oligohydramnios may be suspected antenatally following a history of clear fluid leaking from the vagina; this may represent PPROM (see Chapter 11, Late miscarriage and early birth). Clinically, on abdominal palpation, the fetal poles may be very obviously felt and 'hard', with a small for dates uterus. The possible causes of oligohydramnios and anhydramnios (no amniotic fluid) are described in the box.

The fetal prognosis depends on the cause of oligohydramnios, but both pulmonary hypoplasia and limb deformities (contractures, talipes) are common to severe early-onset (<24 weeks) oligohydramnnios. Renal agenesis and bilateral multicystic kidneys carry a lethal prognosis, as life after birth is impossible without functioning kidneys. In this situation, the fetal lungs would probably be hypoplastic; this may also be true of severe urinary tract obstruction. Oligohydramnios due to FGR/uteroplacental insufficiency is usually of a less severe degree and less commonly causes limb and lung problems.

Polyhydramnios

Polyhydramnios is the term given to an excess of amniotic fluid, i.e. AFI >95th centile for gestation on ultrasound estimation. It may present as severe abdominal swelling and discomfort. On examination, the abdomen will appear distended out of proportion to the woman's gestation (increased SFH). Furthermore, the abdomen may be tense and tender and the fetal poles will be hard to palpate. The condition may be caused by maternal, placental or fetal conditions.

Maternal
- Diabetes

Placental
- Chorioangioma
- Arterio-venous fistula

Possible causes of oligohydramnios and anhydramnios	
Too little production	**Diagnosed by**
Renal agenesis	Ultrasound: no renal tissue, no bladder
Multicystic kidneys	Ultrasound: enlarged kidneys with multiple cysts, no visible bladder
Urinary tract abnormality/ obstruction	Ultrasound: kidneys may be present, but urinary tract dilatation
FGR and placental insufficiency	Clinical: reduced SFH, reduced fetal movements, possibly abnormal CTG Ultrasound: FGR, abnormal fetal Dopplers
Maternal drugs (e.g NSAIDs)	Withholding NSAIDs may allow amniotic fluid to re-accumulate
Post-dates pregnancy	
Leakage	**Diagnosed by**
PPROM	Speculum examination: pool of amniotic fluid on posterior blade

NSAIDs, non-steroidal anti-inflammatory drugs; SFH, symphysis–fundal height.

Fetal

- Multiple gestation (in monochorionic twins, it may be twin-to-twin transfusion syndrome)
- Idiopathic
- Oesophageal atresia/tracheo-oesophageal fistula
- Duodenal atresia
- Neuromuscular fetal condition (preventing swallowing)
- Anencephaly.

The management of polyhydramnios is directed towards establishing the cause (hence determining fetal prognosis), relieving the discomfort of the mother (if necessary by amniodrainage), and assessing the risk of preterm labour due to uterine over-distension. The last-mentioned may require assessment of cervical length by ultrasound. If prior to 24 weeks, following amniotic fluid drainage, the cervical length is less than 25 mm, consideration might be given to cervical suture insertion.

Polyhydramnios due to maternal diabetes needs urgent investigation, as it often suggests high maternal blood glucose levels. In this context, polyhydramnios should correct itself when the mother's glycaemic control is optimized.

Twin-to-twin transfusion syndrome is a rare cause of acute polyhydramnios in the recipient sac of monochorionic twins. It is associated with oligohydramnios and a small baby in the other sac. The condition may be rapidly fatal for both twins; amniodrainage and removal by laser of the placental vascular connections are two therapeutic modalities employed in dealing with this condition. This is discussed further in Chapter 9, Twins and higher multiple gestations.

Fetal malpresentation at term

Malpresentation is a presentation that is not cephalic. Breech presentation is the most commonly encountered malpresentation and occurs in 3–4 per cent of term pregnancies, but is more common at earlier gestations. Similarly, oblique and transverse positions are not uncommon antenatally. They only become a problem if the baby (or first presenting baby in a multiple gestation) is not cephalic by 37 weeks.

Breech presentation

There are three types of breech: the most common is extended (frank) breech (Figure 8.3a); less common is a flexed (complete) breech (Figure 8.3b); and least common is footling breech, in which a foot presents at the cervix (Figure 8.3c). Cord and foot prolapse are risks in this situation.

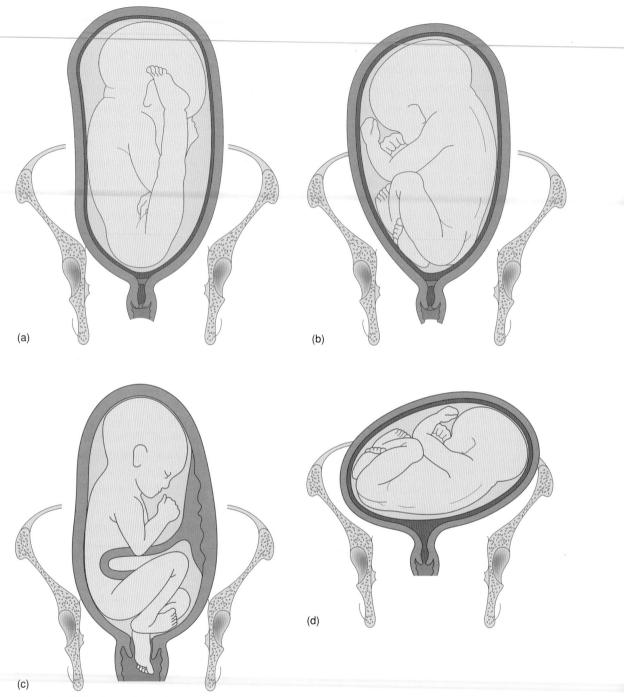

(a)

(b)

(c)

(d)

Figure 8.3 (a) Frank breech (also known as extended breech) presentation with extension of the legs. (b) Breech presentation with flexion of the legs. (c) Footling breech presentation. (d) Transverse lie. (e) Oblique lie

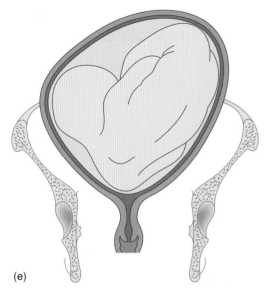

(e)

Figure 8.3 (*continued*)

Predisposing factors for breech presentation

Maternal
- Fibroids
- Congenital uterine abnormalities, e.g. bicornuate uterus
- Uterine surgery

Fetal/placental
- Multiple gestation
- Prematurity
- Placenta praevia
- Abnormality, e.g. anencephaly or hydrocephalus
- Fetal neuromuscular condition
- Oligohydramnios
- Polyhydramnios

Antenatal management of breech presentation

If a breech presentation is clinically suspected at or after 36 weeks, this should be confirmed by ultrasound scan. The scan should document fetal biometry, amniotic fluid volume, the placental site and the position of the fetal legs. The scan should also look for any anomalies previously undetected.

The three management options available at this point should be discussed with the woman. These are external cephalic version (ECV), vaginal breech delivery and elective Caesarean section.

External cephalic version

ECV is a relatively straightforward and safe technique and has been shown to reduce the number of Caesarean sections due to breech presentations. Success rates vary according to the experience of the operator but in most units are around 50 per cent (and are higher in multiparous women who tend to have more lax abdominal musculature).

The procedure is performed at or after 37 completed weeks by an experienced obstetrician at or near delivery facilities. ECV should be performed with a tocolytic (e.g. nifedipine) as this has been shown to improve the success rate. The woman is laid flat with a left lateral tilt having ensured that she has emptied her bladder and is comfortable. With ultrasound guidance, the breech is elevated from the pelvis and one hand is used to manipulate this upward in the direction of a forward role, while the other hand applies gentle pressure to flex the fetal head and bring it down to the maternal pelvis (Figure 8.4).

The procedure can be mildly uncomfortable for the mother and should last no more than 10 minutes. If the procedure fails, or becomes difficult, it is abandoned. A fetal heart rate trace must be performed before and after the procedure and it is important to administer anti-D if the woman is Rhesus-negative.

Contraindications to ECV

- Fetal abnormality (e.g. hydrocephalus)
- Placenta praevia
- Oligohydramnios or polyhydramnios
- History of antepartum haemorrhage
- Previous Caesarean or myomectomy scar on the uterus
- Multiple gestation
- Pre-eclampsia or hypertension
- Plan to deliver by Caesarean section anyway

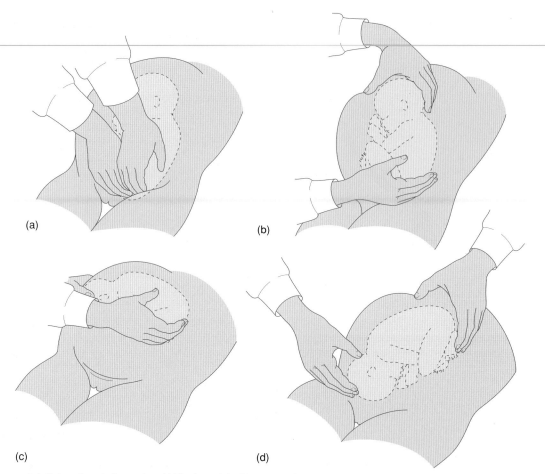

Figures 8.4 External cephalic version. (a) The breech is disengaged from the pelvic inlet. (b) Version is usually performed in the direction that increases flexion of the fetus and makes it do a forward somersault. (c) On completion of version, the head is often not engaged for a time. (d) The fetal heart rate should be checked after the external version has been completed

Risks of ECV

- Placental abruption
- Premature rupture of the membranes
- Cord accident
- Transplacental haemorrhage (remember anti-D administration to Rhesus-negative women)
- Fetal bradycardia

Mode of delivery

If ECV fails, or is contraindicated, and Caesarean section is not indicated for other reasons, then women should be counselled regarding elective Caesarean section and planned vaginally delivery. A recent large multicentre trial (the Term Breech Trial) confirmed that planned vaginal delivery of a breech presentation is associated with a 3 per cent increased risk of death or serious morbidity to the baby. Although this trial did not evaluate long-term outcomes for child or mother, it has led to the recommendation that the best method of delivering a term breech singleton is by planned Caesarean section. Despite this, either by choice or as a result of precipitous labour, a small proportion of women with breech presentations will deliver vaginally. It therefore remains important that clinicians and hospitals are prepared for vaginal breech delivery.

Prerequisites for vaginal breech delivery

Feto-maternal:

- The presentation should be either extended (hips flexed, knees extended) or flexed (hips flexed, knees flexed but feet not below the fetal buttocks).
- There should be no evidence of feto-pelvic disproportion with a pelvis clinically thought to be adequate and an estimated fetal weight of <3500 g (ultrasound or clinical measurement).
- There should be no evidence of hyperextension of the fetal head, and fetal abnormalities that would preclude safe vaginal delivery (e.g. severe hydrocephalus) should be excluded.

Management of labour:

- Fetal well-being and progress of labour should be carefully monitored.
- An epidural analgesia is not essential but may be advantageous; it can prevent pushing before full dilatation.
- Fetal blood sampling from the buttocks provides an accurate assessment of the acid-base status (when the fetal heart rate trace is suspect).
- There should be an operator experienced in delivering breech babies available in the hospital.

Although much emphasis is placed on adequate case selection prior to labour, a survey of outcome of the undiagnosed breech in labour managed by experienced medical staff showed that safe vaginal delivery can be achieved.

Technique

Breech delivery epitomizes the position of 'masterly inactivity' (hands-off). Problems are more likely to arise when the obstetrician tries to speed up the process (by pulling on the baby).

Delivery of the buttocks

In most circumstances, full dilatation and descent of the breech will have occurred naturally. When the buttocks become visible and begin to distend the perineum, preparations for the delivery are made. The buttocks will lie in the anterior–posterior diameter. Once the anterior buttock is delivered and the anus is seen over the fourchette (and no sooner than this), an episiotomy can be cut.

Delivery of the legs and lower body

If the legs are flexed, they will deliver spontaneously. If extended, they may need to be delivered using Pinard's manoeuvre. This entails using a finger to flex the leg at the knee and then extend at the hip, first anteriorly then posteriorly. With contractions and maternal effort, the lower body will be delivered. Usually a loop of cord is drawn down to ensure that it is not too short.

Delivery of the shoulders

The baby will be lying with the shoulders in the transverse diameter of the pelvic mid-cavity. As the anterior shoulder rotates into the anterior–posterior diameter, the spine or the scapula will become visible. At this point, a finger gently placed above the shoulder will help to deliver the arm. As the posterior arm/ shoulder reaches the pelvic floor, it too will rotate anteriorly (in the opposite direction). Once the spine becomes visible, delivery of the second arm will follow. This can be imagined as a 'rocking boat' with one side moving upwards and then the other. Loveset's manoeuvre essentially copies these natural movements (Figure 8.5). However, it is unnecessary and meddlesome to do routinely (one risks pulling the shoulders down but leaving the arms higher up, alongside the head).

Delivery of the head

The head is delivered using the Mauriceau–Smellie–Veit manoeuvre: the baby lies on the obstetrician's arm with downward traction being levelled on the head via a finger in the mouth and one on each maxilla (Figure 8.6). Delivery occurs with first downward and then upward movement (as with instrumental deliveries). If this manoeuvre proves difficult, forceps need to be applied. An assistant holds the baby's body aloft while the forceps are applied in the usual manner (Figure 8.7).

Complications

The greatest fear with a vaginal breech is that the baby will get 'stuck'. Interference in the natural process by the inappropriate use of oxytocic agents or by trying to pull the baby out (breech extraction) will (paradoxically) increase the risk of obstruction occurring. When delay occurs, particularly with

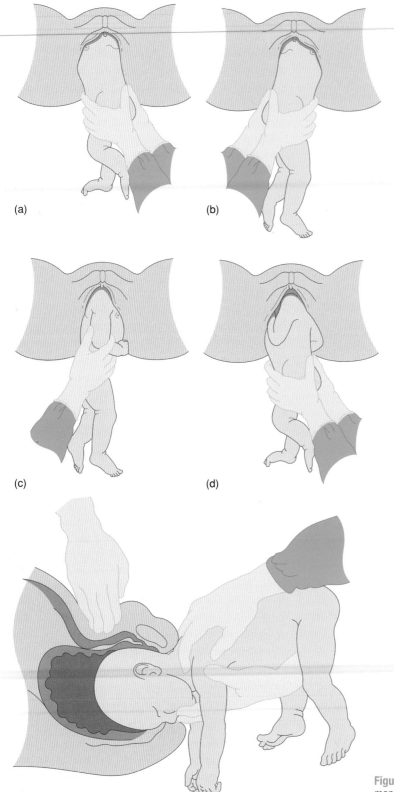

(a)

(b)

(c)

(d)

Figure 8.5 Loveset's manoeuvre.

Figure 8.6 Mauriceau–Smellie–Veit
manoeuvre for delivery of the head

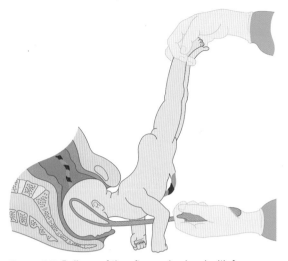

Figure 8.7 Delivery of the aftercoming head with forceps

delivery of the shoulders or head, the presence of an experienced obstetrician will reduce the risk of death or serious injury.

Key points

Breech presentation
- ECV should be offered at 36–37 weeks in selected women.
- Elective Caesarean section is safer than vaginal delivery for a baby presenting by the breech at or close to term.
- Planned or unexpected vaginal breech deliveries should be attended by experienced clinicians.

Other fetal malpresentations

A transverse lie occurs when the fetal long axis lies perpendicular to that of the maternal long axis and classically results in a shoulder presentation (see Figure 8.3d). An oblique lie occurs when the long axis of the fetal body crosses the long axis of the maternal body at an angle close to 45 degrees (see Figure 8.3e).

Any woman presenting at term with a transverse or oblique lie is at potential risk of cord prolapse following spontaneous rupture of the membranes, and prolapse of the hand, shoulder or foot once in labour. In most cases, the woman is multiparous with a lax uterus and

abdominal wall musculature, and gentle version of the baby's head in the clinic or on the ward will restore the presentation to cephalic. If this does not occur, or the lie is unstable (alternating between transverse, oblique and longitudinal), it is important to think of possible uterine or fetal causes of this (see the box describing predisposing factors for breech presentation).

The diagnosis of transverse or oblique lie might be suspected by abdominal inspection: the abdomen often appears asymmetrical. The SFH may be less than expected, and on palpation the fetal head or buttocks may be in the iliac fossa. Palpation over the pelvic brim will reveal an 'empty' pelvis.

It goes without saying that a woman in labour with the baby's lie anything other than longitudinal will not be able to deliver vaginally; this is one situation in which if Caesarean section is not performed both the mother and baby are at considerable risk of morbidity and mortality. The only exception to this is for exceptionally preterm or small babies, where vaginal delivery may occur irrespective of lie or presentation.

A woman with an unstable lie at term should be admitted to the antenatal ward. The normal plan would be to deliver by Caesarean section if the presentation is not cephalic in early labour or if spontaneous rupture of the membranes occurs. In a multiparous woman, an unstable lie will often correct itself in early labour (as long as the membranes are intact).

Post-term pregnancy

A pregnancy that has extended to or beyond 42 weeks gestation is defined as a prolonged or post-term pregnancy. Accurate dating remains essential for the correct diagnosis and should ideally involve a first-trimester ultrasound estimation of crown–rump length.

Post-term pregnancy affects approximately 10 per cent of all pregnancies and the aetiology is unknown. Post-term pregnancy is associated with increased risks to both the fetus and the mother an increased risk of stillbirth and perinatal death, an increased risk of prolonged labour and an increased risk of Caesarean section.

Fetal surveillance and induction of labour are two strategies employed that may reduce the risk of adverse outcome. Unfortunately, there are no known tests that can accurately predict fetal outcome post-term; an ultrasound scan may give temporary reassurance if the amniotic fluid and fetal growth are normal. Similarly, a CTG should be performed at and after 42 weeks.

Immediate induction of labour or delivery post-dates should take place if:

- there is reduced amniotic fluid on scan;
- fetal growth is reduced;
- there are reduced fetal movements;
- the CTG is not perfect;
- the mother is hypertensive or suffers a significant medical condition.

Induction of labour is discussed further in Chapter 14, Labour.

When counselling the parents regarding waiting for labour to start naturally after 42 weeks, it is important that the woman is aware that no test can guarantee the safety of her baby, and that perinatal mortality is increased (at least two-fold) beyond 42 weeks. A labour induced post-term is more likely to require Caesarean section; this may partly be due to the reluctance of the uterus to contract properly, and the possible compromise of the baby leading to abnormal CTG.

Antepartum haemorrhage

This is defined as vaginal bleeding from 24 weeks to delivery of the baby. The causes are placental or local.

Placental causes

- Placental abruption
- Placenta praevia
- Vasa praevia

Local causes

- Cervicitis
- Cervical ectropion
- Cervical carcinoma
- Vaginal trauma
- Vaginal infection

The incidence of antepartum haemorrhage is 3 per cent. It is estimated that 1 per cent is attributable to placenta praevia, 1 per cent is attributable to placental abruption and the remaining 1 per cent is from other causes. Placental causes are obviously the most worrying, as potentially the mother's and/or fetus' life is in danger. However, any antepartum haemorrhage must always be taken seriously, and any woman presenting with a history of fresh vaginal bleeding must be investigated promptly and properly. The key question is whether the bleeding is placental, and is compromising the mother and/or fetus, or whether it has a less significant cause. A pale, tachycardic woman looking anxious with a painful, firm abdomen, underwear soaked in fresh blood and reduced fetal movements needs emergency assessment and management for a possible placental abruption (see Chapter 16, Obstetric emergencies). A woman having had a small postcoital bleed with no systemic signs or symptoms represents a different end of the spectrum.

History

- How much bleeding?
- Triggering factors (e.g. postcoital bleed).
- Associated with pain or contractions?
- Is the baby moving?
- Last cervical smear (date/normal or abnormal)?

Examination

- Pulse, blood pressure.
- Is the uterus soft or tender and firm?
- Fetal heart auscultation/CTG.
- Speculum vaginal examination, with particular importance placed on visualizing the cervix (having established that placenta is not a praevia, preferably using a portable ultrasound machine).

Investigations

- Depending on the degree of bleeding, full blood count, clotting and, if suspected praevia/abruption, crossmatch six units of blood.

- Ultrasound (fetal size, presentation, amniotic fluid, placental position and morphology).

Placental abruption

The premature separation of the placenta is termed 'abruption'. The bleeding is maternal and/or fetal and abruption is acutely dangerous for both the mother and fetus (Figures 8.8 and 8.9; see Chapter 10, Pre-eclampsia and other disorders of placentation and Chapter 16, Obstetric emergencies).

Placenta praevia

A placenta covering or encroaching on the cervical os may be associated with bleeding, either provoked or spontaneous. The bleeding is from the maternal not fetal circulation and is more likely to compromise the mother than the fetus (Figure 8.10).

Risk factors for placenta praevia
• Multiple gestation
• Previous Caesarean section
• Uterine structural anomaly
• Assisted conception

Vasa praevia

Vasa praevia is present when fetal vessels traverse the fetal membranes over the internal cervical os. These vessels may be from either a velamentous insertion of the umbilical cord or may be joining an accessory (succenturiate) placental lobe to the main disk of the placenta. The diagnosis is usually suspected when either spontaneous or artificial rupture of the membranes is accompanied by painless fresh vaginal bleeding

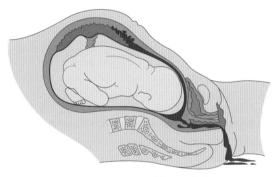

Figure 8.8 Placental abruption with revealed haemorrhage

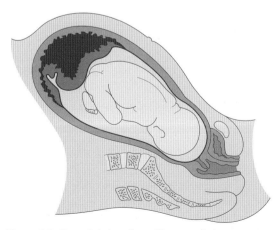

Figure 8.9 Placental abruption with concealed haemorrhage

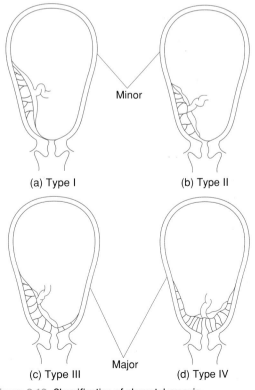

Minor

(a) Type I   (b) Type II

Major

(c) Type III   (d) Type IV

Figure 8.10 Classification of placental praevia

from rupture of the fetal vessels. This condition is associated with a very high perinatal mortality from fetal exsanguination. If the baby is still alive once the diagnosis is suspected, the immediate course of action is delivery by emergency Caesarean section.

Key points

- Placenta praevia is most dangerous for the mother.
- Placental abruption is more dangerous for the fetus than the mother.
- Vasa praevia is not dangerous for the mother but is nearly always fatal for the baby.

Further management

If there is minimal bleeding and the cause is clearly local vaginal bleeding, symptomatic management may be given (for example, antifungal preparations for candidiasis), as long as there is reasonable certainty that cervical carcinoma is excluded by smear history and direct visualization of the cervix. Placental causes of bleeding are a major concern. A large-gauge intravenous cannula is sited, blood sent for full blood count, clotting and crossmatch, and appropriate fetal and maternal monitoring instituted. If there is major fetal or maternal compromise, decisions may have to be made about immediate delivery irrespective of gestation. Emergency management is described in Chapter 16, Obstetric emergencies. If bleeding settles, the ongoing management depends on the underlying cause. If the cause was a suspected placental abruption, the woman must be admitted for 48 hours as the risk of rebleeding is high within this time frame. Steroids should be administered if the gestation is less than 34 weeks. Rhesus status is important: if the mother is Rhesus negative, send a Kleihauer test (to determine whether any, or how much, fetal blood has leaked into the maternal circulation) and administer anti-D. The ongoing management of placenta praevia is more contentious. Many clinicians favour retaining major placenta praevias in hospital until delivery.

Rhesus iso-immunization

Blood group is defined in two ways. First, there is the ABO group, allowing four different permutations of blood group (O, A, B, AB). Second, there is the rhesus system, which consists of C, D and E antigens. The importance of these blood group systems is that a mismatch between the fetus and mother can mean that when fetal red cells pass across to the maternal circulation, as they do to a greater or lesser extent during pregnancy, sensitization of the maternal immune system to these fetal 'foreign' red blood cells may occur and subsequently give rise to haemolytic disease of the fetus and newborn (HDFN).

The Rhesus system is the one most commonly associated with severe haemolytic disease.

The aetiology of Rhesus disease

The Rhesus system is coded on two adjacent genes, which sit within chromosome one. One gene codes for antigen polypeptides C/c and E/e while the other codes for the D polypeptide (Rhesus antigen). Note that the d (little d) antigen has not been identified so it may be that women who are D negative lack the antigen altogether, as opposed to those with c (little c) or e (little e), where c is the allelic antigen of C and e is the allelic antigen of E. Antigen expression is usually dominant, whereas those who have a negative phenotype are either homozygous for the recessive allele or have a deletion of that gene (Figure 8.11). In practice, only anti-D and anti-c regularly cause HDFN. Anti-D is much more common than anti-c and is therefore the focus of this discussion.

Occurrence of HDFN as a result of Rhesus isoimmunization involves three key stages (see Figure 8.12). First, a Rhesus negative mother must conceive a baby who has inherited the Rhesus positive phenotype from the father. Second, fetal cells must gain access to the maternal circulation in a sufficient volume to provoke a maternal antibody response. Finally, maternal antibodies must gain transplacental access and cause immune destruction of red cells in the fetus. Rhesus disease does not affect a first pregnancy as the primary response is usually weak and consists primarily of IgM antibodies that do not cross the placenta. Thereafter IgG antibodies are produced and these can cross the placenta. Rhesus antigens are well expressed by the fetus from as early as 30 days gestation so in a subsequent pregnancy, when maternal resensitization occurs (Rhesus-positive red cells pass from the baby to the maternal circulation; Figure 8.12), IgG antibodies cross from the mother to the fetal circulation. If these antibodies

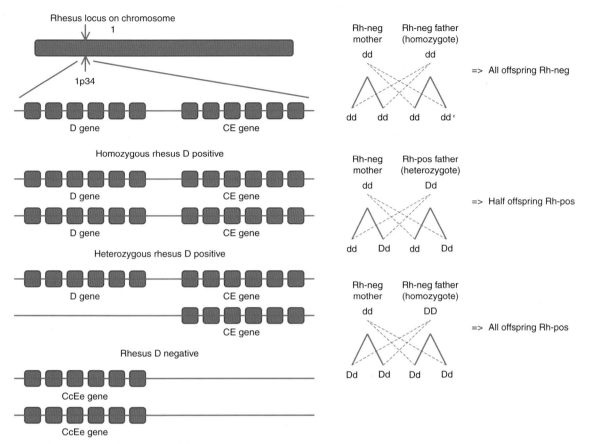

Figure 8.11 The parental genotype determinants of Rhesus group

are present in sufficient quantities, fetal haemolysis may occur, leading to such severe anaemia that the fetus may die unless a transfusion is performed. It is for this reason that Rhesus-negative women have frequent antibody checks in pregnancy; an increasing titre of atypical antibodies may suggest an impending problem.

Potential sensitizing events for Rhesus disease

- Miscarriage
- Termination of pregnancy
- Antepartum haemorrhage
- Invasive prenatal testing (chorion villus sampling, amniocentesis and cordocentesis)
- Delivery
- Ectopic pregnancy

Prevalence of Rhesus disease

The prevalence of D Rhesus negativity is 15 per cent in the Caucasian population, but lower in all other ethnic groups. It is very uncommon in Orientals. Rhesus disease is most common in countries where anti-D prophylaxis is not widespread, such as the Middle East and Russia.

Preventing Rhesus iso-immunization

The process of iso-immunization can be 'nipped in the bud' by the intramuscular administration of anti-D immunoglobulins to a mother, preferably within 72 hours of exposure to fetal red cells. Anti-D immunoglobulins 'mop up' any circulating rhesus-positive cells before an immune response is excited in the mother. The practical implications of this are that anti-D immunoglobulin must be

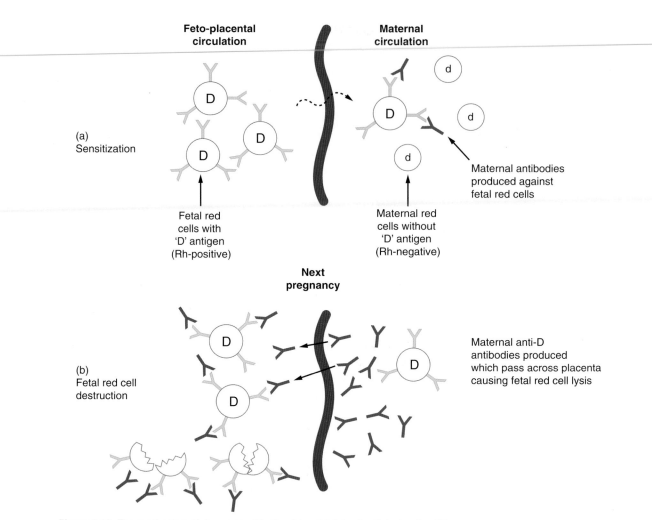

Figure 8.12 The mechanism of rhesus sensitization (a) and fetal red cell destruction (b)

given intramuscularly as soon as possible after any potentially sensitizing event. It is normal practice to administer anti-D after any of these events; the exact dose is determined by the gestation at which sensitization has occurred and the size of the feto-maternal haemorrhage.

In the first trimester of pregnancy, because the volume of fetal blood is so small, it is unlikely that sensitization would occur, and a 'standard' dose of anti-D (the exact dose varies from country to country) is given; this will more than cover even the largest feto-maternal transfusion. In the second and third trimesters, fetal blood volume is greater and because there is a possibility of a feto-maternal transfusion of several millilitres, a larger dose is given and a Kleihauer test performed.

A Kleihauer is a test of maternal blood to determine the proportion of fetal cells present (relying on their ability to resist denaturation by alcohol or acid); it will allow calculation of the amount of extra anti-D immunoglobulin required should a large transfusion have occurred.

In many countries, Rhesus-negative women are given anti-D at 28 and/or 34 weeks routinely. This is based on the finding that a small number of Rhesus-negative women become sensitized during pregnancy despite the administration of anti-D at delivery and without a clinically obvious sensitizing event. The likelihood is that a small feto-maternal haemorrhage occurs without any obvious clinical signs; therefore, prophylactic anti-D would reduce the risk of iso-immunization from this event.

Signs of fetal anaemia

Note: Clinical and ultrasound features of fetal anaemia do not usually become evident unless fetal haemoglobin is more than 5 g/dL less than the mean for gestation. Usually, features are not obvious unless the fetal haemoglobin is less than 6 g/dL.

- Polyhydramnios.
- Enlarged fetal heart.
- Ascites and pericardial effusions.
- Hyperdynamic fetal circulation (can be detected by Doppler ultrasound by measuring increased velocities in the middle cerebral artery or aorta).
- Reduced fetal movements.
- Abnormal CTG with reduced variability, eventually a 'sinusoidal' trace.

The management of Rhesus disease in a sensitized woman

Once a woman who is D Rhesus negative has been sensitized to the D Rhesus antigen, no amount of anti-D will ever turn the clock back. In a subsequent pregnancy, close surveillance is required. Rhesus disease gets worse with successive pregnancies, so it is important to note the severity of the disease in previous pregnancies. The management depends on the clinical scenario.

- The father of the next baby is D Rhesus negative. In this situation, there is no risk that the baby will be D Rhesus positive and therefore there is no chance of Rhesus disease.

- The father of the next baby is D Rhesus positive. He may be heterozygous and in this situation determining the paternal phenotype is useful in anticipating the likely fetal phenotype and, thus, the potential for development of HDFN. However, it is important to bear in mind that there are issues regarding paternal testing, and assuming paternity runs the risk of false prediction. Not withstanding this issue, paternal blood grouping is frequently used and often useful.

- In a sensitized woman, if the father is D Rhesus positive or unknown, standard management involves monitoring antibody levels every 2–4 weeks from booking. Antibody levels or quantity can be described using the titre or by using

IU (international units) as a standard quantification method. The titre simply refers to the number of times a sample has been diluted before the amount of antibody becomes undetectable; titre of 2, 4, 8, 16, 32, 64, 128, etc. Each time a sample is tested, it should be checked in parallel with the previous sample to ensure the detection of significant changes in the antibody level. It has been found that titrations of anti-D do not correlate well with the development of HDFN, and that the standard quantification method (IU/mL) gives more clinically relevant levels.

Anti-D level	Outcome
<4 IU/mL	HDFN unlikely
4–15 IU/mL	Moderate risk of HDFN
>15 IU/mL	High risk of hydrops fetalis

- If antibody levels rise, the baby should be examined for signs of anaemia. In the past, the bilirubin concentration of amniotic fluid was determined optically to give an indirect measure of fetal haemolysis. This involved an invasive procedure with the attendant risks of miscarriage/preterm labour and further boosting of the alloimmune response. In the last decade, middle cerebral artery (MCA) Dopplers (peak velocity measurement) have been shown to correlate reliably with fetal anaemia. In practice, this means that the use of invasive tests to monitor disease progression (once a critical antibody level has been reached) have been replaced by non-invasive assessment using MCA Doppler. There is now substantial data to support the use of peak MCA velocity as a correlate of fetal anaemia. The sensitivity is reported at 100 per cent with a false positive rate of 12 per cent (see figure 6.17 in Chapter 6, Antenatal imaging and assessment of fetal well-being).

- A fetus with raised MCA Dopplers has a high probability of anaemia. These cases are not common and the treatment should be in, or guided by, tertiary fetal medicine centres. Treatment options include delivery or fetal blood transfusion. Delivery of the fetus is an option if the fetus is sufficiently mature. However, delivery of an anaemic, rapidly haemolysing premature baby is a significant risk and should not be undertaken lightly. Delivery must take place in a unit where adequate neonatal support and expertise is available and generally delivery should not be before 36–37 weeks of gestation unless there are specific reasons, such as special difficulty with fetal transfusion.

- Fetal blood transfusion is life saving in a severely anaemic fetus that is too premature for delivery to be contemplated. The aim is to restore haemoglobin levels, reversing or preventing hydrops or death. A side effect is that transfusion will also suppress fetal erythropoesis, which reduces the concentration of antigen positive cells available for haemolysis. Blood can be transfused into a fetus in various ways depending on the gestation, the site of the cord insertion and the clinical situation.

- Routes of administration:
  - into the umbilical vein at the point of the cord insertion (ideally through the placenta and not through the amniotic sac);
  - into the intrahepatic vein;
  - into the peritoneal cavity (not as effective but some blood is absorbed and this may be the only option, for example in low gestations);
  - into the fetal heart.

Once a decision has been made that the fetus is severely anaemic and requires a blood transfusion, the invasive procedure aims to first take a sample to confirm the anaemia and then infuse the blood during a single puncture.

- Transfused blood is:
  - RhD negative;
  - crossmatched with a maternal sample;
  - densely packed (Hb usually around 30 g/L) so that small volumes are used;
  - white cell depleted and irradiated;
  - screened for infection including CMV.

At delivery

If the baby is known to be anaemic or has had multiple transfusions, a neonatologist must be present at delivery should exchange transfusion be required.

Blood must therefore always be ready for the delivery. All babies born to Rhesus-negative women should have cord blood taken at delivery for a blood count, blood group and indirect Coomb's test.

Key points

D Rhesus disease
- Rhesus disease gets worse with successive pregnancies.
- If the father of the fetus is Rhesus negative, the fetus cannot be Rhesus positive.
- If the father of the fetus is Rhesus positive, he may be a heterozygote (50 per cent likelihood that the baby is D Rhesus positive) or a homozygote (100 per cent likelihood).
- Anti-D is given only as prophylaxis and is useless once sensitization has occurred.
- Prenatal diagnosis for karyotype, or attempts at determining fetal blood group by invasive testing (e.g. chorion villus sampling), may make the antibody levels higher in women who are already sensitized.

ABO

ABO blood group iso-immunization may occur when the mother is blood group O and the baby is blood group A or B. Anti-A and anti-B antibodies are present in the maternal circulation naturally, usually secondary to sensitization against A or B substances in food or bacteria. This means that ABO incompatibility may occur in a first pregnancy. In this situation, anti-A or anti-B antibodies may pass to the fetal circulation, causing fetal haemolysis and anaemia. However, most anti-A and anti-B are mainly IgM and do not cross the placenta. In addition, A and B antigens are not fully developed in the fetus. Therefore ABO incompatibility generally causes only mild haemolytic disease of the baby, but may sometimes explain unexpected jaundice in an otherwise healthy term infant.

Additional reading

James DK, Steer PJ, Weiner CP, Gonik B. *High risk pregnancy*, 3rd end. London: WB Saunders, 2005.

Lewis, G (ed.). The Confidential Enquiry into Maternal and Child Health (CEMACH). Saving Mothers' Lives: reviewing maternal deaths to make motherhood safer – 2003–2005. The Seventh Report on Confidential Enquiries into Maternal Deaths in the United Kingdom. London: CEMACH, 2007.

CHAPTER 9

TWINS AND HIGHER MULTIPLE GESTATIONS

Griffith Jones

OVERVIEW

In 1–2 per cent of pregnancies, there is more than one fetus. The chances of miscarriage, fetal abnormalities, poor fetal growth, preterm delivery and intrauterine or neonatal death are considerably higher in twin than in singleton pregnancies. In about two-thirds of twins the fetuses are non-identical, or dizygotic, and in one-third they are identical, or monozygotic. In all dizygotic pregnancies there are two functionally separate placentae (dichorionic). In two-thirds of monozygotic pregnancies there are vascular communications within the two placental circulations (monochorionic) and in the other one-third of cases there is dichorionic placentation. Monochorionic, compared to dichorionic, twins have a much higher risk of abnormalities and death. The maternal risks are also increased in multiple gestations, including adverse symptoms such as nausea and vomiting, tiredness and discomfort, and the risk of serious complications, including hypertensive and thromboembolic disease, and antepartum and postpartum haemorrhage.

Definitions

In general terms, multiple pregnancies consist of two or more fetuses. There are rare exceptions to this, such as twin gestations made up of a singleton viable fetus and a complete mole. Twins make up the vast majority (nearly 99 per cent) of multiple gestations. Pregnancies with three or more fetuses are referred to as 'higher multiples'.

Prevalence

Risk factors for multiple gestations include assisted reproduction techniques (both ovulation induction and *in vitro* fertilization (IVF)), increasing maternal age, high parity, black race and maternal family history.

In the UK, twins currently account for approximately 1.5 per cent of all pregnancies, up from 1 per cent in 1984.

Since the mid-1980s, the incidence of multiple pregnancy has been increasing. Two related and overlapping trends are contributors to this. Delay in childbearing results in increased maternal age at conception. The increased use of infertility treatments, also often by older women, is another factor.

Traditionally, the expected incidence was calculated using Hellin's rule. Using this rule, twins were expected in 1 in 80 pregnancies, triplets in 1 in 80^2 and so on. Based upon the number of births in the UK in 2007, 9555 twins would have been predicted. In fact, 11 573 were delivered, 21 per cent higher than expected. The figures for triplets are similar; 119 sets may have been expected but in actuality 149 were delivered. Now seen in just over 1 in 5000 UK pregnancies, this represents a 25 per cent excess over expected; however, these figures for triplets have actually fallen dramatically since the late 1990s. At that time, the Human Fertilisation and Embryology Authority placed restrictions on fertility centres, limiting the number of embryos that could be routinely transferred per cycle. More recently, they have promoted single embryo transfers for the majority of patients, hoping to cap or even reduce the incidence of iatrogenic twinning.

In contrast, there is scant regulation of fertility services in the USA. Figures from 2006 suggest an incidence of twin births 31 per cent above expected with triplets increased by a remarkable 211 per cent (although this had fallen slightly compared to the previous year). Even more staggering is the 355 quadruplet pregnancies seen in the USA, compared to seven in the UK the same year.

Classification

The classification of multiple pregnancy is based on:

- number of fetuses: twins, triplets, quadruplets, etc.
- number of fertilized eggs: zygosity
- number of placentae: chorionicity
- number of amniotic cavities: amnionicity.

Non-identical or fraternal twins are dizygotic, having resulted from the fertilization of two separate eggs. Although they always have two functionally separate placentae (dichorionic), the placentae can become anatomically fused together and appear to the naked eye as a single placental mass. They always have separate amniotic cavities (diamniotic) and the two cavities are separated by a thick three-layer membrane (fused amnion in the middle with chorion on either side). The fetuses can be either same-sex or different-sex pairings.

Identical twins are monozygotic – they arise from fertilization of a single egg and are always same-sex pairings. They may share a single placenta (monochorionic) or have one each (dichorionic). If dichorionic, the placentae can become anatomically fused together and appear to the naked eye as a single placental mass, as mentioned above. The vast majority of monochorionic twins have two amniotic cavities (diamniotic) but the dividing membrane is thin, as it consists of a single layer of amnion alone. Monochorionic twins may occasionally share a single sac (monoamniotic). Figure 9.1 shows the relative contributions of the different types of twins to a hypothetical random selection of 1000 twin pairs.

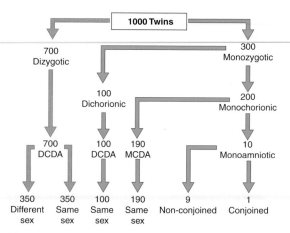

Figure 9.1 Incidence of monozygotic and dizygotic twin pregnancies. (DCDA, dichorionic diamniotic; MCDA, monochorionic diamniotic; MCMA, monochorionic monoamniotic.)

Key points

- Not all dichorionic pregnancies are dizygotic.
- All monochorionic pregnancies are monozygotic.

Aetiology

Dizygotic twins may arise spontaneously from the release of two eggs at ovulation. This tendency to release more than one egg can be familial or racial in origin and increases with maternal age. Ovulation induction treatments may also cause the release of more than one egg. With assisted conception techniques such as IVF, two or more embryos fertilized in the laboratory may be replaced in the uterus, although single embryo transfer is becoming more frequent.

Monozygotic twins arise from a single fertilized ovum that splits into two identical structures. The type of monozygotic twin depends on how long after conception the split occurs. When the split occurs within 3 days of conception, two placentae and two amniotic cavities result, giving rise to a dichorionic diamniotic (DCDA) pregnancy. When splitting occurs between days 4 and 8, only the chorion has differentiated and a monochorionic diamniotic (MCDA) pregnancy results. Later splitting after the amnion has differentiated leads to both twins developing in a single amniotic cavity, a monochorionic monoamniotic (MCMA) pregnancy. If splitting is delayed beyond day 12, the embryonic disc has also formed, and conjoined, or 'Siamese' twins will result.

The incidence of monozygotic or identical twins is generally accepted to be constant at 1 in 250. It is not influenced by race, family history or parity. There is some evidence of a small increase in monozygotic twinning after IVF, for reasons that are unclear.

Other physiology

Maternal

All the physiological changes of pregnancy (increased cardiac output, volume expansion, relative haemodilution, diaphragmatic splinting, weight gain, lordosis, etc.) are exaggerated in multiple gestations. This results in much greater stresses being placed on maternal reserves. The 'minor' symptoms of pregnancy may be exaggerated; however, for women with pre-existing health problems, such as cardiac disease, a multiple pregnancy may substantially increase their risk of morbidity.

Fetal

Monochorionic placentae have the unique ability to develop vascular connections between the two fetal circulations. These anastomoses carry the potential for complications, discussed in the next section.

Complications relevant to twin pregnancy

Miscarriage and severe preterm delivery

General

Spontaneous preterm delivery is an ever-present risk in any twin pregnancy (Figure 9.2) where the average gestation at delivery is 37 weeks. Therefore, about half of all twins deliver preterm. With two or more babies resulting from each delivery, multiple gestations account for 20–25 per cent of NICU admissions. Due to their associated high mortality and/or morbidity rates, the births that attract the most interest are births below 32 weeks gestation. In singleton pregnancies,

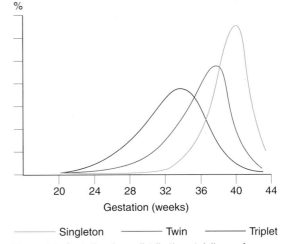

Figure 9.2 Gestational age distribution at delivery of singleton, twin and triplet pregnancies

each of these outcomes has a frequency of about 1 per cent.

Dichorionic/monochorionic differences

In a dichorionic pregnancy, the chance of late miscarriage is 2 per cent. In 15 per cent of cases, delivery will be very preterm. For monochorionic twins, the chance of early birth is increased even further, with 12 per cent born before viability and 25 per cent delivering between 24 and 32 weeks (Table 9.1).

Perinatal mortality in twins

General

The overall infant mortality rate for twins is around 5.5 times higher than for singletons. The biggest contributor to this high rate is complications related to preterm birth. Data from the UK suggest that the survival at any given gestation is identical for singletons and multiples.

Dichorionic/monochorionic differences

UK birth registration data for 2007 show at least one twin is stillborn in 20 per 1000 twin maternities. This is in contrast to a figure of 5 per 1000 singleton births. However, the rate for different-sex pairs (who must be dichorionic) is 12 per 1000, while that for same-sex pairs (roughly one-third of whom will be monochorionic) is 23 per 1000. As two-thirds of these same-sex pairs are dichorionic (and should have a stillbirth rate of 12 per 1000), the true stillbirth rate for monochorionic pairs must be substantially higher.

Table 9.1 Common pregnancy complications in twin pregnancies according to chorionicity, compared with singleton pregnancies

Complication		Twins	
	Singleton (%)	Dichorionic (%)	Monochorionic (%)
Miscarriage at 12–23 weeks	1	2	12
Delivery at 24–32 weeks		15	25
Small for gestation	10	25	50
Fetal defects	1	2	4

Some of this increase in perinatal mortality will be due to the excess of preterm delivery in monochorionic twins, but monozygotic twins also have both additional risks and unique complications that further increase their chance of death and handicap, as discussed below.

Death of one fetus in a twin pregnancy

General

With the more liberal use of early pregnancy scanning, it has been recognized that up to 25 per cent of twins may suffer an early demise and subsequently 'vanish' well before they would have previously been detected. After the first trimester, the intrauterine death of one fetus in a twin pregnancy may be associated with a poor outcome for the remaining co-twin. Maternal complications such as disseminated intravascular coagulation have been reported, but the incidence of this appears to be very low.

Dichorionic/monochorionic differences

In dichorionic twins, the second or third trimester intrauterine death of one fetus may be associated with the onset of labour, although in some cases the pregnancy may continue uneventfully and even result in delivery at term. Careful fetal and maternal monitoring is required. By contrast, fetal death of one twin in monochorionic twins may result in immediate complications in the survivor. These include death or brain damage with subsequent neurodevelopmental handicap. Acute hypotensive episodes, secondary to placental vascular anastomoses between the two fetuses, result in haemodynamic volume shifts from the live to the dead fetus. The acute release of vasoactive substances into the survivor's circulation may also play a role. Death or handicap of the co-twin occurs in up to 30 per cent of cases.

Fetal growth restriction

General

Compared to singletons, the risk of poor growth is higher in each individual twin alone and substantially raised in the pregnancy as a whole.

When a fetus is growth restricted, the main aims of antenatal care become prediction of the severity of impaired fetal oxygenation and selecting the appropriate time for delivery. In singletons, this is a balance between the relative risks of intrauterine death versus the risk of neonatal death or handicap from elective preterm delivery. The situation is much more complicated in twin pregnancies. The potential benefit of expectant management or elective delivery for the small fetus must also be weighed against the risk of the same policy for the normally grown co-twin.

Dichorionic/monochorionic differences

In a dichorionic pregnancy, each fetus runs twice the risk of a low birth weight and there is a 25 per cent chance that at least one of the fetuses will be small for gestational age. The chance of suboptimal fetal growth for monochorionic twins is almost double that for dichorionic twins (see Table 9.1).

In dichorionic twin pregnancies where one fetus has fetal growth restriction (FGR), elective preterm delivery may lead to iatrogenic complications of prematurity in the previously healthy co-twin. In general, delivery should be avoided before 28–30 weeks gestation, even if there is evidence of imminent intrauterine death of the smaller twin; however, this may not be applicable in the management of monochorionic twins. The death of one of a monochorionic twin pair may result in either death or handicap of the co-twin because of acute hypotension secondary to placental vascular anastomoses between the two circulations (see earlier discussion under

Death of one fetus in a twin pregnancy). As the damage potentially happens at the moment of death of the first twin, the timing of delivery may be a very difficult decision. Below 30 weeks gestation, the aim is to prolong the pregnancy as far as possible without risking the death of the growth-restricted twin.

Fetal abnormalities

General

Compared to singletons, twin pregnancies carry at least twice the risk of the birth of a baby with an anomaly. There are, however, important differences in both risk and management, based upon chorionicity.

Dichorionic/monochorionic differences

Each fetus of a dichorionic twin pregnancy has a risk of structural anomalies, such as spina bifida, that is similar to that of a singleton. Therefore, the chance of finding an anomaly within a dichorionic twin pregnancy is twice that of a singleton. In contrast, each fetus in a monochorionic twin pregnancy carries a risk for abnormalities that is four times that of a singleton. This is presumably due to a higher risk of vascular events during embryonic development (see Table 9.1).

Multiple gestations with an abnormality in one fetus can be managed expectantly or by selective fetocide of the affected twin. In cases where the abnormality is non-lethal but may well result in handicap, the parents may need to decide whether the potential burden of a handicapped child outweighs the risk of loss of the normal twin from fetocide-related complications, which occur after 5–10 per cent of procedures. In cases where the abnormality is lethal, it may be best to avoid such risk to the normal fetus, unless the condition itself threatens the survival of the normal twin. Anencephaly is a good example of a lethal abnormality that can threaten the survival of the normal twin. At least 50 per cent of pregnancies affected by anencephaly are complicated by polyhydramnios, which can lead to the spontaneous preterm delivery of both babies.

Fetocide in monochorionic pregnancies carries increased risk and requires a different technique. As there are potential vascular anastomoses between the two fetal circulations, intracardiac injections cannot be employed. Methods have evolved that employ cord occlusion techniques. These require significant instrumentation of the uterus and are therefore associated with a higher complication rate.

Chromosomal defects and twinning

General

In twins, as in singletons, the risk for chromosomal abnormalities increases with maternal age. The rate of spontaneous dizygotic twinning also increases with maternal age. Many women undergoing assisted conception techniques (which increase the chance of dizygotic twinning) are also older than the mean maternal age. Chromosomal defects may be more likely in a multiple pregnancy for various reasons, and couples should be counselled accordingly.

Dichorionic/monochorionic differences

Monozygotic twins arise from a single fertilized egg and therefore have the same genetic make up. It is clear that in monozygotic twin pregnancies, chromosomal abnormalities such as Down's syndrome affect neither fetus or both. The risk is based upon maternal age.

In dizygotic twins, the maternal age-related risk for chromosomal abnormalities for each individual twin remains the same as for a singleton pregnancy. Therefore, at a given maternal age, the chance that at least one of the twin pair is affected by a chromosomal defect is twice as high as for a singleton pregnancy. For example, a 40-year-old woman with a singleton pregnancy has a fetal risk of trisomy 21 of 1 in 100. If she has a dizygotic twin pregnancy, the risk that one fetus would be affected is 1 in 50 (1 in 100 plus 1 in 100).

Complications unique to monochorionic twinning

In all monochorionic twin pregnancies there are placental vascular anastomoses present, which allow communication between the two fetoplacental circulations. In approximately 15 per cent of monochorionic twin pregnancies, imbalance in the flow of blood across these arteriovenous communications results in twin-to-twin transfusion syndrome (TTTS). One fetus becomes overperfused and the other underperfused. The development of mild, moderate or severe TTTS depends on the degree of imbalance. The growth-restricted donor fetus suffers from hypovolaemia and becomes oliguric. As fetal urine is the major component of amniotic fluid, this fetus develops oligohydramnios. The recipient fetus becomes hypervolaemic, leading to polyuria and polyhydramnios. There is also a risk of myocardial damage and high output cardiac failure. Severe disease may become apparent in the second trimester. The mother often complains of a sudden increase in abdominal girth associated with extreme discomfort. Clinical examination shows tense polyhydramnios and ultrasound confirms the diagnosis.

More than 90 per cent of pregnancies complicated by TTTS end in miscarriage or very preterm delivery. With treatment, one or both babies survive in about 70 per cent of pregnancies.

The long-standing method of treatment has been amniocentesis every 1–2 weeks with the drainage of large volumes of amniotic fluid. Exactly how this treatment improves the underlying pathophysiology is uncertain, but it appears to prolong the pregnancy and improve survival. More recently, a small number of centres have used fetoscopically guided laser coagulation to disrupt the placental blood vessels that connect the circulations of the two fetuses. Initial randomized studies suggest that laser therapy is associated with delivery at later gestational ages, higher survival rates and lower levels of handicap at six months of age. It remains, however, a highly specialized procedure with limited availability.

Complications unique to monoamniotic twinning

Monoamniotic twins share a single amniotic cavity, with no dividing membrane between the two fetuses. They are at increased risk of cord accidents, predominantly through their almost universal cord entanglement. Many clinicians advocate elective delivery by Caesarean section at 32–34 weeks gestation, as this complication is usually acute, fatal and unpredictable.

Differential diagnosis

The differential diagnosis of a multiple gestation includes all the other causes of a 'large for dates' uterus: polyhydramnios, uterine fibroids, urinary retention and ovarian masses.

Antenatal management

Routine antenatal care for all women involves screening for hypertension and gestational diabetes. These conditions occur more frequently in twin pregnancies and there is also a higher risk of other problems (such as antepartum haemorrhage and thromboembolic disease); however, the management is the same as for a singleton. Due to the increased fetoplacental demand for iron and folic acid, many would recommend routine (as opposed to selective) supplementation in multiple pregnancies. Minor symptoms of pregnancy are more common, but management is again unchanged compared to singletons.

Elements of antenatal care that have specific importance in multiple pregnancies include the following.

Determination of chorionicity

As described, there are important differences in risk and outcome between dichorionic and monochorionic pregnancies. Therefore, determination of chorionicity is critical to 'good' management, and this is done most reliably by ultrasound in the late first trimester. In dichorionic twins, there is a V-shaped extension of placental tissue into the base of the inter-twin membrane, referred to as the 'lambda' or 'twin-peak' sign. In monochorionic twins, this sign is absent and the inter-twin membrane joins the uterine wall in a T shape (Figure 9.3).

Assessment of chorionicity later in pregnancy is less reliable and relies upon the assessment of fetal gender, number of placentae and characteristics of the membrane between the two amniotic sacs. The 'lambda' sign becomes less accurate, and membrane thickness must be utilized. Different-sex twins must be dizygotic and therefore dichorionic. In same-sex twins, two separate placentae mean dichorionic, although the babies may still be monozygotic. However, monozygotic dichorionic twins do not carry the additional risks of vascular anastomoses.

Screening for fetal abnormalities

Screening for trisomy 21 using maternal serum biochemistry has been described in twin pregnancies but has not come into widespread use, in part due to its lower sensitivity. Normal ranges for serum alpha-fetoprotein have been established and allow detection of increased risk for neural tube defects. The measurement of nuchal translucency at 12 weeks gestation allows each fetus to have an individualized

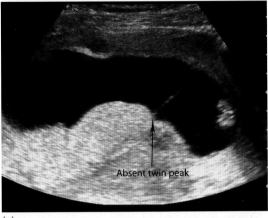

(a)

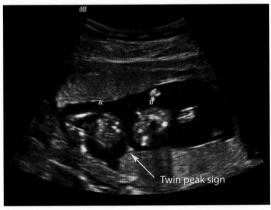

(b)

Figure 9.3 Ultrasound appearance of monochorionic (a) and dichorionic (b) twin pregnancies at 12 weeks gestation. Note that in both types there appears to be a single placental mass, but in the dichorionic type there is an extension of placental tissue into the base of the inter-twin membrane forming the lambda sign

assessment of risk. The NHS Fetal Anomaly Screening Programme has recommended it as the screening test of choice for multiple pregnancies. If prenatal diagnosis is required (see Chapter 7, Prenatal diagnosis), knowledge of chorionicity is essential. Monochorionic twins are monozygotic and therefore only one sample is needed for karyotyping.

Both amniocentesis and chorion villus sampling (CVS) can be performed in twin pregnancies, but in dichorionic pregnancies, it is essential that both fetuses are sampled. As the placentae are often fused together, CVS has special challenges. With amniocentesis, dye-injection techniques have previously been used to prevent sampling the same sac twice; however, to avoid this, many practitioners now rely on direct puncture of the inter-twin membrane.

Screening for fetal structural anomalies is done using second trimester ultrasound, with optimal detection rates seen at 20 weeks gestation. More time must be allowed for each appointment. As monochorionic twins have a significantly increased risk of fetal anomalies, many argue that they should be screened within specialized fetal medicine units.

Monitoring fetal growth and well-being

Measurement of symphysis–fundal height and maternal reporting of fetal movements are unreliable, as the individual contribution of each twin cannot be assessed. Monitoring for fetal growth and well-being in twins is principally by ultrasound. Each assessment should include fetal measurements, fetal activity, fetal lies and amniotic fluid volumes. In monochorionic twins, features of TTTS should be sought, including discordances between fetal size, fetal activity, bladder volumes, amniotic fluid volumes and cardiac size. In any twin pregnancy, when one or both fetuses are small, additional information about fetal well-being can be obtained from Doppler assessment of the fetal circulations and cardiotocography (CTG). Specialized twin monitors should be used to ensure each twin's heart rate is sampled.

It is reasonable to plan 4- to 6-weekly ultrasound scans in uncomplicated dichorionic twins. However, due to their higher background risk, fortnightly ultrasound is appropriate in monochorionic pregnancies. These are approximate guidelines that should be modified around individual pregnancy circumstances.

Threatened preterm labour

As in singleton pregnancies, neither bed rest nor prophylactic administration of tocolytics is useful in preventing preterm delivery. Despite this, screening for preterm birth may be worthwhile. Antenatal strategies in those identified as at high risk may include maternal steroid therapy to enhance fetal lung maturation, supplementary education as to the signs and symptoms of preterm labour, advance planning regarding intrapartum care, screening for group B streptococcus (GBS) (intrapartum antibiotics reduce neonatal infection) and additional medical and midwifery support.

At present, transvaginal cervical ultrasound shows the most promise as a predictor of very preterm delivery (see Chapter 11, Late miscarriage and early birth). As regular ultrasound examination is already part of the care of multiple pregnancy, there is little impact on health-care resources. Once preterm labour is diagnosed, neonatal unit staff must be promptly involved. The use of tocolytic drugs in this situation, particularly the beta-agonists, carries risks of serious maternal morbidity.

Multiple pregnancy support groups

Twin pregnancies are associated with a number of financial, personal and social costs for families, that continue long beyond the neonatal period. A significant contribution to these costs comes from the increased incidence of handicap, largely secondary to preterm delivery. Several specialized support groups for multiple pregnancy exist. In the UK, these include the Twins and Multiple Birth Association (TAMBA) and the Multiple Birth Foundation. All parents expecting twins should be given contact details for such resources locally.

Intrapartum management

Complications in labour are more common with twin gestations. These include premature birth, abnormal presentations, prolapsed cord, premature separation of the placenta and postpartum haemorrhage. Judiciously managed, labour is generally considered to be safe. It may require considerable expertise and is the only situation in which internal podalic version is still practised in obstetrics.

Preparation

This should begin long before labour, with antenatal education and an intrapartum care plan. A twin CTG machine should be used for fetal monitoring and a portable ultrasound machine should be available during the delivery. A standard oxytocin solution for augmentation should be prepared, run through an intravenous giving-set and clearly labelled 'for augmentation', for use for delivery of the second twin, if required. A second high-dose oxytocin infusion should also be available for the management of postpartum haemorrhage. However, it is advisable to keep this separate, not run through a giving-set until needed and clearly labelled 'for postpartum use only'. It is essential that two neonatal resuscitation trolleys, two obstetricians and two paediatricians are available and that the special care baby unit and anaesthetist are informed well in advance of the delivery.

Analgesia during labour

Epidural analgesia is recommended. Indeed, if the presentation of twins is anything other than vertex–vertex, the use of an epidural can be justified in terms of analgesia for possible intrauterine manipulations required in the second stage for delivery of the second twin. Contrary to recommendations for the management of a singleton labour, the epidural should be kept running throughout the second stage, as it is most likely to be required after the delivery of the first twin. Having an anaesthetist present and ready to administer anaesthesia if complications arise is a satisfactory alternative. However, many obstetric units now opt to deliver twins in the operating theatre.

Fetal well-being in labour

Fetal heart rate monitoring should be continuous throughout labour, ideally using a specialized twin monitor. An abnormal fetal heart rate pattern in the first twin may be assessed using fetal scalp sampling, as for a singleton pregnancy. However, a non-reassuring pattern in the second twin will usually necessitate delivery by Caesarean section. The condition of the second twin must be carefully monitored after the delivery of the first twin, as acute complications such as cord prolapse and placental separation are well recognized.

Vaginal delivery of vertex–vertex

Although this combination is considered low risk, an obstetrician should be present, as complications with delivery of the second twin can occur. Delivery of the first twin is undertaken in the usual manner and thereafter the majority of second twins will be delivered within 15 minutes. However, there is no urgency to deliver the second twin within a set time period, providing both mother and baby remain well.

After the delivery of the first twin, abdominal palpation should be performed to assess the lie of the second twin. It is helpful to use ultrasound for confirmation, which is also useful for checking the fetal heart rate. If the lie is longitudinal with a cephalic presentation, one should wait until the head is descending and then perform amniotomy with a contraction. If contractions do not ensue within 5–10 minutes after delivery of the first twin, an oxytocin infusion should be started. The indications for instrumental delivery of the second twin are as for singletons (see Chapter 15, Operative intervention in obstetrics).

Delivery of vertex–non-vertex

If the second twin is non-vertex, which occurs in about 40 per cent of twins, numerous studies have shown that vaginal delivery can be safely considered.

If the second twin is a breech, the membranes can be ruptured once the breech is fixed in the birth canal. A total breech extraction may be performed if fetal distress occurs or if a footling breech is encountered, but this requires considerable expertise. Complications are less likely if the membranes are not ruptured until the feet are held by the operator. Where the fetus is transverse, external cephalic version can be successful in more than 70 per cent of cases. The fetal heart rate should be closely monitored, and ultrasound can be helpful to demonstrate the final position of the baby. If external cephalic version is unsuccessful, and assuming that the operator is experienced, an internal podalic version can be undertaken (Figure 9.4).

A fetal foot is identified by recognizing a heel through intact membranes. The foot is grasped and pulled gently and continuously into the birth canal. The membranes are ruptured as late as possible. This procedure is easiest when the transverse lie is with the back superior or posterior. If the back is inferior or if the limbs are not immediately palpable, ultrasound may help to show the operator where they would be found. This will minimize the unwanted experience of bringing down a fetal hand in the mistaken belief that it is a foot.

Non-vertex first twin

When the first twin presents as a breech, clinicians usually recommend delivery by elective Caesarean section. This is largely because of the increased risks associated with singleton breech vaginal delivery. Other factors include dwindling experience of breech delivery and the rarely seen phenomenon of 'locked twins'.

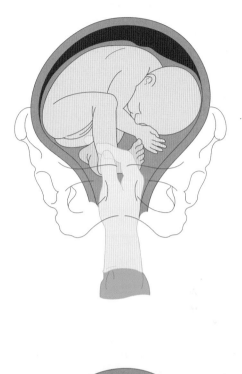

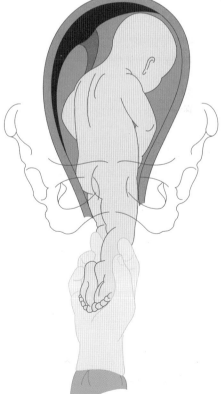

Figure 9.4 Internal podalic version

In this latter case, the chin of the first (breech) baby locks against the chin of the second (cephalic) twin.

Preterm twins

Even in low birth weight twin gestations, the method of delivery in relation to fetal presentation will have little or no effect on neonatal mortality and subsequent neonatal developmental outcome. No significant differences in perinatal outcome exist when comparing breech-extracted second twins to those delivered by Caesarean section.

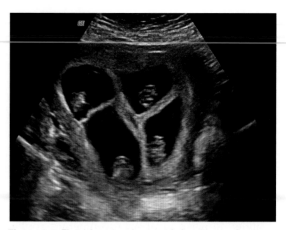

Figure 9.5 First trimester ultrasound showing quadruplet pregnancy

Requirements for twin delivery

- Large delivery room
- Operating theatre and staff ready
- Anaesthetist present
- Senior obstetrician present
- At least two midwives present
- Twin resuscitaires
- Ventouse/forceps to hand
- Blood grouped and saved
- Intravenous access
- Neonatologists present
- Pre-mixed oxytocin infusion ready

Postpartum haemorrhage

The risk of postpartum haemorrhage is increased in twin pregnancies due to the larger placental site and uterine over-distension. For that reason, all multiple gestations should have an intravenous line and blood grouped and saved during labour.

Management is generally no different from that of postpartum haemorrhage complicating singleton delivery (see Chapter 16, Obstetric emergencies). However, ideally, the third stage should be actively managed and a high-dose oxytocin infusion commenced following delivery as prophylaxis.

Higher multiples

A consequence of the widespread introduction of assisted reproductive techniques has been an exponential increase in the incidence of higher multiple gestations (Figure 9.5), mostly triplets. At least 75 per cent of triplet pregnancies are secondary to assisted conception. They are associated with increased risks of miscarriage, perinatal death and handicap. The median gestational age at birth is 33 weeks and long-term complications are primarily a consequence of extremely preterm delivery. Although the demands on maternal physiology are greater still, antenatal care is essentially no different from that for a twin gestation. Caesarean section is usually advocated for delivery due to the difficulties of intrapartum fetal monitoring; however, the evidence to support this strategy is weak, and several case series of vaginal birth have reported comparable neonatal outcomes.

In an attempt to reduce the morbidity and mortality associated with extremely preterm delivery, the procedure of multi-fetal reduction was introduced. Iatrogenic fetal death is achieved by the ultrasound-guided puncture of the fetal heart and injection of potassium chloride. Although it is technically feasible to perform reduction from as early as 7 weeks gestation, it is usually delayed until around 11–12 weeks. This allows for spontaneous reduction to occur and for the screening and diagnosis of major fetal abnormalities and chromosomal defects. Following reduction, there is gradual resorption of the dead fetuses and their placentae.

A triplet pregnancy managed expectantly has a 4 per cent chance of loss prior to 24 weeks and a

25 per cent risk of extremely preterm delivery between 24 and 32 weeks. After multi-fetal reduction, usually to twins, the risk of loss before viability is increased to 8 per cent. However, the chance of a very preterm birth drops to 10 per cent. The risks of subsequent miscarriage and extremely preterm delivery have been found to increase with the number of fetuses reduced.

CASE HISTORY

Miss C is a 19-year-old woman who is single. She is unemployed. She has no active medical problems. She was discovered to have a twin pregnancy at 12 weeks gestation, after presenting to the A&E deptartment with an episode of bleeding. The pregnancy was classified as DCDA. She had no further prenatal care until she presented to the Maternity Unit with reduced fetal movements at 28 weeks.

An ultrasound was organized and showed one fetus (twin A) to be growth restricted (with an estimated weight on the fifth centile) and have oligohydramnios. The other fetus was on the 40th centile.

Could this be TTTS?

One-third of monozygotic twins will be dichorionic. However, it is the monochorionic placentation that carries a risk of unbalanced vascular anastamoses between the two fetuses. Therefore, TTTS is unlikely.

What other useful information should you seek from this ultrasound?

Miss C must have missed her review of fetal anatomy at 19–20 weeks. As anomalies can be associated with intrauterine growth restriction (IUGR), a careful anatomy review should be performed. Doppler studies of the fetal circulation may also aid in diagnosis, with increased resistance in the umbilical arteries and a 'brain-sparing' effect in the fetal circulation seen in true IUGR. As the patient presented with reduced fetal movement, some assessment of individual fetal activity could be undertaken, such as a biophysical profile.

If fetal activity was not assessed during the ultrasound, which test is indicated?

A CTG should be performed. Although there may be only slight differences in the heart rate patterns of the two fetuses, a special twin monitor allows them to be clearly identified.

Although the umbilical Doppler for twin A is abnormal, the CTG is reactive with accelerations. Should delivery be organized?

Delivery would subject the healthy and well-grown twin B to the risks of iatrogenic prematurity. The risk of death or serious morbidity to twin A by remaining in utero has to be balanced against this.

With a normal CTG and no evidence of acute compromise, delivery would not be appropriate at this time.

What other antenatal measures should be taken?

Close follow-up of fetal well-being should be organized, at least on a weekly basis. Steroids should be considered for fetal lung maturity, as early delivery is a possibility. All the routine antenatal tests should now be organized, as Miss C has missed a large component of her prenatal care. Miss C may be at risk for anaemia. Social work involvement may be appropriate, to discover the underlying factors behind her failure to obtain antenatal care.

New developments

- Transvaginal ultrasound measurement of cervical length at 20–24 weeks may be used to assess the risk of very preterm delivery.
- The interrelated phenomena of delayed childbearing and increased use of assisted conception techniques have dramatically increased the incidence of multiple pregnancy.
- The optimal way to screen for Down's syndrome in multiple pregnancy is by nuchal translucency at 12 weeks gestation. Chorionicity can also be reliably determined at this time.
- Multi-fetal reduction is increasingly accepted as improving overall outcomes in higher multiples.

Key points

- Twins account for about 1.5 per cent of pregnancies but up to 25 per cent of special care baby unit admissions.
- Perinatal mortality rate in twins is nearly six times higher than in singletons, primarily due to spontaneous preterm births.
- Both serious maternal complications and minor discomforts are increased in multiple gestation.
- The determination of chorionicity is very important – the highest risks are seen in monochorionic twins.

CHAPTER 10

PRE-ECLAMPSIA AND OTHER DISORDERS OF PLACENTATION

Louise C Kenny

OVERVIEW

Pre-eclampsia is a leading cause of maternal death. The World Health Organization estimates that globally between 50 000 and 75 000 women die of this condition each year. Furthermore, pre-eclampsia is frequently accompanied by fetal growth restriction (FGR), which is responsible for considerable perinatal morbidity and mortality. Although fetal growth is controlled by a number of factors including genetic predisposition and maternal nutritional status, it is now apparent that the origins of both pre-eclampsia and much of FGR seen in clinical practice lie in defective placentation. A further condition frequently related to impaired placentation is abruptio placentae or placental abruption. This is the premature separation of a normally sited placenta, which is usually of sudden onset and associated with a high fetal mortality and substantial maternal morbidity and mortality. Knowledge of the early events in the invasion of the maternal uterine wall by placental trophoblast cells is therefore helpful in understanding the aetiology of these important clinical conditions.

The placenta

The placenta is a fetomaternal organ. The functional unit of the placenta is the fetal cotyledon. The mature human placenta has about 120 fetal cotyledons grouped into visible lobes (frequently and somewhat confusingly termed 'maternal cotyledons'). Each cotyledon contains a primary villus stem arising from the chorionic plate and supplied by primary branches of fetal vessels. The primary stems divide to form secondary and tertiary stems from which arise the terminal villi, where maternal–fetal exchange takes place. The fetal cotyledons appear to develop around the entries of the maternal spiral arteries from the decidual plate. The centre of each cotyledon is hollow and during maternal systole, blood spurts from the spiral arteries and enters the intercotyledon space. Blood rises high to the chorionic plate then disperses laterally between and over the surface of the terminal villi, becoming increasingly desaturated of oxygen and nutrients and picking up carbon dioxide and waste products. The blood then filters into narrow venous channels between the cotyledons, before falling back to the maternal decidual plate, where the maternal veins return the desaturated blood to the maternal circulation (Figure 10.1). Maternal and fetal blood is separated by three microscopic tissue layers: trophoblastic tissue, connective tissue and the endothelium of the fetal capillaries. However, microscopic examination of the terminal villi surrounding the intracotyledon space shows numerous vasculosyncytial membranes where the fetal capillaries and trophoblast fuse to form a very thin membrane, where most of the transfer of nutrients and blood gases takes place.

Normal placentation

The maternal blood flow to the placenta increases throughout pregnancy from 50 mL/min in the first trimester to 500–750 mL/min at terms. This increase in perfusion is accomplished by anatomical conversion of the maternal spiral arteries by trophoblast. Trophoblast cells invade the spiral arterioles within the first 12 weeks of pregnancy and replace the smooth muscle of the wall of the vessels, thus converting them to wide bore, low resistance, large capacitance vessels (Figure 10.2). This process is normally complete by 20 weeks gestation.

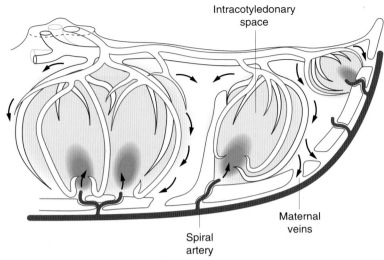

Figure 10.1 Anatomy and distribution of blood flow through the intracotyledonary space

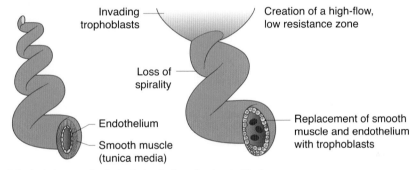

Figure 10.2 Physiological change of spiral arteries by invading trophoblast

Abnormal placentation

In pregnancies destined to be complicated by pre-eclampsia, FGR and/or abruptio placentae, there is a complete or partial failure of trophoblast invasion of the myometrial segments of the spiral arteries. Hence, spiral arteries retain some of their pre-pregnancy characteristics being relatively narrow bore and of low capacitance and high resistance and resulting in impaired perfusion of the fetoplacental unit. The mechanism underlying decreased trophoblast invasion in complicated pregnancies is poorly understood but it may reflect an 'immune intolerance' of the mother to the invading trophoblast. Affected placentae have gross morphological changes, which include infarcts and basal haematomas. An infarct represents an area of ischaemic necrosis of a cotyledon resulting from a spiral artery occlusion, usually by thrombosis. A placenta

with multiple infarcts is significantly associated with intrauterine fetal death and growth restriction. Basal haematomas consist of a mass of blood in the centre of the fetal cotyledon due to the rupture of a damaged spiral artery. This lesion is associated with maternal hypertension and increased perinatal mortality.

Pre-eclampsia

Definition

In the past, the definition of pre-eclampsia has been inconsistent and this has led to difficulty in comparing studies on treatments or outcomes. There is now a widely accepted classification system of hypertensive disorders in pregnancy (see Chapter 12, Medical diseases complicating pregnancy), which defines *pre-eclampsia* as hypertension of at least 140/90 mmHg recorded on at least two separate occasions and at least 4 hours apart and in the presence of at least 300 mg protein in a 24 hour collection of urine, arising *de novo* after the 20th week of pregnancy in a previously normotensive woman and resolving completely by the sixth postpartum week.

Chronic hypertension (with or without renal disease) existing prior to pregnancy can predispose to the later development of superimposed pre-eclampsia. Even in the absence of superimposed pre-eclampsia, chronic hypertension is associated with increased maternal and fetal morbidity (see Chapter 12, Medical diseases complicating pregnancy) and pregnancies complicated by chronic hypertension should therefore be regarded as high risk.

Non-proteinuric gestational hypertension, i.e. hypertension arising for the first time in the second half of pregnancy and in the absence of proteinuria, is not associated with adverse pregnancy outcome. Every effort therefore should be made to clearly distinguish it from pre-eclampsia.

Incidence

Pre-eclampsia complicates approximately 2–3 per cent of pregnancies, but the incidence varies depending on the exact definition used and the population studied. In the most recent Confidential Enquiry (2003–2005), there were 18 deaths due to pre-eclampsia, making this the second most common cause of direct death in pregnancy and the puerperium in the UK.

Epidemiology

Pre-eclampsia is more common in primigravid women. It is thought that the normal fetal–maternal transfusion that occurs during pregnancy and particularly during delivery exposes the mother to products of the fetal (and hence paternal) genome, protecting her in subsequent pregnancies. In line with this, the protective effect of first pregnancy seems to be lost if a woman has a child with a new partner. Overall the recurrence risk in a subsequent pregnancy is 20 per cent, but is much higher if severe pre-eclampsia developed at an extremely early gestation in the first pregnancy. There also appears to be a maternal genetic predisposition to pre-eclampsia as there is a three- to four-fold increase in the incidence of pre-eclampsia in the first degree relatives of affected women. Finally,

there are a number of general medical conditions and pregnancy-specific factors that predispose to the development of pre-eclampsia.

Risk factors for pre-eclampsia

- First pregnancy
- Multiparous with:
  - pre-eclampsia in any previous pregnancy
  - ten years or more since last baby
- Age 40 years or more
- Body mass index of 35 or more
- Family history of pre-eclampsia (in mother or sister)
- Booking diastolic blood pressure of 80 mmHg or more
- Booking proteinuria (of ≥1+ on more than one occasion or quantified at ≥0.3 g/24 hour)
- Multiple pregnancy
- Certain underlying medical conditions:
  - pre-existing hypertension
  - pre-existing renal disease
  - pre-existing diabetes
  - antiphospholipid antibodies

Aetiology and pathophysiology

Pre-eclampsia only occurs in pregnancy, but has been described in pregnancies lacking a fetus (molar pregnancies) and in the absence of a uterus (abdominal pregnancies) (see Chapter 9, Problems in early pregnancy, in *Gynaecology by Ten Teachers*, 19th edn), suggesting that it is the presence of trophoblast tissue that provides the stimulus for the disorder. Placental bed biopsies have demonstrated that trophoblast invasion is patchy in pre-eclampsia and the spiral arteries retain their muscular walls. This is thought to prevent the development of a high flow, low impedance uteroplacental circulation. The reason why trophoblast invades less effectively in these pregnancies is not known but may reflect an abnormal adaptation of the maternal immune system.

It is widely believed that defective trophoblast invasion results in relative under-perfusion of the placenta and that this releases a factor(s) into the maternal circulation that targets the vascular endothelium (Figure 10.3). The nature of this factor

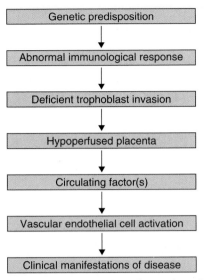

Genetic predisposition

↓

Abnormal immunological response

↓

Deficient trophoblast invasion

↓

Hypoperfused placenta

↓

Circulating factor(s)

↓

Vascular endothelial cell activation

↓

Clinical manifestations of disease

Figure 10.3 The proposed aetiology of pre-eclampsia

has not been identified, although numerous candidates have been proposed including a variety of growth factors, cytokines and products of oxidative stress caused by hypoxic-reperfusion injury in the placenta.

As the target cell of the disease process, the vascular endothelial cell, is so ubiquitous, pre-eclampsia is a truly multisystem disease, affecting multiple organ systems, often concurrently.

Cardiovascular system

Normal pregnancy is characterized by marked peripheral vasodilatation resulting in a fall in total peripheral resistance despite an increase in plasma volume and cardiac rate. Pre-eclampsia is characterized by marked peripheral vasoconstriction, resulting in hypertension. The intravascular high pressure and loss of endothelial cell integrity results in greater vascular permeability and contributes to the formation of generalized oedema.

Renal system

In the kidney, a highly characteristic lesion called 'glomeruloendotheliosis' is seen. This is relatively specific for pre-eclampsia (it is not seen with other hypertensive disorders) and is associated with impaired glomerular filtration and selective loss of intermediate weight proteins, such as albumin and transferrin, leading to proteinuria. This, in turn, causes a reduction in plasma oncotic pressure and exacerbates the development of oedema.

Haematological system

In the event of endothelial damage, platelets adhere to the damaged area. Furthermore, diffuse vascular damage is associated with the laying down of fibrin. Pre-eclampsia in association with increased fibrin deposition and a reduction in the platelet count may accompany and occasionally predate the onset of disease.

The liver

In the liver, subendothelial fibrin deposition is associated with elevation of liver enzymes. This can be associated with haemolysis and a low platelet count due to platelet consumption (and subsequent widespread activation of the coagulation system). The presence of these findings is called HELLP syndrome (haemolysis, elevation of liver enzymes and low platelets). HELLP syndrome is a particularly severe form of pre-eclampsia, occurring in just 2–4 per cent of women with the disease. It is associated with a high fetal loss rate (of up to 60 per cent). The management of HELLP syndrome is discussed further in Chapter 16, Obstetric emergencies.

Neurological system

The development of convulsions in a woman with pre-eclampsia is defined as eclampsia. Vasospasm and cerebral oedema have both been implicated in the pathogenesis of eclampsia. Retinal haemorrhages, exudates and papilloedema are characteristic of hypertensive encephalopathy and are rare in pre-eclampsia, suggesting that hypertension alone is not responsible for the cerebral pathology.

Clinical presentation

The classic symptoms of pre-eclampsia include a frontal headache, visual disturbance and epigastric pain. However, the majority of women with pre-eclampsia are asymptomatic or merely complain of general, vague 'flu-like' symptoms.

Clinical examination should include a complete obstetric and neurological examination. Hypertension is usually the first sign, but occasionally is absent or transient until the late stages of the disease. Dependent oedema of the feet is very common in healthy pregnant women. However, rapidly progressive oedema of the face and hands may suggest pre-eclampsia. Epigastric tenderness is a worrying sign and suggests liver involvement. Neurological examination may reveal hyperreflexia and clonus in severe cases. Urine testing for protein should be considered part of the clinical examination.

Testing for proteinuria

Dipstick urinalysis
- Instant result but quantitatively inaccurate
- Results: trace: seldom significant; 1+: possible significant proteinuria, warrants quantifying; ≥2+: probable significant proteinuria, warrants quantifying

Protein:creatinine ratio
- Fast (within an hour)
- Results semi-quantitative: >30 mg/mol – probable significant proteinuria

24 hour collection
- Slow
- Results: >0.3 g/24 hour represents confirmed significant proteinuria

---

Management and treatment

There is no cure for pre-eclampsia other than to end the pregnancy by delivering the baby (and placenta). This can be a significant problem if pre-eclampsia occurs early in pregnancy, particularly at gestations below 34 weeks. Therefore, management strategies are aimed at minimizing risk to the mother in order to permit continued fetal growth. In severe cases, this is often not possible.

The principles of management of pre-eclampsia are:

- early recognition of the symptomless syndrome;
- awareness of the serious nature of the condition in its severest form;
- adherence to agreed guidelines for admission to hospital, investigation and the use of antihypertensive and anticonvulsant therapy;
- well-timed delivery to pre-empt serious maternal or fetal complications;
- post-natal follow up and counselling for future pregnancies.

A diagnosis of pre-eclampsia usually requires admission. Patients with mild hypertension, minimal protein and normal haematological and biochemical parameters may be monitored as outpatients but will require frequent attendance for fetal and maternal assessment. Women with moderate or severe hypertension, significant proteinuria or abnormal haematological or biochemical parameters require admission and inpatient management. Investigations indicated in the ongoing management of pre-eclampsia are listed in the following box.

Investigations for pre-eclampsia

To monitor maternal complications:
- Full blood count (with particular emphasis on falling platelet count and rising haematocrit)
- If platelet values are normal, additional clotting studies are not indicated
- Serum renal profile (including serum uric acid levels)
- Serum liver profile
- Frequent repeat proteinuria quantification is probably unhelpful once a diagnosis of pre-eclampsia has been made

To monitor fetal complications
- Ultrasound assessment of:
  - fetal size
  - amniotic fluid volume
  - maternal and fetal Dopplers
- Antenatal cardiotocography used in conjunction with ultrasound surveillance, provides a useful but by no means infallible indication of fetal well-being. A loss of baseline variability or decelerations may indicate fetal hypoxia

---

The aim of antihypertensive therapy is to lower the blood pressure and reduce the risk of maternal cerebrovascular accident without reducing uterine blood flow and compromising the fetus. There are a variety of antihypertensives used in the management of pre-eclampsia. Methyldopa is a centrally acting antihypertensive agent. It has a long established safety record in pregnancy. However, it can only be given orally, it takes upwards of 24 hours to take effect and has a range of unpleasant side effects, including sedation and depression. These properties limit its usefulness. Labetalol is an alpha-blocking and beta-blocking agent. It too has a good safety record in pregnancy and can be given orally and intravenously. Nifedipine is a calcium-channel blocker with a rapid onset of action. It can, however, cause severe headache that may mimic worsening disease.

In severe cases of fulminating disease, an intravenous infusion of hydralazine or labetalol can be titrated rapidly against changes in the blood pressure. The drug of choice for the treatment of eclampsia is magnesium sulphate. This is given intravenously and has been shown to reduce the incidence of further convulsions in women with eclampsia. Magnesium sulphate should also be used in women with severe pre-eclampsia to prevent the onset of convulsions.

In the UK, over half of all women who died of pre-eclampsia or eclampsia in the last Confidential Enquiry into Maternal and Child Health (2003–2005) died from intracranial haemorrhage. This illustrates the importance of obtaining adequate blood pressure control in women with pre-eclampsia. In women who develop serious multisystem complications, the importance of a multidisciplinary approach involving clinicians from other specialties (e.g. intensive care, haematology, nephrology) cannot be overstated.

Screening and prevention

The accurate prediction of women at risk of developing pre-eclampsia will facilitate targeting of increased antenatal surveillance while allowing women at low risk to participate in community-based antenatal care. In addition, a predictive test would in turn facilitate the development of novel therapeutic preventative interventions. Unfortunately, there is currently no screening test for pre-eclampsia. Despite intensive research in this area, no single blood biomarker has emerged that either alone or in combination with other biomarkers or clinical data possesses sufficient sensitivity and specificity to be clinically useful.

The ability of Doppler ultrasound uterine artery waveform analysis to identify women at risk of pre-eclampsia (and other adverse pregnancy outcomes) has been investigated with varying success. In pregnancies with incomplete trophoblast remodelling of the spiral arteries, a characteristic 'notch' can often be seen in the waveform pattern which frequently also demonstrates high resistance (see Chapter 6, Antenatal imaging and assessment of fetal well-being, and Figure 6.20). This screening test may have a role in the women who have already been identified as being at risk of the disease because of their medical or past obstetric history. However, it is not of value in screening low risk women.

Established preventative interventions include low-dose aspirin (typically 75 mg daily), which modestly reduces the risk of pre-eclampsia in high-risk women, and calcium supplementation may also reduce risk, but only in women with dietary intake. Despite encouraging preliminary studies, its now appears certain that vitamins C and E do not lower the risk of pre-eclampsia.

Additional points in management

Iatrogenic premature delivery of the fetus is often required in severe pre-eclampsia. If her condition allows, the mother should be transferred to a centre with adequate facilities to care for her baby and prior to 34 weeks gestation steroids should be given intramuscularly to the mother to reduce the chance of neonatal respiratory distress syndrome. Delivery before term is often by Caesarean section. Such patients are at particularly high risk for thromboembolism and should be given prophylactic subcutaneous heparin and issued with antithromboembolic stockings. In the case of spontaneous or induced labour and if clotting studies are normal, epidural anaesthesia is indicated as it helps control blood pressure. Ergometrine is avoided in the management of the third stage as it can significantly increase blood pressure.

Post-natally, blood pressure and proteinuria will resolve; however, in a minority of cases one or both persist beyond 6 weeks and this suggests the presence of underlying chronic hypertension or renal disease. Additionally, a careful search should be made post-natally for underlying medical disorders in women who present with severe pre-eclampsia before 34 weeks gestation.

Fetal growth restriction

There are a wide variety of reasons why a baby may be born small including congenital anomalies, fetal infections and chromosomal abnormalities. However, most babies that are born small are either constitutionally small (i.e. healthy, but born to small parents and fulfilling their genetic growth potential) or are small secondary to abnormal placenta function and have FGR.

FGR is a major cause of neonatal and infant morbidity and mortality. There is a significant cost associated with providing adequate facilities to look after these babies. In addition, there is an increasing body of evidence that certain adult diseases (such as diabetes and hypertension) are more common in adults who were born with FGR.

Definition and incidence

FGR is defined as a failure of a fetus to achieve its genetic growth potential. This usually results in a fetus that is small for gestational age (SGA). SGA means that the weight of the fetus is less than the tenth centile for its gestation. Other cut-off points (e.g. the third centile) can be used. The terms SGA and FGR are not synonymous. It is important to remember that most SGA fetuses are constitutionally small and are not compromised. Intrauterine growth restriction (IUGR) indicates that there is a pathological process operating to restrict the growth rate of the fetus. Consequently, some FGR fetuses may not actually be SGA, but nevertheless will have failed to fulfil their growth potential.

Aetiology

The common causes of FGR are listed in Table 10.1. They are grouped into two main categories: factors that directly affect the intrinsic growth potential of the fetus and external influences that reduce the support for fetal growth. Chromosome abnormalities, genetic syndromes and fetal infections can alter intrinsic fetal growth potential. External influences that affect fetal growth can be subdivided into maternal systemic factors and placental insufficiency.

Maternal under-nutrition is globally the major cause of FGR. Low maternal oxygen saturation, which can occur with cyanotic heart disease or at high altitude, will reduce fetal PO_2 levels and fetal metabolism. Smoking, by increasing the amount of carboxyhaemoglobin in the maternal circulation, effectively reduces the amount of oxygen available to the fetus, thus causing FGR. A wide variety of drugs other than tobacco can affect fetal growth including alcohol and cocaine, probably through multiple mechanisms affecting fetal enzyme systems, placental blood flow and maternal substrate levels.

In developed countries, the most common cause of FGR is poor placental function secondary to inadequate trophoblast invasion of the spiral arteries. This results in reduced perfusion of the intracotyledon space which in turn leads to abnormal development of the terminal villi and impaired transfer of oxygen and nutrients to the fetus. Less frequently, reduced perfusion can occur from other conditions such as maternal sickle cell disease and the antiphospholipid syndrome (see Chapter 12, Medical diseases complicating pregnancy). Multiple pregnancy usually results in a sharing of the uterine vascularity, which causes a relative reduction in the blood flow to each placenta. On the fetal side of the placental circulation, abnormalities of the umbilical cord, such as a single umbilical artery, are associated with FGR as are the intraplacental vascular connections found in monochorionic twinning.

Pathophysiology

FGR is frequently classified as symmetrical or asymmetrical. Symmetrically small fetuses are

Table 10.1 Causes of fetal growth restriction

Reduced fetal growth potential	Aneuploidies, e.g. trisomy 18
	Single gene defects, e.g. Seckel's syndrome
	Structural abnormalities, e.g. renal agenesis
	Intrauterine infections, e.g. cytomegalovirus, toxoplasmosis
Reduced fetal growth support	
Maternal factors	Under-nutrition, e.g. poverty, eating disorders
	Maternal hypoxia, e.g. living at altitude, cyanotic heart disease
	Drugs, e.g. alcohol, cigarettes, cocaine
Placental factors	Reduced uteroplacental perfusion, e.g. inadequate trophoblast invasion, sickle cell disease, multiple gestation
	Reduced fetoplacental perfusion, e.g. single umbilical artery, twin–twin transfusion syndrome

normally associated with factors that directly impair fetal growth, such as chromosomal disorders and fetal infections. Asymmetrical growth restriction is classically associated with uteroplacental insufficiency which leads to reduced oxygen transfer to the fetus and impaired excretion of carbon dioxide by the placenta. A fall in PO_2 and a rise in pCO_2 in the fetal blood induces a chemoreceptor response in the fetal carotid bodies with resulting vasodilatation in the fetal brain, myocardium and adrenal glands, and vasoconstriction in the kidneys, splanchnic vessels, limbs and subcutaneous tissues. The liver circulation is also severely reduced. Normally, 50 per cent of the well-oxygenated blood in the umbilical vein passes to the right atrium through the ductus venosus, eventually to reach the fetal brain, with the remainder going to the portal circulation in the liver. When there is fetal hypoxia, more of the well-oxygenated blood from the umbilical vein is diverted through the ductus venosus, which means that the liver receives less. The result of all these circulatory changes is an asymmetrical fetus with relative brain sparing, reduced abdominal girth and skin thickness. The vasoconstriction in the fetal kidneys results in impaired urine production and oligohydramnios. The fetal hypoxaemia also leads to severe metabolic changes in the fetus reflecting intrauterine starvation. Antenatal fetal blood sampling has shown reduced levels of nutrients such as glucose and amino acids (especially essential amino acids) and of hormones such as thyroxine and insulin. There are increased levels of corticosteroids and catecholamines, which reflect the increased perfusion of the adrenal gland. Haematological changes also reflect the chronic hypoxia, with increased levels of erythropoietin and nucleated red blood cells.

Chronic fetal hypoxia in FGR may eventually lead to fetal acidaemia, both respiratory and metabolic, which if prolonged can lead to intrauterine death if the fetus is not removed from its hostile environment. FGR fetuses are especially at risk from profound asphyxia in labour due to further compromise of the uteroplacental circulation by uterine contractions.

Management

The assessment of fetal well-being is described in detail in Chapter 6, Antenatal imaging and assessment of fetal well-being.

In brief, the detection of an SGA infant contains two elements: first, the accurate assessment of gestational age and second, the recognition of fetal smallness.

Early measurement of the fetal crown–rump length before 13 weeks plus 6 days gestation or head circumference between 13+6 and 20 weeks remains the method of choice for confirming gestational age. Thereafter, the most precise way of assessing fetal growth is by ultrasound biometry (biparietal diameter, head circumference, abdominal circumference and femur length) serially at set time intervals (usually of 4 weeks and no less than 2 weeks). As resources in most units do not permit comprehensive serial ultrasound in all pregnancies, serial ultrasound biometry is usually performed in 'at risk' pregnancies (see box below).

Pregnancies at risk of FGR

- Multiple pregnancies (see Chapter 9, Twins and higher multiple gestations)
- History of FGR in previous pregnancy
- Current heavy smokers
- Current drug users
- Women with underlying medical disorders:
  - hypertension
  - diabetes
  - cyanotic heart disease
  - antiphospholipid syndrome
- Pregnancies where the symphysis-fundal height is less than expected

---

When a diagnosis of SGA has been made, the next step is to clarify whether the baby is normal and simply constitutionally small or whether it is FGR. A comprehensive ultrasound examination of the fetal anatomy should be made looking for fetal abnormalities that may explain the size. Even if the anatomy appears normal, the presence of symmetrical growth restriction in the presence of a normal amniotic fluid volume raises the suspicion of a fetal genetic defect and the parents should be counselled accordingly. Amniocentesis and rapid fetal karyotype should be offered. Features suspicious of uteroplacental insufficiency are an asymmetrically growth restricted fetus with a relatively small abdominal circumference, oligohydramnios and a high umbilical artery resistance (see Chapter 6, Antenatal imaging and assessment of fetal well-being, Figures 6.8 and 6.16).

At present, there are no widely accepted treatments available for FGR related to uteroplacental insufficiency. Obvious contributing factors, such as smoking, alcohol and drug abuse, should be stopped and the health of the women should be optimized. Low-dose aspirin may have a role in the prevention of FGR in high-risk pregnancies but is not effective in the treatment of established cases.

When growth restriction is severe and the fetus is too immature to be delivered safely, bed rest in hospital is usually advised in an effort to maximize placental blood flow although the evidence supporting this practice is limited. The aim of these interventions is to gain as much maturity as possible before delivering the fetus, thereby reducing the morbidity associated with prematurity. However, timing the delivery in such a way that maximizes gestation without risking the baby dying *in utero* demands intensive fetal surveillance. The most widely accepted methods of monitoring the fetus are discussed in detail in Chapter 6, Antenatal imaging and assessment of fetal well-being, and summarized briefly in the following box.

Surveillance of the FGR fetus

- Serial biometry and amniotic fluid volume measurement performed at no less than 2-weekly intervals
- In the FGR fetus dynamic tests of fetal well-being including:
  - Umbilical artery Doppler wave form analysis
  - Absence or reversed flow of blood in the umbilical artery during fetal diastole requires delivery in the near future
  - In extremely pre-term or pre-viable infants with absent or reversed end diastolic flow in the umbilical artery, other fetal arterial and venous Doppler studies can be performed although their use has not yet been proven by large prospective trials.
  - Fetal cardiotocography

Prognosis

The prognosis of FGR is highly dependent upon the cause, severity and the gestation at delivery. When FGR is related to a congenital infection or chromosomal abnormality, subsequent development of the child will be determined by the precise abnormality.

Of babies with FGR secondary to uteroplacental insufficiency, some babies will suffer morbidity or mortality as a result of prematurity. For the survivors, the long-term prognosis is good with low incidences of mental and physical disability and most infants demonstrate 'catch-up growth' after delivery when feeding is established.

A link between FGR and the adult onset of hypertension and diabetes has been established. It remains to be seen whether other associations will be found in the future.

Placental abruption

Definition

This is the premature separation of a normally sited placenta from the uterine wall. In more than two-thirds of cases, the separation is at the edge of the placenta and the blood tracks down to the cervix and is revealed as vaginal bleeding. The remaining cases are concealed and present as uterine pain and potentially maternal shock, fetal distress or fetal death without obvious or with minimal bleeding.

Incidence

This has been documented as between 0.4 and 2.0 per cent of pregnancies, but varies depending upon the criteria used for diagnosis. Histological examination of the placenta suggest that the actual incidence is much higher (4 per cent), but obviously many of these cases are clinically silent.

Aetiology

This is unknown in the majority of cases, although there is an association with defective trophoblastic invasion, as with pre-eclampsia and FGR. Other associations include direct abdominal trauma, high parity, uterine over-distension (polyhydramnios and multiple gestation), sudden decompression of the uterus (e.g. after delivery of the first twin or after rupture of the membrane in polyhydramnios). The association with hypertension may reflect a direct cause, or may be a manifestation of poor trophoblast invasion.

Clinical presentation and diagnosis

The classical presentation is that of abdominal pain, vaginal bleeding and uterine contractions, often close to term or in established labour. Bleeding may be concealed so its absence does not preclude the diagnosis. Large abruptions may present with maternal shock and/or collapse. Abdominal palpation typically reveals a tender, tense uterus that is often described as being 'woody hard'. The fetus is often difficult to palpate. Depending on the size and location of the abruption, the fetus may be dead, in distress or unaffected. The diagnosis is usually made on clinical grounds. Occasionally, ultrasound demonstrates the presence of retroplacental clot, but this is not a reliable diagnostic tool.

Management

A large placental abruption is a life-threatening emergency for both mother and baby. The management is described in detail in Chapter 16, Obstetric emergencies. Where smaller degrees of abruption have occurred and there is no fetal distress, particularly where gestational age favours delaying the delivery to allow greater fetal maturity, conservative management may be instituted. This will require close monitoring of fetal well-being, using ultrasound scans of fetal growth, amniotic fluid volume, umbilical artery Doppler and cardiotocography. As with many complicated obstetric problems, the timing of delivery will be based on when the perceived risks of leaving the fetus undelivered outweigh the risks of premature delivery and the decision is best taken in conjunction with paediatricians.

Mrs B was a 34-year-old Caucasian primigravid teacher. At a gestation of 11 weeks, she was seen in the hospital antenatal clinic for the first time. She was noted to be a non-smoker. There was no relevant past history, but family history revealed that her mother has had hypertension since her late forties. Mrs B was 1.56 m tall and weighed 83 kg. Her booking blood pressure was 110/74 mmHg and urinalysis was normal.

The antenatal period was uneventful until 37 weeks. At 37 weeks gestation, a community midwife noted that Mrs B's blood pressure had risen to 150/100 mmHg and that there was 1+ of protein in the urine. Mrs B was referred to the hospital as an emergency admission.

On arrival at the hospital, Mrs B's blood pressure was 160/110 mmHg and there was 3+ of protein in the urine. She was complaining of some upper abdominal pain and there was hyperreflexia. The fetal heart rate was normal.

What are the risks in this case?

Mrs B was hypertensive and had marked proteinuria, having previously been normotensive. The diagnosis is pre-eclampsia. The level of the blood pressure denotes severe disease. The pregnancy is at term.

Mrs B is at risk of developing a worsening condition. A further rise in her blood pressure will put her at risk of intracranial haemorrhage. She may have an eclamptic fit, develop a coagulopathy and HELLP syndrome, and possibly renal failure. There is a further risk of placental abruption and severe haemorrhage. The fetus is at risk secondary to the mother's condition.

Plan of action

- The patient does not require resuscitation.
- The fetus does not require emergency delivery.
- Call for help.
- Establish an intravenous line with a wide-bore cannula.
- Take blood for clotting studies, full blood count and blood biochemistry and save serum.
- Prevent an eclamptic fit from occurring.
- Give magnesium sulphate intravenously 4 g bolus over 20 minutes. Continue with 1 g/hour.
- At these doses, monitoring blood levels is not necessary unless the urine output falls to less than 20 mL/hour (magnesium sulphate is excreted via the kidneys).
- Lower the blood pressure. The aim is to achieve a diastolic blood pressure of 90–100 mmHg and the systolic blood pressure should be treated if above 160 mmHg. Check the blood pressure every 5 minutes. Oral labetalol or nifedipine can be used to treat blood pressure. If unsuccessful, intravenous hydrallazine or labetalol, as a bolus followed by an infusion will be needed.
- Measure input and output of fluids.
  - Put a Foley catheter into the bladder.
  - Restrict input from all sources to 80 mL/hour (or 1 mL/kg/hour).
  - A CVP line may be needed.
- If the clotting becomes deranged (platelets <50 × 10^9/L), contact a consultant haematologist for advice.

Management of the case

In this case, the blood pressure fell to 145/96 mmHg on treatment with labetalol. Treatment with magnesium sulphate was started and the urine output averaged 35 mL/hour. Clotting studies, full blood count and biochemistry remained normal. The cardiotocograph showed a normal fetal heart pattern.

Once stabilization had been achieved, delivery was planned. Because the clotting studies were normal, an epidural was put in place. Vaginal examination showed that the cervix was favourable, with the fetus presenting by the head. Therefore, induction of labour was commenced, and after a rapid labour a 3.2 kg boy was delivered, with normal Apgar scores. The estimated blood loss was 600 mL.

After delivery, Mrs B was nursed in the delivery suite for 36 hours. The magnesium sulphate infusion was continued for 24 hours after delivery. The labetalol infusion was stopped and labetalol was continued orally to control blood pressure. There was initial concern with regard to the urine output, which remained at 25 mL/hour for the first 6 hours after delivery. The position was watched, but no active steps were taken to redress the issue and, between 6 and 12 hours after delivery, the patient began to have a marked diuresis. Seven days after delivery, Mrs B's blood pressure had returned to normal without medication.

Conclusion

This case demonstrates appropriate management of moderate to severe pre-eclampsia at term. Major problems were prevented by swift action. Mrs B is at risk of pre-eclampsia in her next pregnancy, although it is likely to be less severe. She is also at risk of developing hypertension later in life.

Additional reading

Confidential Enquiry into Maternal and Child Health. Saving Mothers' Lives: Reviewing maternal deaths to make motherhood safer – 2003–2005: The Seventh Report of the Confidential Enquiries into Maternal Deaths in the United Kingdom. London: CEMACH.

Milne F, Redman C, Walker J *et al*. The pre-eclampsia community guideline (PRECOG): how to screen for and detect onset of pre-eclampsia in the community. *BMJ* 2005; **330**: 576–80.

CHAPTER 11

LATE MISCARRIAGE AND EARLY BIRTH

Griffith Jones

OVERVIEW

Preterm or early delivery occurs after viability but before 37 weeks gestation. Spontaneous preterm labour and preterm pre-labour rupture of membranes account for approximately two-thirds of preterm births with the remainder resulting from medical or obstetric complications. Second trimester or late miscarriage occurs prior to viability. It is particularly distressing to the woman and her family because the pregnancy has become obvious abdominally and the mother may have started to notice fetal movements. Currently, the 'grey zone' for viability is around 23 weeks. Early births remain the predominant cause of perinatal mortality and morbidity, particularly those occurring between viability and 32 weeks gestation. The aetiology underlying late miscarriage and spontaneous preterm delivery varies with gestational age.

Definition

In pregnancy, term refers to the gestational period from 37+0 to 41+6 weeks. Preterm births occur between 24+0 and 36+6 weeks. Although births earlier than this are referred to as miscarriages, occasional survivors are seen after delivery at 23 weeks, which has become the 'grey zone' for viability. A 'late' or second trimester miscarriage occurs between 12 and 23 weeks gestation. The predominant causes of losses at 12–16 weeks are those of first trimester miscarriage, namely fetal chromosomal and structural anomalies and some implantation abnormalities. A more practical definition of late miscarriage is one occurring between 17 and 23 weeks.

Early births occur either because delivery is felt to be in the best interests of the mother or baby (indicated deliveries) or because the mother develops spontaneous contractions or membrane rupture earlier than normal (spontaneous deliveries). After viability, the latter group has two subdivisions: spontaneous preterm labour (PTL) and preterm pre-labour rupture of membranes (PPROM). Indicated deliveries, PTL and PPROM each account for approximately one-third of early births (Figure 11.1).

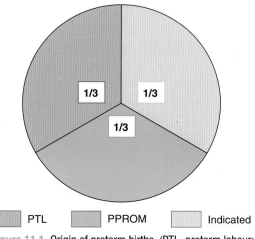

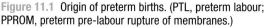

Figure 11.1 Origin of preterm births. (PTL, preterm labour; PPROM, preterm pre-labour rupture of membranes.)

Prevalence

In 2005, there were just over 645 000 live births in the UK. Of these 7.4 per cent were preterm, delivering between 24 and 36 weeks. Significantly higher rates of preterm birth of 12 per cent are reported from the USA. Conversely, many Nordic countries with very reliable data collection quote rates around 5 per cent. This must reflect, at least in part, differing socioeconomic and cultural factors. There is no evidence that the incidence of preterm birth is declining. In fact, the rate appears to be slowly increasing, in part due to an increasing incidence of multiple pregnancy.

In most countries, including the UK, there are no formal records of miscarriages. The exact incidence of late miscarriages is unknown, but is estimated to be approximately 1 per cent.

Preterm births contribute significantly to perinatal mortality, half of which results from babies born before 32 weeks. UK infant mortality figures in 2005 for live births at each gestational age are shown in Figure 11.2.

Predicted survival can be modified if accurate information concerning fetal sex, weight and well-being is available. Parents are particularly anxious about the risks of later disability and handicap. These risks are especially significant below 26 weeks gestation. When assessed at six years of age, nearly half the survivors at 23–25 weeks gestation have a moderate or severe disability. Furthermore, many of these disabilities only become apparent after two to three years of age. Survival with no disability is only seen in 1, 3 and 8 per cent of live births at <24, 24 and 25 weeks, respectively. There are other long-term worries after very preterm births, including subsequent growth, educational needs and social behaviour. There may also be influences on later

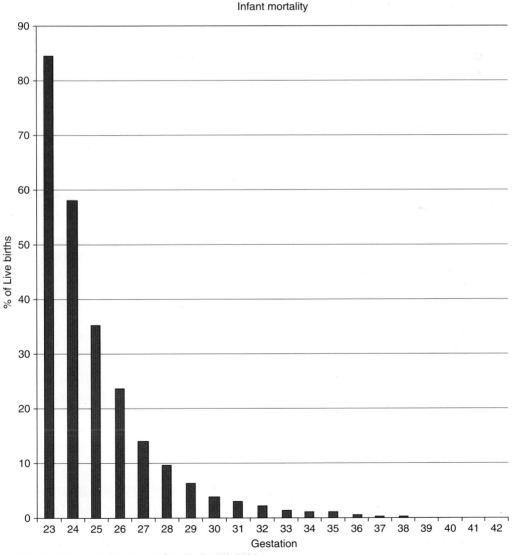

Figure 11.2 Infant mortality of live born infants in the UK, 2005

adult health. Fortunately, both morbidity and mortality fall dramatically with increasing gestation.

It is important to recognize the effect of denominator differences in survival figures, especially at the earliest gestations. If the figures are based on fetuses alive at the start of labour, the survival rates will be lower, as there is an inherent risk of intrapartum death. If the figures are based on NICU admissions, the figures will be higher, as some live births will succumb during initial resuscitation in the maternity unit. At 25 weeks or less, such statistical manipulations may lead to a change of nearly 10 per cent in the quoted survival figures.

Classification

For reasons related to aetiology, outcome and recurrence risk, preterm births should be divided into three gestational periods: mildly preterm births at 32+0 to 36+6 weeks (incidence 6.1 per cent), very preterm births at 28+0 to 31+6 weeks (incidence 0.9 per cent) and extremely preterm births at 24+0 to 27+6 weeks (incidence 0.4 per cent).

Late miscarriages occur across a broad gestational age range. At the latter part of the second trimester, between 17 and 23 weeks, the commonest factors underlying such losses will be those linked to extremely preterm births. Indeed, research shows that women who have such a late second trimester delivery are at increased risk of a very preterm birth in their next pregnancy.

As the interval between symptom onset and delivery can occasionally be measured in weeks, some 'inevitable' or 'threatened' second trimester miscarriages may result in preterm deliveries. Pre-viable membrane rupture represents the most common precedent for this scenario. Before 22 weeks gestation, membrane rupture with severe oligohydramnios carries a significant risk of lethal fetal lung hypoplasia. Unfortunately, this complication cannot be reliably predicted antenatally. The parents should be counselled as to the poor prognosis but if there are no signs of infection, there is no urgency to interfere. Some may want to wait for nature to take its course; others may want more immediate action. In both cases, continuing support is important. No harm will come from conservative management as long as careful observation is made for signs of infection. Established chorioamnionitis usually declares itself with contractions and delivery. Rarely do the membranes seal and fluid reaccumulate. This is usually only seen when membrane rupture follows amniocentesis.

Aetiology

Labour at term and prior to it share a common pathway involving uterine contractility, cervical effacement and dilatation and membrane rupture. At term, the activation of this pathway is physiological. However, a variety of pathologies underlie labour remote from term. It has been suggested by some authors that preterm labour be considered a syndrome, in order to emphasize its multifactorial nature.

Infection

Subclinical intrauterine infection of the choriodecidual space and amniotic fluid is the most widely studied aetiological factor underlying spontaneous preterm births. The uterine cavity is normally sterile but the vagina contains commensal bacteria. Depending on the bacterial load and cervical resistance, the bacteria may ascend through the cervix and reach the fetal membranes. This may activate the decidua, increase prostaglandin release and trigger contractions. Alternatively, it may weaken the membranes, leading to rupture. Early-onset neonatal sepsis, maternal postpartum endometritis and histological chorioamnionitis are all significantly more common after preterm birth, particularly those very early deliveries before 32 weeks.

Over-distension

The commonest cause of uterine over-distension is multiple gestation. Polyhydramnios has a similar effect. Overstretching of the myometrium (and possibly the membranes) leads to increased contractile activity and premature shortening and opening of the cervix.

Vascular

Disturbance at the uteroplacental interface may lead to intrauterine bleeding. The blood can track down behind the membranes to the cervix and be revealed. Alternatively, it may track away from the cervix and be concealed. Either way, the blood irritates the uterus, leading to contractions, and damages the membranes, leading to early rupture.

Surgical procedures and intercurrent illness

Serious maternal infective illnesses such as pyelonephritis, appendicitis and pneumonia are associated with preterm labour. In these cases, preterm labour is presumed to be due either to direct blood-borne spread of infection to the uterine cavity or indirectly to chemical triggers, such as endotoxins or cytokines. Many other illnesses, such as cholestasis of pregnancy, and non-obstetric surgical procedures are associated with preterm labour, although the mechanisms for this remain obscure.

Amniocentesis is a pregnancy-specific procedure associated with an increased risk of late miscarriage and early birth. It is most commonly performed at 15–18 weeks gestation. It is associated with a 0.5 per cent chance of subsequent pregnancy loss before viability. This may happen in the days after the procedure but many losses occur several weeks later and a small increased chance of preterm delivery persists after reaching viability.

Abnormal uterine cavity

A uterine cavity that is distorted by congenital malformation may be less able to accommodate the developing pregnancy. Associated abnormal placentation and cervical weakness may also contribute. Fibroids in a low position may also lead to complications. However, fibroids are common and most pregnancies are successful despite their presence.

Cervical weakness

Due to previous surgical damage or a congenital defect, the cervix may shorten and open prematurely. The membranes then prolapse and may be damaged by stretching or by direct contact with vaginal pathogens. These same pathogens may ascend and trigger contractions. Often referred to as 'cervical incompetence', weakness may be a better term. The evidence suggests that gradations of deficiency exist, rather than an 'all-or-nothing' phenomenon.

This remains a notoriously difficult diagnosis to make, as dilatation of the cervix remains the final common pathway for all late miscarriages and early births. Reliably distinguishing between such dilatation being the primary event or secondary to other pathologies is challenging.

Idiopathic

In many cases, especially mildly preterm births between 34 and 36 weeks, no cause will be found. In these cases, the physiological pathways to parturition may simply have been turned on too early.

Risk factors for preterm labour/PPROM

Non-modifiable, major
- Last birth preterm: 20 per cent risk
- Last two births preterm: 40 per cent risk
- Twin pregnancy: 50 per cent risk
- Uterine abnormalities
- Cervical anomalies:
  - cervical damage (cone biopsy, repeated dilatation)
  - fibroids (cervical)
- Factors in current pregnancy:
  - recurrent antepartum haemorrhage
  - intercurrent illness (e.g. sepsis)
  - any invasive procedure or surgery

Non-modifiable, minor
- Teenagers having second or subsequent babies
- Parity (0 or >5)
- Ethnicity (black women)
- Poor socioeconomic status
- Education (not beyond secondary)

Modifiable
- Smoking: two-fold increase of PPROM
- Drugs of abuse: especially cocaine
- Body mass index (BMI) <20: underweight women
- Inter-pregnancy interval <1 year

Clinical features of preterm labour

History

Always check the dating of the pregnancy by reviewing the menstrual history and, if possible, any prior ultrasound examinations. This is critical at gestations near viability.

Less than 50 per cent of all women presenting with symptoms suggesting a risk of early delivery will deliver within 7 days. Too much emphasis is often placed on the contraction frequency. In isolation, it correlates poorly with the risk of preterm birth. Markers of intensity, such as analgesic requirements or simple bedside clinical impression, may add refinement. Vague complaints such as increased discharge, pelvic pressure or low backache are sometimes reported, with the latter two often showing a cyclical pattern. Nonetheless, the diagnosis of preterm labour remains notoriously difficult unless contractions are accompanied by advanced dilatation (>3 cm), ruptured membranes or significant vaginal bleeding.

Examination

A brief general examination is important to assess overall health. This will include pulse, blood pressure, temperature and state of hydration.

Abdominal examination may reveal the presence of uterine tenderness, suggesting abruption or chorioamnionitis. A careful speculum examination by an experienced clinician may yield valuable information; pooling of amniotic fluid, blood and/ or abnormal discharge may be observed. A visual assessment of cervical dilatation is usually possible and has been shown to be as accurate as digital examination findings. Digital exams should be limited, as they are known to stimulate prostaglandin production and may introduce organisms into the cervical canal.

Differential diagnosis
• Urinary tract infection
• Red degeneration of fibroid
• Placental abruption
• Constipation
• Gastroenteritis

Investigations

Bedside fibronectin

Fetal fibronectin (fFN) is a 'glue-like' protein binding the choriodecidual membranes. It is rarely present in vaginal secretions between 23 and 34 weeks. Any disruption at the choriodecidual interface results in fFN release and possible detection in the cervicovaginal secretions.

Bedside fibronectin testing offers a rapid assessment of risk in symptomatic women with minimal cervical dilatation. If performed correctly, the test has a greater predictive value than digital examination. In one study, 30 per cent of women with a positive fibronectin test delivered within 7 days, compared with only 10 per cent of women who were 2–3 cm dilated. Only 1 per cent of those women who test negative for fibronectin will deliver within 1 week. Aggressive intervention can be avoided in these women.

Cervical length

Cervical length measurement by transvaginal ultrasound has also been shown to improve diagnostic accuracy. A normal cervix measures approximately 35 mm in length (Figure 11.3a). Significant cervical shortening is often accompanied by dilatation and funnelling of the membranes down the cervical canal (Figure 11.3b). Although measurements can be repeated frequently and with little expense, skilled ultrasonographers and suitable machines with transvaginal probes are required.

Repeat vaginal examination

Repeat vaginal examination in 1–4 hours should be considered essential in the absence of specialized tests. The interval between assessments should be guided by the severity of the symptoms.

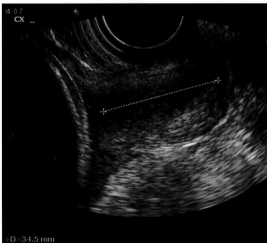

(a)

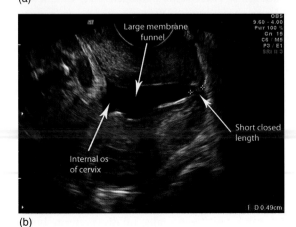

(b)

Figure 11.3 (a) Normal cervix. (b) Cervical length and funnelling on ultrasound

Clinical features of preterm pre-labour rupture of the membranes

History

The most reliable diagnostic feature of PPROM from the history is the report of a 'gush of fluid' vaginally, usually followed by a more-or-less continuous dribble. This must be distinguished from leaking urine (ask about frequency, urgency, leakage and dysuria), as incontinence or a urinary tract infection (UTI) may present in a similar way. The presence of any vaginal discharge should be ascertained. Fetal movements may be reduced in strength or frequency after PPROM, and occasionally uterine irritability or contractions may be reported.

Examination

Infection may lead to an increased pulse and temperature and a flushed appearance. Abdominal examination may reveal a clinical suspicion of oligohydramnios or uterine tenderness if chorioamnionitis is present. The definitive diagnosis of PPROM can only be made by performing a sterile speculum examination, preferably after the patient has been resting supine for 20–30 minutes. A pool of amniotic fluid in the posterior vagina is diagnostic. It is also important at this point to visualize the cervix. Fluid may be seen trickling through the external os and dilatation can be assessed. Digital vaginal examinations should be avoided if possible in PPROM, as they are associated with a significant reduction in the latent interval before labour. This reduction is most dramatic at the earliest gestations.

Differential diagnosis

- Urine loss: incontinence and UTIs are both more common in pregnancy
- Vaginal infection
- Leukorrhoea: the cervical glands often become overactive during pregnancy

---

Investigations

Nitrazine testing

Amniotic fluid is alkaline, whereas the vaginal secretions are usually acidic. An elevated pH turns a nitrazine stick black. Some units use nitrazine sticks to define the presence of amniotic fluid. Unfortunately, false positives occur, with blood, semen and even urine limiting its usefulness. However, the predictive value of a negative test is very high.

Genital tract swabs

A high vaginal swab may help to guide antibiotic therapy, if subsequently required. Screening for group B streptococcus (GBS) can also be performed, as there is a substantial risk of labour in the next few days.

Maternal well-being

This should include regular assessment of the mother's blood pressure, pulse and temperature. Some advise serial white cell counts and C-reactive proteins as early markers of infection, although this has not been shown to improve management.

Fetal well-being

Serial antepartum cardiotocography is important after PPROM, as a gradually increasing baseline heart rate or fetal tachycardia can be the first sign of intrauterine infection.

Ultrasound

Ultrasound can give valuable information about the amniotic fluid volume. The presence or absence of oligohydramnios provides further diagnostic support. In established PPROM, there is a direct correlation between the amount of amniotic fluid remaining and the latency period. Unlike preterm labour, cervical length measurements do not have predictive ability in PPROM.

Amniocentesis

A sample of amniotic fluid can be sent for Gram stain, microscopy and culture, to establish whether there is an intrauterine infection (chorioamnionitis). There is, however, a risk of stimulating preterm labour by performing an invasive test, and amniocentesis can be technically very difficult when there is little amniotic fluid.

Clinical features of late miscarriage

The clinical presentation of second trimester miscarriage is diverse, encompassing those of both

PTL and PPROM. Commonly, there will be uterine cramping and bleeding. The membranes may be intact or ruptured. However, events may progress rapidly without significant pain, the mother complaining of relatively minor backache or abdominal discomfort. Some women report only a sudden increase in mucous vaginal discharge.

History

As per PTL and PPROM.

Examination

Prior to 24 weeks, fetal parts cannot be reliably felt. A hand-held Doppler device (often referred to as a Sonicaid) should be used to auscultate the fetal heart. There is no role for CTG assessment.

Initially, a speculum examination should be performed. A good light and proper positioning are important. The cervix should be visualized. It may have started to dilate and the membranes may be seen bulging through the external os.

Investigations

As per PTL and PPROM.

Management of symptomatic women

Communication and support

A holistic approach to the situation is essential. Sympathy, explanations and reassurance are mandatory. There are two vital areas of communication in the management of threatened preterm labour or PPROM. Communication with the woman and her family ensures that they have a full understanding of the risks involved and enables a clear management plan to be discussed. Communication with the neonatal unit staff ensures that adequate and appropriate resources are available at the time of delivery. Parents often also appreciate the opportunity to have discussed the care of their baby with the neonatology staff in advance of delivery.

While women in preterm labour need to be on an acute care unit, the ideal place for women experiencing a late miscarriage is a purpose-designed area, away from a busy labour and delivery unit or gynaecological ward. Despite a gestational age of 23 weeks or less, some babies will show signs of life at delivery. The parents should be made aware of this beforehand to avoid unnecessary distress. Comfort care should be offered to all of these newborns. If there is any uncertainty as to the gestation or the pregnancy is close to 24 weeks, a paediatrician should be briefed and may need to attend the delivery to assess viability at birth. The mother should view the fetus as a baby. She may want to touch or hold the baby, and this should be encouraged. Appropriate sensitivities should be exercised according to the choice of the woman and her partner. Follow up by a senior member of staff and specialist midwife should be organized after a late miscarriage; this will lead to discussion about a future pregnancy. Contact details of local or national support groups, such as the Stillbirth and Neonatal Death Society (SANDS), should also be given.

Maternal steroids

Current evidence shows that a single course of maternal steroids (two injections 12–24 hours apart) given between 28 and 34 weeks gestation and received within 7 days of delivery results in markedly improved neonatal outcomes. This is primarily due to a reduction in neonatal respiratory distress syndrome (RDS). Maximum benefit from the injection is seen after 48 hours. Courses received less than 48 hours or more than 7 days before delivery still lead to benefit, as may courses given between 24 and 28 weeks. They are not indicated below 24 weeks.

There is considerable reassuring evidence about the long-term safety of single courses of maternal steroids, with paediatric follow-up into the teenage years. However, there is growing concern about adverse consequences of multiple dosing. Like antibiotics, steroids have the potential for harm in pregnancy and should be used carefully.

Tocolytics

The Canadian Preterm Labor Trial remains the most influential tocolytic trial to date. It concluded that ritodrine, a beta-agonist that relaxes smooth muscle, had no significant benefit on perinatal mortality or the prolongation of pregnancy to term; however, it was able to reduce the number of women delivering within 2 days by 40 per cent. This 48-hour window of opportunity is the sole reason for using tocolytics. Beta-agonists have significant maternal side effects, and maternal deaths from acute cardiopulmonary compromise are described. Other smooth muscle relaxants used to treat preterm labour include nifedipine and glyceryl trinitrate. The former has become popular, as it is inexpensive, given orally and has a low side-effect profile. The oxytocin antagonist atosiban now has a UK product licence. Although side effects are seen less frequently than with ritodrine, the cost is much higher. As prostaglandins appear to be one of the pivotal chemicals involved in parturition, non-steroidal anti-inflammatories, such as indomethacin have attracted considerable interest as tocolytics. They have been associated with significant fetal cardiovascular side effects, although these can be mitigated by limiting them to short-term use below 30 weeks gestation only.

Unfortunately, despite a multitude of pharmacological approaches, no tocolytic medication has yet been shown to have increased efficacy in comparison to ritodrine or to improve neonatal outcomes. At the time of writing, the role for tocolysis is to allow a course of steroids for fetal lung maturation to be completed and to facilitate transfer of the undelivered mother to a unit able to provide appropriate neonatal care, should delivery occur. As neither of these aims is appropriate before 24 weeks, tocolysis has no role in late miscarriage.

Antibiotics

Broad-spectrum antibiotics offering aerobic and anaerobic coverage are necessary in the presence of overt clinical infection, such as chorioamnionitis. The role of antibiotics in the absence of clinical signs of infection is much less clear.

The MRC Oracle Study initially concluded that the use of prophylactic antibiotics in uncomplicated preterm labour before 37 weeks with intact membranes did not confer any short-term neonatal benefit. Worryingly, subsequent long-term follow up of survivors actually showed a significant increase in neurodevelopmental handicap in those who received either erythromycin or co-amoxiclav.

In PPROM, the same study concluded that a 10-day course of erythromycin led to improved short-term neonatal outcomes. A much smaller US study that only enrolled women below 32 weeks with

PPROM also confirmed the benefit of antibiotics in the short term.

Most North American centres continue to give intrapartum antibiotics to women in preterm labour unless GBS status is known to be negative. For reasons that are unclear, the risk of early-onset neonatal disease appears much less in the UK and this approach has not been widely adopted.

Emergency cervical cerclage

When a patient presents with an open cervical os and bulging membranes before viability, the idea of closing the cervix by passing a stitch around it seems logical. However, the results of emergency cervical cerclage are poor and are related to the cervical dilatation at insertion. The procedure itself can be technically challenging. A dilatation of more than 3 cm with an effaced cervix poses extreme difficulties, even for the most experienced operator. Every effort should be made to detect and treat other causes of the uterine instability. If persistent placental bleeding is leading to secondary opening of the cervix, suturing the cervix clearly does not address the primary issue and is unlikely to be successful. Bleeding, contractions and infection are all contraindications to cerclage. Depending on the initial dilatation of the cervix, the chance of the pregnancy proceeding beyond 26 weeks may be less than 50 per cent.

Induction or augmentation

In some cases, it may be judged appropriate to hasten delivery, either because a late miscarriage appears inevitable or because the maternal or fetal risks of continuing the pregnancy are judged too high. Before 24 weeks, this would be carried out by inducing contractions with prostaglandins, such as Cervagem® or Cytotec®. A high-dose oxytocin infusion may be necessary later in the process. After 24 weeks, if there is no evidence of acute maternal or fetal compromise, induction with milder prostaglandins, such as Cervidil®, or conventional-dose oxytocin can be considered as an alternative to a planned Caesarean. Great care must be exercised if there is already clinical evidence of chorioamnionitis. In these cases, delay in ending the pregnancy may lead to worsening infection and consequent morbidity for both mother and baby. Augmenting labour may be the most appropriate management.

Mode of delivery

With a late miscarriage, vaginal delivery will almost always occur, even if there is a transverse lie or fetal malformation. This is because of the relatively small size of the fetus. Unfortunately, retention of the placenta or part of it is more common under these circumstances, and manual removal under anaesthetic may be required.

Many clinicians feel that the combination of high fetal morbidity and mortality, difficulty in diagnosing intrapartum hypoxia/acidosis and maternal risk of operative complications do not justify Caesarean section for fetal indications below 26 weeks. As gestation advances, both neonatal outcomes and the ability to diagnose fetal compromise improve, and intervention for fetal reasons becomes appropriate. The safety of preterm breech vaginal delivery is often questioned and Caesarean section commonly performed, although evidence to support this policy is weak.

Type of Caesarean section

At the earliest gestations and in the presence of oligohydramnios, the lower segment is often poorly formed. Vertical uterine incisions may be necessary. This 'classical' uterine incision carries an up to 5 per cent risk of uterine rupture in subsequent pregnancies, some of which will occur antenatally.

Fetal assessment

At pre-viable gestations, no intrapartum fetal monitoring is required. After 24 weeks, maternal steroid therapy can suppress both fetal activity and heart rate variability, although Doppler studies are not influenced. Whenever possible, the presentation in preterm labour should be confirmed by ultrasound, as clinical palpation is notoriously unreliable. An estimated fetal weight, particularly below 28 weeks, can be helpful. Preterm infants have less reserve to tolerate the stress of labour, particularly in the presence of oligohydramnios. Therefore, continuous fetal monitoring may be required, although there may be considerable difficulties interpreting the fetal heart rate pattern in extremely preterm infants. At the extremes of viability, parents may decline intervention for suspected fetal compromise or aggressive resuscitation of the newborn. In these cases, continuous monitoring may be inappropriate.

Analgesia

For intrapartum analgesia, an epidural is frequently advocated. Postulated benefits include avoiding expulsive efforts before full dilatation or a precipitous delivery, a relaxed pelvic floor and perineum and the ability to proceed quickly to abdominal delivery.

Adequate pain relief must also be ensured for late miscarriage. These deliveries are usually quick, but there is no contraindication to epidural anaesthesia. Patient-controlled analgesia often works well in this situation.

In utero transfer

If local resources are unable to care for a viable neonate, in utero transfer to a unit with adequate neonatal facilities is recommended. It is generally accepted that this will improve the outcome for babies, particularly below 30 weeks of gestation.

Management of high-risk asymptomatic women

Due to limited resources, most aspects of prematurity prevention are targeted at asymptomatic women with known risk factors for preterm birth. After a preterm birth, especially those before 32 weeks, a post-natal visit should be organized to review both the events leading to the delivery and any subsequent investigations, such as placental pathology. Ideally, a management plan for the next pregnancy should be made. This should include smoking cessation and a discussion regarding the optimal inter-pregnancy interval. However, if first seen in early pregnancy, the main priority will be a careful analysis of events surrounding the last birth.

Early dating scan

A first trimester dating scan ensures the precise assessment of gestational age in the current pregnancy.

Genital tract infection

Many vaginal pathogens, including bacterial vaginosis (BV), *Trichomonas vaginalis*, ureaplasm and chlamydia, have been associated with an increased risk of preterm birth in observational studies. Unfortunately, randomized studies of targeted antibiotics continue to give conflicting results. Some studies have demonstrated worse outcomes with active treatment. At present, there is some suggestion that early treatment of BV prior to 20 weeks gestation may lower the risk of late miscarriage and early birth.

Asymptomatic bacteriuria

This also carries an increased risk of preterm birth. Short courses of antibiotics based on culture sensitivities reduce the risk of pyelonephritis and early delivery.

GBS genital colonization

Preterm infants are more susceptible to early-onset GBS infection, acquired during passage through the birth canal. In women known to be at increased risk of early delivery, testing for GBS antenatally with a combined low vaginal/rectal swab allows consideration of intrapartum prophylaxis. Attempts at antenatal eradication has repeatedly been shown to be of no benefit.

Fetal fibronectin

Fetal fibronectin testing can only be undertaken after 23 weeks, as high levels may be physiological before then. In high-risk asymptomatic women with a positive fibronectin test at 24 weeks gestation, nearly half will deliver before 30 weeks gestation. Conversely, the chance of such an early birth is less than 1 per cent with a negative test. This negative predictive value may be its main use, as interventions based upon positive test results have not been shown to be helpful.

Progestational agents

Many studies, meta-analyses and reviews have shown no evidence of benefit from prophylactic or maintenance therapy with conventional oral or intravenous tocolytics.

Progesterone has long been recognized as a hormone involved in the support of pregnancy through uterine quiescence. However, it is also believed to affect cervical ripening and mucous production. It may also have anti-inflammatory properties. It appears to have a good safety profile when used in pregnancy. Initial trials using intramuscular or intravaginal progesterone have shown some promise, with reductions in the incidence of preterm birth. None have yet had the power to show an improvement in neonatal outcome, but many further studies are currently underway. Uncertainty remains over which subgroups of women are most likely to benefit and the ideal dosing regimes.

Lifestyle modification

Randomized trials of social support in the UK failed to improve pregnancy outcomes. In some studies, hospitalization for bed rest led to an increase in preterm birth. Roles for sexual abstinence and/or psychological support are no clearer.

Cervical ultrasound

Cervical length can be accurately and repeatedly measured by transvaginal ultrasound. In asymptomatic women with a short cervix at 23 weeks, the risk of very preterm delivery rises to 4 per cent with lengths of 11–20 mm. At 10 mm, the risk is 15 per cent, and it increases dramatically with further decreases in length. In the presence of a normal cervical length, intervention can usually be deferred. When significant cervical shortening is found at or beyond 24 weeks, women should be educated as to the signs and symptoms that should provoke hospital attendance. Prophylactic steroids should be considered. A small trial has suggested that vaginal progesterone reduces the risk of preterm delivery in cases where the cervix is short. Additional studies are currently investigating this further. Although many of the other strategies described earlier are commonly performed, definitive evidence of usefulness is often lacking. Before 24 weeks gestation, cervical cerclage is an option.

Cerclage

Elective cerclage may be advised solely based on a woman's past obstetric history. Randomized trials suggest benefit when a woman has had three or more late miscarriages or very preterm deliveries. In this situation, the procedure is usually performed at 12–14 weeks gestation. This is because the risk of first trimester miscarriage has passed and an initial assessment of fetal well-being can be performed with nuchal translucency.

In selective cerclage, surgery is based upon serial transvaginal ultrasound measurements of cervical length. Various thresholds have been used to define a weak cervix that may benefit from cerclage. Although randomized trials have failed to show a reduction in preterm births using this approach, many women with normal cervical appearances can avoid intervention, due to their low risk of early birth.

Cervical cerclage can be done under general or regional anaesthesia. The commonest procedure, a McDonald cerclage, is also the simplest and quickest to perform. A Mersilene tape purse-string suture (Mersilene RS22; Ethicon, Edinburgh, UK; Figure 11.4) is placed around the cervix. Tissue bites are taken at all four quadrants. Due to the reflections of the vaginal epithelium being situated around the upper third of the cervical body, the suture usually ends up halfway along the canal (Figure 11.5). Although more invasive cerclage techniques can result in higher suture placement, they have not been definitively associated with better outcomes and are generally reserved for atypically high-risk cases. A further advantage of the McDonald technique is that removal later in pregnancy does not usually require an anaesthetic.

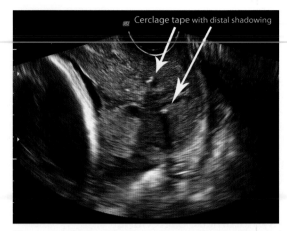
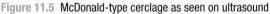
Cerclage tape with distal shadowing

Figure 11.5 McDonald-type cerclage as seen on ultrasound

Key points

- Preterm delivery complicates about 7.5 per cent of UK pregnancies.
- Major risk factors are a previous early birth and multiple pregnancy.
- The diagnosis of spontaneous preterm labour is difficult before advanced cervical dilatation.
- Histological chorioamnionitis is much more common after spontaneous preterm birth than after either term birth or indicated preterm deliveries.
- Ninety per cent of histologically proven cases of chorioamnionitis are subclinical with no overt clinical signs of infection.
- The most beneficial treatment in preterm labour is a course of maternal steroids, which substantially improve neonatal outcomes.

New developments

- Epidemiological studies are beginning to investigate genetic susceptibilities to preterm birth. Initial work is focusing on polymorphisms related to inflammatory cytokines, such as tumour necrosis factor.
- Inflammatory cytokines are now thought to be involved in the aetiology of many neonatal injuries, such as bronchopulmonary dysplasia and cerebral palsy. High levels of these chemicals are found in preterm births complicated by chorioamnionitis.
- Initial research suggests a possible role for progesterone supplementation in the prevention of preterm birth. Numerous studies are now underway to more precisely define its role and hopefully confirm that neonatal morbidity and mortality are improved.

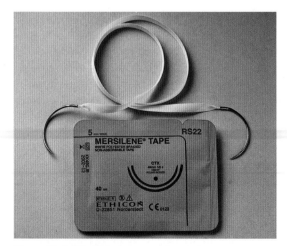

Figure 11.4 Mersilene tape used for cerclage

CASE HISTORY

Mrs A, a 39-year-old Caucasian woman, works as a secretary in a bank. She has no known medical problems but is a smoker. This is her fifth pregnancy. At the age of 18, she had a termination of pregnancy at 10 weeks gestation. She had two spontaneous first trimester miscarriages, aged 36 and 37. Both required D&C for retained products of conception. Just over 1 year ago, she had a late miscarriage at 22 weeks. She has been trying to conceive since the last miscarriage.

She is now 8 weeks pregnant, fit and well, and is taking iron supplements. When seen in the antenatal booking clinic, concerns were raised about her risks of an early delivery.

What risk factors does Mrs A have for preterm labour?

Her greatest risk factor is the 22-week loss in her last pregnancy. Although a single operative cervical dilatation is unlikely to lead to any significant degree of cervical weakness, there is some evidence that three or more such procedures pose a risk for early delivery.

Finally, smoking is associated with increased risks of antepartum haemorrhage and spontaneous membrane rupture, either of which can lead to early birth.

What care should Mrs A receive?

In view of her high risk of preterm delivery, she should receive consultant-led care in a hospital. It may be a good idea for her to meet a neonatologist and to be shown around the neonatal unit, particularly if any antenatal investigations further elevate her risk.

Discuss specific elements of her antenatal care that may be beneficial

A careful history should be taken regarding the events surrounding her last delivery. Presentation in advanced labour or with bulging membranes despite little or no pain may suggest a degree of cervical weakness. Although cerclage could be contemplated for such a history, the use of ultrasound assessment of cervical length may allow her to avoid surgery. Even if cerclage is not contemplated, cervical length measurements can guide interventions such as maternal steroids. Cervicovaginal fFN may allow even greater predictive accuracy. Screening for BV between 12 and 18 weeks may allow a specific intervention (i.e. targeted antibiotics) that reduces risk and improves outcome.

CHAPTER 12

MEDICAL DISEASES COMPLICATING PREGNANCY

Keelin O'Donoghue

OVERVIEW

Pregnancy is a normal physiological event during which most women remain fit and well. However, it may cause specific medical conditions. There are few medical disorders that are associated with sterility, although some may reduce a woman's fertility. Therefore it is not uncommon to encounter pregnant women with pre-existing medical diseases. Both pregnancy-specific and pre-existing medical conditions may in some circumstances be associated with significant maternal and fetal morbidity and, more rarely, mortality.

A multidisciplinary approach is vital in helping to ensure appropriate levels of care for pregnant women with medical problems. Members of such a team include specialist midwives, obstetricians, physicians and obstetric anaesthetists, and dieticians and physiotherapists will often provide support. Ideally, assessment of medical conditions and discussion regarding any implications for pregnancy should be available and offered and a plan of care documented before pregnancy. Such pre-conception counselling does occur, but it is not universal and often takes place either once the woman becomes pregnant or after a first pregnancy has ended in failure. For example, women with insulin-dependent diabetes should only embark on pregnancy when their diabetic control is very tight; failure to do so is associated with a significantly increased risk of pregnancy failure, complications and fetal abnormality. Counselling prior to the pregnancy allows women with, for example, severe heart or renal disease to understand the possible risks in pregnancy and the level of antenatal care they will require.

What the pregnant woman wants to know:

- Will I have a normal healthy baby?
- Will pregnancy make my disease worse?
- Will my disease be worse after pregnancy?
- Is there a risk of my children inheriting my condition?

- What treatment is safe during pregnancy?
- Can I have an epidural?
- Should I be delivered by Caesarean section?
- Is breastfeeding advisable?

Haematological abnormalities

Haemoglobinopathies

Clinically significant variants of haemoglobin:

- Sickle cell trait (Hb AS)
- Sickle cell disease (Hb SS)
- Sickle cell/haemoglobin C disease (Hb SC)
- Sickle cell/beta thalassaemia

Sickle cell anaemia

Sickle cell disease (SCD) is an autosomally inherited genetic condition, where abnormal haemoglobin (HbS) contains beta-globin chains with an amino acid substitution that results in it precipitating when in its reduced state. The red blood cells become sickle shaped and occlude small blood vessels. There is severe anaemia, chronic hyperbilirubinaemia, a predisposition to infection, vaso-occlusive complications including the acute chest syndrome, and chronic kidney disease. Pulmonary hypertension is found in 30 per cent of patients and is associated with a high mortality rate.

Advances in treatment of SCD have resulted in the average lifespan in the Western world extending past 50 years, which means many more women with the condition are now becoming pregnant. Like other medical disorders, ideal management begins with pre-pregnancy optimization of maternal health and education about the risks in pregnancy. High-dose folate supplements (5 mg daily) are recommended and the majority of women are also managed from early pregnancy on low-dose aspirin (75 mg daily). The disease response to pregnancy varies and there is no treatment to prevent crises. Pregnancy seems to be associated with an increased incidence of sickle cell crises that may result in episodes of severe pain, typically affecting the bones or chest. The acute chest syndrome may result from an initial uncomplicated crisis and is responsible for around 25 per cent of all deaths in sickle cell disease. Crises in pregnancy may be precipitated by hypoxia, stress, infection and haemorrhage. Mothers are also at increased risk of miscarriage, pre-eclampsia, fetal growth restriction (FGR) and premature labour, with three times the risk of eclampsia compared to women without SCD. Thromboembolic events including cerebral vein thrombosis and deep venous thrombosis are implicated in the higher rates of maternal deaths reported in SCD.

Management of sickle cell crisis in pregnancy

- Prompt treatment
- Adequate hydration
- Oxygen
- Analgesia
- Screen for infection (urinary, respiratory)
- Antibiotics
- Blood transfusion (leukocyte depleted and phenotype specific)
- Exchange transfusion
- Prophylaxis against thrombosis (heparin)
- Fetal monitoring

Sickle cell carriers have a 1:4 risk of having a baby with SCD if their partner also has sickle cell trait. Carriers are usually fit and well, but are at increased risk of urinary tract infection, and rarely suffer from crises. Although sickle cell haemoglobin C disease may cause only mild degrees of anaemia, it is associated with very severe crises that occur more often in pregnancy. In this condition, women are not as anaemic as those with SS disease and the severity of crises may be underestimated.

Thalassaemia

The thalassaemia syndromes are the commonest genetic blood disorders. The defect is a reduced production of normal haemoglobin and the syndromes are divided into alpha and beta types, depending on which globin chain is affected. In alpha-thalassaemia minor, there is a deletion of one of the two normal alpha genes required for haemoglobin production. Although the affected individual is chronically anaemic, this condition rarely produces obstetric complications except in cases of severe blood loss. It is important to screen the woman's partner for thalassaemia and to consider prenatal diagnosis; if he is also affected, there is a 1:4 chance of the fetus having alpha-thalassaemia major, which is lethal.

The beta-thalassaemias result from defects in the normal production of the beta chains. Beta-thalassaemia minor/trait is more commonly found in people from the eastern Mediterranean, but may also occur sporadically in other communities. Consequently, all pregnant women should be offered electrophoresis as part of the antenatal screening process. Beta-thalassaemia minor is not a problem antenatally, although women tend to be mildly anaemic and have a low MCV. Iron and folate supplements should be given and partners should also be screened. However, if both partners have beta-thalassaemia minor, there is a 1:4 chance that the fetus could have beta-thalassaemia major, which is associated with profound anaemia in post-natal life.

Thrombocytopenia

Thrombocytopenia is defined as a platelet count $<150 \times 10^9$/L. Incidental or gestational thrombocytopenia is common and is found in 7–8 per cent of pregnant women. Mild falls in platelet counts to between 100 and 150×10^9/L are only very rarely associated with poor maternal outcome.

Bleeding is rarely a complication unless the count is <50×10^9/L. However, the diagnosis of gestational thrombocytopenia is a diagnosis of exclusion and can only be made when autoimmune and other causes have been excluded. It usually occurs in late pregnancy, with no prior history of thrombocytopenia outside pregnancy and a normal platelet count recorded at the start of pregnancy. No intervention is required other than monitoring of the platelet count during and after pregnancy. There is no association with fetal thrombocytopenia and spontaneous resolution occurs after delivery.

Causes of thrombocytopenia in pregnancy

- Idiopathic
- Increased consumption or destruction
  - autoimmune (ITP)
  - antiphospholipid syndrome
  - pre-eclampsia
  - HELLP syndrome (haemolysis, elevation of liver enzymes and low platelets)
  - disseminated intravascular coagulation
  - thrombotic thrombocytopenic purpura
  - hypersplenism
- Decreased production
  - sepsis
  - HIV infection
  - malignant marrow infiltration

Autoimmune thrombocytopenia

In immune thrombocytopenic purpura (ITP), autoantibodies are produced against platelet surface antigens, leading to platelet destruction by the reticuloendothelial system. The incidence in pregnancy is around 1 in 5000. The maternal platelet count may fall at any stage of pregnancy and can reach levels of <50×10^9/L. Maternal haemorrhage at delivery is very unlikely if the platelet count is >50×10^9/L, and spontaneous bleeding during pregnancy very unlikely if the platelet count is >20×10^9/L. There is a 5–10 per cent chance of associated fetal thrombocytopenia (<50×10^9/L), which cannot be predicted using maternal counts or antibody tests.

Management in pregnancy should include serial monitoring of platelet counts and, provided the count remains above 80×10^9/L, no complications are likely. If the count falls below 50×10^9/L approaching term, treatment should be considered. Corticosteroids act by suppressing platelet autoantibodies; however, high doses are often required to improve the platelet count, and long-term use is associated with weight gain, hypertension and diabetes. Corticosteroids also take 2–3 weeks to have a significant effect. Although more expensive, the use of intravenous immunoglobulin G (IgG) has been a major advance in the treatment of autoimmune thrombocytopenia. The mechanism of action is unclear, but the response is usually rapid. IgG is the preferred option where a rapid platelet increase is required close to term, if the duration of treatment is likely to be prolonged, or if unacceptably high maintenance doses of prednisolone are required. Vaginal delivery should be facilitated and regional anaesthesia avoided if the platelet count is <80×10^9/L. Fetal blood sampling in labour and instrumental delivery by ventouse are best avoided because of the risk of fetal thrombocytopenia. A cord blood sample must be collected for platelet counting, but the nadir of the neonatal platelet count occurs 2–5 days after delivery.

Bleeding disorders

Bleeding disorders during pregnancy and delivery

- Inherited
  - vascular abnormalities
  - platelet disorders
  - coagulation disorders
- Acquired
  - thrombocytopenia
  - disseminated intravascular coagulation
  - acquired coagulation disorders
  - marrow disorders

Inherited coagulation disorders

Von Willebrand disease, carriers of haemophilia A and B and factor XI deficiency account for over 90 per cent of all women with inherited bleeding disorders.

Haemophilia A (FVIII deficiency) and haemophilia B (FIX deficiency) are X-linked defects with a prevalence of 1 in 10 000 and 1 in 100 000, respectively, in the population. Carriers of haemophilia A or B usually have clotting factor activity about 50 per cent of normal, but while factor VIIIC levels increase in pregnancy, factor IXC levels increase only slightly. Factor XI deficiency is a rare autosomal dominant bleeding disorder, where the bleeding risk does not relate well to the severity of the deficiency of the factor. FXI levels do not rise significantly during pregnancy. Von Willebrand disease is the most common inherited bleeding disorder with an estimated prevalence of 1 per cent. It results from either a qualitative or quantitative defect in von Willebrand factor (VWF). The inheritance of von Willebrand disease is usually autosomal dominant and while increases in factor VIIIC and VWF antigen activity usually occur during normal pregnancy, they cannot be relied on to buffer the effects of the disease, particularly in severe cases.

Where possible, carriers of haemophilia and women with von Willebrand disease should be identified and counselled prior to pregnancy. Baseline coagulation factor assays should be performed as soon as pregnancy is confirmed and repeated in the third trimester. In haemophilia carriers, fetal sex should be determined either on ultrasound or through sampling fetal DNA in maternal blood. Invasive procedures during pregnancy may require clotting factor cover.

Planning for delivery is done on the basis of the third trimester clotting factor levels, taking into account the individual's bleeding tendency. Those with low factor levels should receive prophylactic treatment (factor concentrate, tranexamic acid, desmopressin) to cover labour and delivery. A clotting factor activity greater than 40 IU/dL is usually safe for vaginal delivery and a level greater than 50 IU/dL is usually adequate for Caesarean section. In haemophilia carriers, epidurals may be permitted if the clotting factor is greater than 40 IU/dL. Invasive fetal monitoring, ventouse and rotational forceps should be avoided if the fetus may be affected, and cord blood samples collected for coagulation tests. Women with bleeding disorders are at significant risk of primary and secondary postpartum haemorrhage, and this risk can be minimized by appropriate prophylactic treatment.

Desmopressin (DDAVP) can be administered intravenously to increase factors VIII and VWF in those known to be responders pre-pregnancy, and is most effective in haemophilia A carriers and type 1 von Willebrand disease. DDAVP is usually reserved for postpartum treatment, due to concerns about inducing uterine contractions or causing vasoconstriction in pregnancy.

Neurological disorders

Epilepsy

Approximately 30 per cent of those with epilepsy are women in their childbearing years, which means 1 in 200–250 pregnancies occur in women with a history of epilepsy. Pregnancy has no consistent effect on epilepsy: some women will have an increased frequency of fits, others a decrease, and some no difference. Nonetheless, there is a ten-fold increase in mortality among pregnant women with epilepsy, and 1 in 26 maternal deaths occur in women with epilepsy. The principles of epilepsy management are that while the risks to pregnancy from seizures outweigh those from anticonvulsant medication, seizures should still be controlled with the minimum possible dose of the optimal drug.

Pre-pregnancy counselling

- Alter medication according to seizure frequency
- Reduce to monotherapy where possible
- Stress importance of compliance with medication
- Pre-conceptional folic acid 5 mg
- Explain risk of congenital malformation
- Explain risk from recurrent seizures

The principal concern related to epilepsy in pregnancy is the increased risk of congenital abnormality caused by anticonvulsant medications. All of these drugs are associated with a two- to three-fold increased risk of fetal abnormality (5–6 per cent) compared to the general population, and an approximate doubling of the risk compared to unexposed epileptic mothers.

Polytherapy further increases the risk (15–25 per cent). The major fetal abnormalities associated with anticonvulsant drugs (including sodium valproate, carbamazepine, phenytoin, phenobarbitone) are neural tube defects, facial clefts and cardiac defects. Many of these abnormalities are detectable by ultrasound and therefore all women should be offered detailed anomaly scanning. In addition, each drug is associated with a specific syndrome that includes developmental delay, nail hypoplasia, growth restriction and mid-face abnormalities. In the case of valproate, the likelihood of these effects is dose dependent (>1000 mg/day) and it should be generally avoided in women, with the exception of idiopathic generalized epilepsy where it controls tonic-clonic seizures. Despite the risks of continuing anticonvulsants in pregnancy, failure to do so may lead to an increased frequency of epileptic seizures that may result in both maternal and fetal hypoxia. Therefore, women on multiple drug therapy should, wherever possible, be converted to monotherapy before pregnancy, and all epileptic women should be advised to start taking a 5 mg daily folic acid supplement prior to conception. In women who have been free of seizures for two years, consideration may be given pre-pregnancy to discontinuing medication.

Many factors contribute to altered drug metabolism in pregnancy and result in a fall in anticonvulsant drug levels. The reasons for increased fit frequency in pregnancy therefore include the effect of pregnancy on the metabolism of anticonvulsant drugs, as well as sleep deprivation or stress and poor compliance with medication. Monitoring of drug levels in pregnancy is difficult. An increase in dosage to combat the anticipated fall may lead to an increased fetal risk. In the majority of cases, provided there is no increase in frequency of seizures, the prenatal drug dosage can be continued. However, an increase in seizure frequency or a recurrence of seizures, especially in the context of subtherapeutic drug levels, should prompt an increase in dosage.

Delivery mode and timing is largely unaltered by epilepsy, unless there has been accelerated seizure frequency in pregnancy, and anticonvulsant medication should be continued during labour. Breastfeeding can be encouraged, although feeding is best avoided for a few hours after taking medication. Information on safe handling of the neonate should be given to all epileptic mothers.

Causes of seizures in pregnancy

- Epilepsy
- Eclampsia
- Encephalitis or meningitis
- Space-occupying lesions (e.g. tumour, tuberculoma)
- Cerebral vascular accident
- Cerebral malaria or toxoplasmosis
- Thrombotic thrombocytopenic purpura
- Drug and alcohol withdrawal
- Toxic overdose
- Metabolic abnormalities (e.g. hypoglycaemia)

Multiple sclerosis

Multiple sclerosis (MS) causes disability through demyelination of the white matter, leading to weakness, lack of co-ordination, numbness in the hands or feet, blurred vision, tremor, spasticity and voiding dysfunction. Like most autoimmune diseases, more women than men are affected, and two-thirds of MS patients are women. One in 1000 pregnancies is estimated to occur in a woman with MS, and the onset of MS during pregnancy is unusual, with optic neuritis reported as the predominant symptom, usually postpartum. Pregnant women with MS are no more likely to experience complications in their pregnancy than those unaffected, nor are there increased risks of preterm delivery, intrauterine growth restriction or congenital malformation. The course of MS during pregnancy changes – a lower relapse rate has been shown, while the rate of relapse rises significantly during the first three months postpartum. Interestingly, pregnancy after MS onset may be associated with a lower risk of progression of the condition. Certainly, pregnancy has no adverse effect on the progression of long-term disability.

Apart from methotrexate and cyclophosphamide, pregnant women can safely take most drugs used regularly to treat MS. However, while it is unclear whether interferon-beta is teratogenic in humans, it is recommended that it be discontinued before pregnancy. Steroids are the treatment of choice for acute relapses and should be used where clinically indicated. Delivery is not more complicated in MS patients and the mode of delivery should be decided on the usual obstetric criteria. Regional anaesthesia is not contraindicated and no effect on the subsequent risk of relapse has been found.

Bell's palsy

Bell's palsy is a unilateral neuropathy of the seventh cranial nerve leading to paralysis of the forehead and lower face. Its incidence is increased ten-fold during the third trimester of pregnancy. The outcome is generally good and complete recovery may be anticipated if the time of onset is within 2 weeks of delivery. The role of corticosteroids and antiviral agents for Bell's palsy is controversial, but they may hasten recovery if given within the first 24 hours of the onset of symptoms. A reducing dose regime of steroids is used over a 10-day period. Bell's palsy does not affect pregnancy outcome.

Migraine

Migraine is influenced by cyclical changes in the sex hormones, and attacks often occur during the menstrual period, attributed to a fall in oestrogen levels. Migraine is generally seen to improve in pregnancy, with worsening of headache occurring very infrequently, although a considerable recurrence rate postpartum has been reported. Throughout pregnancy around 20 per cent of pregnant women will experience migraine, many of whom do not get migraines outwith pregnancy. Obstetric complications are not increased in migraine sufferers. Migraine during pregnancy should be treated with analgesics, anti-emetics and, where possible, avoidance of factors that trigger the attack. Low-dose aspirin or beta-blockers may be used to prevent attacks. If migraine occurs frequently, either low-dose aspirin or beta-blockers can be considered for prophylaxis.

Respiratory disease

Asthma

The worldwide prevalence of asthma is increasing, and with 3–12 per cent of pregnant women affected by asthma, it is the most common chronic disease in pregnancy. Asthma is not consistently affected by pregnancy and it is reported that, during pregnancy, the severity of asthma remains stable in one-third of women, worsens in another third and improves in the remaining third. However, prospective studies show that exacerbations of asthma are more likely to occur in women with severe asthma than mild asthma and that most episodes occur between 24 and 36 weeks of pregnancy.

It is not clear how asthma control before pregnancy impacts on pregnancy outcome. In contrast, there is evidence that adequate management during pregnancy decreases maternal and fetal morbidity. Asthma severity and suboptimal control are associated with adverse pregnancy outcomes. The effects of asthma on the fetus are still controversial and while systematic reviews report that FGR is more common in women with symptomatic asthma than in non-asthmatic women, the historic increased risk of preterm delivery is not borne out by prospective studies. Prolonged maternal hypoxia can lead to FGR and, ultimately, to fetal brain injury. An association between hypertension and asthma has also been suggested, and although there is an increase in gestational hypertension, asthma does not seem to be a risk factor for pre-eclampsia. Labour and delivery are not usually affected by asthma and attacks are uncommon in labour. Parenteral steroid cover may be needed for those who are on regular steroids, regular medications should be continued throughout labour and bronchoconstrictors, such as ergometrine or prostaglandin F2α, should be avoided. Adequate hydration is important in labour, and regional anaesthesia favoured over general, to decrease the risk of bronchospasm, provide adequate pain relief and to reduce oxygen consumption and minute ventilation. The inheritance risk of asthma for the fetus ranges from 6 to 30 per cent. Postpartum, there is no increased risk of exacerbations and those whose asthma deteriorated during pregnancy have usually returned to pre-pregnancy levels by three months after birth.

Features of severe life-threatening asthma
• Peak expiratory flow rate <35 per cent of predicted
• pO_2 <8 kPa
• pCO_2 >4.6 kPa
• Silent chest
• Cyanosis
• Bradycardia
• Arrhythmia
• Hypotension
• Exhaustion
• Confusion

Many women with asthma are concerned about the effect of drugs on the fetus, and this can lead to inappropriate cessation of treatment in early pregnancy. However, it is safer to take asthma drugs in pregnancy than to leave asthma uncontrolled. Inhaled beta-sympathomimetics are safe, as is theophylline, although its metabolism is altered and drug levels need to be monitored. Long-acting β_2 agonists like salmetrerol do not cause fetal malformation or FGR in prospective studies and there is limited systemic absorption. Inhaled corticosteroids prevent asthma exacerbations in pregnancy and have been shown to be safe with no association with fetal malformations or perinatal morbidity in large studies and reviews. Oral corticosteroid use in the first trimester has been associated with an increased risk of fetal cleft lip or palate in epidemiological studies, but the increase in risk is small and not confirmed in other work. Data are scarce on the safety of the relatively newer leukotriene antagonists, although no adverse outcomes have been reported.

Management of asthma in pregnancy

- Pregnancy is a time to improve asthma care
- Encourage smoking cessation
- Ensure patient education regarding condition and adequate use of medications
- Ensure optional control and response to therapy throughout pregnancy
- Manage exacerbations aggressively and avoid delays in treatment
- Manage acute attacks as in non-pregnant individual
- Offer a multidisciplinary team approach

Cystic fibrosis

Cystic fibrosis (CF) is an inherited autosomal recessive condition, with a carrier frequency of around 1 in 25 in the general population. The abnormal gene controls the movement of salt in the body, and as a result the internal organs become clogged with thick mucus, leading to infections and chronic inflammation, particularly affecting the lungs, gut and pancreas. Life expectancy is increasing, with over half the current CF population expected to live over 35 years. Therefore, more women are surviving to an age at which pregnancy is possible, and the estimates of pregnancy rates among women with CF range from 5 to 10 per cent.

Women with a higher FEV_1 and higher body weight have been shown to be more likely to become pregnant. The live birth rate ranges from 70 to 90 per cent and the rate of spontaneous miscarriage is no different to the general population. However, the prematurity rate is around 25 per cent, due to iatrogenic delivery where maternal health deteriorates, as well as a higher rate of spontaneous preterm labour with poorer maternal lung function. Pregnancy itself is probably not deleterious but the maternal prognosis is poor if there is pulmonary hypertension, infection with *Burkholderia cepacia*, if FEV_1 is <50 per cent predicted or if there is chronic hypoxia (pO_2 <7.3 kPa). Pre-existing diabetes also increases the risk of pregnancy complications, including preterm birth and stillbirth. While pregnancy does not significantly shorten survival, the long-term prognosis still needs consideration, as around 20 per cent of mothers will not live for ten years after delivery and 40 per cent of those with poor lung function at the start of pregnancy will die in this time period.

Pregnant women with CF should be jointly managed between the obstetrician and a respiratory physician with expertise in CF. Most women will have a daily physiotherapy regime and require prolonged antibiotic therapy and hospital admission during infective exacerbations. Close attention should be paid to maternal nutritional status and weight gain during pregnancy, with screening for gestational diabetes also indicated. Fetal growth and well-being should be monitored by serial ultrasound scans, as there is an association with FGR. It is also important to check the cystic fibrosis carrier status of the woman's partner, and the couple should be offered genetic counselling regarding the risks of the fetus having CF or being a carrier. Ideally, a vaginal delivery should be the aim and epidural analgesia offered.

Sarcoidosis

Sarcoidosis is a non-caseating granulomatosis that may affect any organ, but principally affects the lung and skin. Complications include severe progressive lung problems with pulmonary fibrosis, hypoxaemia and pulmonary hypertension, and these features are associated with a poor prognosis. Treatment is with corticosteroids. Sarcoidosis usually improves and is uncommonly diagnosed in pregnancy, although erythema nodosum, which may occur in both normal pregnancy and in sarcoidosis, may cause diagnostic confusion. Pregnancy does not influence the long-term natural history of sarcoidosis.

Pneumonia

Viral pneumonia follows a more complicated course in pregnancy, while bacterial pneumonia is not affected. The latter should be treated as in the non-pregnant state with penicillin or cephalosporins usually the first choice antibiotics, and erythromycin used if atypical organisms are suspected. Pneumonia complicates varicella infection in 10 per cent of pregnant women and can be severe, with complications increased in late gestation. Mortality rates of 20–40 per cent were reported before antiviral agents were used, but treatment with acyclovir >20 weeks gestation has reduced these rates to 1–3 per cent. Interestingly, both influenza A and severe acute respiratory syndrome (SARS) appear to be associated with more complications in pregnant women, with increased mortality rates and prolonged ventilation reported.

Pneumonia: warning signs

- Respiratory rate >30/minute
- Hypoxaemia; pO_2 <7.9 kPa on room air
- Acidosis; pH <7.3
- Hypotension
- Disseminated intravascular coagulation
- Elevated blood urea
- Evidence of multiple organ failure

Heart disease

Pre-pregnancy counselling

Most women with heart disease will be aware of their condition prior to becoming pregnant. Ideally, these women should be fully assessed before embarking on a pregnancy and the maternal and fetal risks carefully explained. A cardiologist should be involved in this assessment, which should include maternal echocardiography. Any concurrent medical problems should be aggressively treated, dental problems should be resolved and medical therapy optimized. If there is a possibility that the heart disease will require surgical correction, it is recommended that this should be undertaken before a pregnancy.

Issues in pre-pregnancy counselling of women with heart disease

- Risk of maternal death
- Possible reduction of maternal life expectancy
- Effects of pregnancy on cardiac disease
- Mortality associated with high risk conditions
- Risk of fetus developing congenital heart disease
- Risk of preterm labour and FGR
- Need for frequent hospital attendance and possible admission
- Intensive maternal and fetal monitoring during labour
- Other options – contraception, adoption, surrogacy
- Timing of pregnancy

Antenatal management

Experienced physicians and obstetricians should manage pregnant women with significant heart disease in a joint obstetric/cardiac clinic. Continuity of care makes the detection of subtle changes in maternal well-being more likely. In trying to distinguish between 'normal' symptoms of pregnancy and impending cardiac failure, it is important to ask the pregnant woman if she has noted any breathlessness, particularly at night, any change in her heart rate or rhythm, any increased tiredness or a reduction in exercise tolerance. Routine physical examination should include pulse rate and pressure, blood pressure, jugular venous pressure, ankle and sacral oedema, and presence of basal crepitations (Table 12.1).

Most women will remain well during the antenatal period and outpatient management is usually possible, although women should be advised to have a low threshold for reducing their normal physical activities (Tables 12.1 and 12.2). Echocardiography is non-invasive and useful in its ability to serially assess function and valves, and an echocardiogram at the booking visit and at around 28 weeks is usual. Any

Table 12.1 The stages of heart failure – New York Heart Association (NYHA) classification

Class	Patient symptoms
1: Mild	No limitation of physical activity. Ordinary physical activity does not precipitate fatigue, palpitations, dyspnoea, angina
2: Mild	Slight limitation of physical activity. Comfortable at rest, but ordinary physical activity results in fatigue, palpitation or dyspnoea
3: Moderate	Marked limitation of physical activity. Comfortable at rest, but less than ordinary activity causes fatigue, palpitation or dyspnoea
4: Severe	Unable to carry out any physical activity without discomfort. Symptoms of cardiac insufficiency at rest. If any physical activity is undertaken, discomfort is increased

Table 12.2 Toronto risk markers for maternal cardiac events

	Markers
1	Prior episode of heart failure, arrhythmia or stroke
2	NYHA class >II or cyanosis
3	Left heart obstruction
4	Reduced left ventricular function (EF <40 per cent)

0 predictors: risk of cardiac event is 5 per cent; 1 predictor: risk of cardiac event is 37 per cent; >1 predictors: risk of cardiac event is 75 per cent.

High-risk cardiac conditions

- Systemic ventricular dysfunction (ejection fraction <30 per cent, NYHA class III–IV)
- Pulmonary hypertension
- Cyanotic congenital heart disease
- Aortic pathology (dilated aortic root >4 cm, Marfan syndrome)
- Ischaemic heart disease
- Left heart obstructive lesions (aortic, mitral stenosis)
- Prosthetic heart valves (metal)
- Previous peripartum cardiomyopathy

Fetal risks of maternal cardiac disease

- Recurrence (congenital heart disease)
- Maternal cyanosis (fetal hypoxia)
- Iatrogenic prematurity
- FGR
- Effects of maternal drugs (teratogenesis, growth restriction, fetal loss)

signs of deteriorating cardiac status should be carefully investigated and treated. Hospital admission for bed rest will reduce the workload of the heart. The use of anticoagulants during pregnancy is a complicated issue because warfarin is teratogenic if used in the first trimester, and is linked with fetal intracranial haemorrhage in the third trimester (mainly at doses >5 mg daily). Low molecular weight heparin may be insufficient at preventing thrombosis in women with mechanical prosthetic heart valves, where the risk of valve thrombus is >10 per cent. Anticoagulation is essential in patients with congenital heart disease who have pulmonary hypertension, or artificial valve replacements, and in those in or at risk of atrial fibrillation. The options are either to continue warfarin for the pregnancy, or replace it with heparin between 6 and 12 weeks gestation to avoid the teratogenic risk.

Management of labour and delivery

In most cases, the aim of management is to await the onset of spontaneous labour, as this will minimize the risk of intervention and maximize the chances of a normal delivery. Induction of labour should be considered for the usual obstetric indications and in very high-risk women to ensure that delivery occurs at a reasonably predictable time when all the relevant personnel are present or available (Table 12.2). Epidural anaesthesia is often recommended, as this reduces the pain-related stress, and thereby some of the demand on cardiac function. However, regional anaesthesia is not without some risk to both the mother and baby in some cardiac conditions, principally because of the potential complication of maternal hypotension. The input of a senior anaesthetist to formulate and document an anaesthetic management plan and minimize the procedure-related risks is essential. Prophylactic antibiotics should be given to any woman with a structural heart defect to reduce the risk of bacterial endocarditis. Depending on the severity of the condition, other forms of monitoring may be appropriate during labour, including oxygen saturation and continuous arterial blood pressure monitoring.

Assuming normal progress in labour, the second stage may deliberately be kept short, with an elective forceps or ventouse delivery if normal delivery does not occur readily. This reduces maternal effort and the requirement for increased cardiac output. Caesarean section should only be performed for the normal obstetric indications. Caesarean delivery is associated with an increased risk of haemorrhage, thrombosis and infection; conditions that are likely to be much less well tolerated in women with cardiac disease. Postpartum haemorrhage in particular can lead to major cardiovascular instability. Ergometrine may be associated with intense vasoconstriction, hypertension and heart failure, and therefore active management of the third stage is usually with Syntocinon alone. Syntocinon is a vasodilator and therefore should be given slowly to patients with significant heart disease, with low-dose infusions preferable. High-level maternal surveillance is required until the main haemodynamic changes following delivery have passed.

Management of labour in women with heart disease

- Avoid induction of labour if possible
- Use prophylactic antibiotics
- Ensure fluid balance
- Avoid the supine position
- Discuss regional/epidural anaesthesia/analgesia with senior anaesthetist
- Keep the second stage short
- Use Syntocinon judiciously

Treatment of heart failure in pregnancy

The development of heart failure in pregnancy is dangerous, but the principles of treatment are the same as in the non-pregnant individual. The woman should be admitted and the diagnosis confirmed by clinical examination for signs of heart failure, and by echocardiography. Drug therapy may include diuretics, vasodilators and digoxin. Oxygen and morphine may also be required. Arrhythmias also require urgent correction and drug therapy, including adenosine for supraventricular tachycardias, and selective beta-adrenergic blockade may be required. In all cases, assessment of fetal well-being is essential and should include fetal ultrasound to assess fetal growth and regular cardiotocography (CTG). If there is evidence of fetal compromise, premature delivery may be considered. Similarly, in cases of intractable cardiac failure, the risks to the mother of continuing the pregnancy and the risks to the fetus of premature delivery must be carefully balanced.

Risk factors for the development of heart failure

- Respiratory or urinary infections
- Anaemia
- Obesity
- Corticosteroids
- Tocolytics
- Multiple gestation
- Hypertension
- Arrhythmias
- Pain-related stress
- Fluid overload

Specific conditions

Ischaemic heart disease

Up to 10 per cent of women who experience myocardial infarction (MI) are currently under the age of 35 years. The risk of MI during pregnancy is estimated as 1 in 10 000, and the peak incidence is in the third trimester, in parous women older than 35. The underlying pathology is frequently not atherosclerotic, and coronary artery dissection is the primary cause in the postpartum period. Before the current practice of percutaneous transluminal coronary angioplasty (PTCA), mortality was reported as 20–37 per cent for the mother and 17 per cent for the fetus. PTCA is now considered acceptable but should still be only used when absolutely necessary, avoiding the time when the fetus is most susceptible to radiation (8–15 weeks). There is little experience with thrombolytic therapy in pregnancy, and although not apparently teratogenic, there are risks of fetal and maternal haemorrhage. The diagnosis of MI in pregnant women is often missed, and prompt diagnosis and therapy are necessary to reduce the high associated maternal and perinatal mortality.

Mitral and aortic stenosis

Obstructive lesions of the left heart are well-recognized risk factors for maternal morbidity and mortality, as they result in an inability to increase cardiac output to meet the demands of pregnancy. Aortic stenosis is usually congenital and mitral stenosis usually rheumatic in origin. For those with known mitral stenosis, 40 per cent experience worsening symptoms in the pregnancy with the average time of onset of pulmonary oedema at 30 weeks. The aim of treatment is to reduce the heart rate, achieved through bed rest, oxygen, beta-blockade and diuretic therapy. Balloon mitral valvotomy is the treatment of choice after delivery, but can be considered in pregnancy depending on the clinical condition and gestation. Maternal mortality is reported at 2 per cent and the risk of an adverse fetal outcome is directly related to the severity of mitral stenosis. Pregnancy is usually well tolerated in women with isolated and mild and moderate aortic stenosis, with normal exercise capacity and good ventricular function. However, the risk of maternal death in those with severe aortic stenosis is reported as 17 per cent, with fetal mortality of 30 per cent. As with mitral stenosis, bed rest and medical treatment aims to reduce the heart rate to allow time for ventricular filling. If the woman's condition deteriorates before delivery is feasible, surgical intervention such as balloon or surgical aortic valvotomy can be considered, although there is less experience and success than with mitral stenosis.

Marfan syndrome

Marfan syndrome is an autosomal dominant connective tissue abnormality that may lead to mitral valve prolapse and aortic regurgitation, aortic root dilatation and aortic rupture or dissection. Pregnancy increases the risk of aortic rupture or dissection and has been associated with maternal mortality of up to 50 per cent where there is marked aortic root dilatation. Echocardiography is the principal investigation, as it is able to determine the size of the aortic root, and should be performed serially throughout pregnancy, especially in women who enter pregnancy with an aortic root that is already dilated (>4 cm). Women with an aortic root <4 cm should be reassured that their risks are lower, and the risk of an adverse cardiac event is around 1 per cent. A number of obstetric complications have also been described in women with Marfan syndrome: early pregnancy loss, preterm labour, cervical weakness, uterine inversion and postpartum haemorrhage.

Pulmonary hypertension

Pulmonary hypertension (PH) is characterized by an increase in the pulmonary vascular resistance resulting in an increased workload placed on the right side of the heart. The main symptoms are fatigue, breathlessness and syncope, and clinical signs are those of right heart failure. A median survival of less than three years from diagnosis has been reported. Specific treatments shown to improve symptoms and survival include endothelin blockers, such as bosentan, and phosphodiesterase inhibitors, such as sildenafil. More complex therapies include nebulized, subcutaneous and intravenous prostaglandins.

In women with pulmonary hypertension, pregnancy is associated with a high risk of maternal death. The demands of increasing blood volume and cardiac output may not be met by an already compromised right ventricle, and any decline in cardiac performance in pregnancy represents a life-threatening event. Women may deteriorate early (second trimester) or in the immediate postpartum period. Disease progress can be assessed with echocardiography and exercise capacity using the incremental walking test, which correlates well with cardiac output and mortality in pulmonary hypertension, but the natural history of the disease in pregnancy is still unpredictable.

Close monitoring by a multidisciplinary team is crucial. A variety of approaches to management are reported but despite this, the mortality of the condition remains high at 30–50 per cent. It is currently recommended that women with pulmonary hypertension should be strongly advised against pregnancy and given clear contraceptive advice, with early termination advised in the event of pregnancy. When women who are fully informed of the risks choose to continue their pregnancy, targeted pulmonary vascular therapy is an option, with timely admission to hospital and delivery according to the progress of the woman and condition of the fetus.

Classification of PH

- Pulmonary arterial hypertension
  - Idiopathic – sporadic or familial
  - Persistent PH of the newborn
  - Associated with:
    - collagen vascular disease
    - congenital pulmonary to systemic shunts
    - drugs or toxins
    - portal hypertension
- PH with left heart disease
- PH with lung disease
- PH due to thrombosis and/or embolic disease

Hypertensive disorders

Hypertensive disease complicates 5–7 per cent of all pregnancies. It can be categorized into pre-existing hypertension, pregnancy-induced hypertension and pre-eclampsia. Pre-existing hypertension may be diagnosed before gestation or assumed when a woman is found to be hypertensive in early pregnancy. Pregnancy-induced hypertension occurs when new-onset hypertension develops in the second half of pregnancy (usually defined as after the 20th week) but in the absence of significant proteinuria or any other features of pre-eclampsia.

Classification of hypertension in pregnancy

- Gestational hypertension
  - gestational hypertension (no proteinuria)
  - gestational proteinuria (no hypertension)
  - pre-eclampsia (proteinuria and hypertension)
- Pre-existing hypertension and/or renal disease
  - chronic hypertension (no proteinuria)
  - chronic renal disease (hypertension and/or proteinuria)
  - chronic hypertension with superimposed pre-eclampsia
- Unclassified hypertension and proteinuria

Definition

Hypertension is defined as changes of blood pressure recorded on at least two occasions:

- diastolic blood pressure 90 mmHg, or
- systolic blood pressure 140 mmHg.

Chronic hypertension

Essential hypertension is the underlying cause in 90 per cent of cases. However, before a diagnosis is made, other causes need to be excluded. Appropriate investigations include serum creatinine, electrolytes and urate, liver function tests, urine analysis (blood, protein and glucose), 24-hour urinary protein/creatinine clearance, renal ultrasound, autoantibody screen and cardiac investigations including electrocardiography (ECG) and echocardiography. Renal causes account for over 80 per cent of cases of secondary hypertension.

Causes of chronic hypertension

- Idiopathic
  - essential hypertension
- Renal disease
  - polycystic disease
  - diabetic nephropathy
  - chronic glomerulonephritis
  - nephrotic and nephritic syndrome
- Vascular disorders
  - renal artery stenosis
  - coarctation of the aorta
- Collagen vascular disease
  - systemic sclerosis
  - systemic lupus erythematosus
  - rheumatoid disease
- Endocrine disease
  - phaeochromocytoma
  - Conn's syndrome
  - Cushing's syndrome
  - diabetes mellitus

The maternal risks of pre-existing hypertension include pre-eclampsia, abruption, heart failure and intracerebral haemorrhage. Pre-eclampsia may develop in around one-third of women with pre-existing hypertension and is more likely to occur in those with severe hypertension and/or renal disease.

Management of chronic hypertension

In mild cases (<150/100 mmHg) there is no immediate indication to treat; however, the pregnancy should be monitored carefully to detect rising blood pressure or features of pre-eclampsia, as well as FGR by serial ultrasound scans. Women who are receiving antihypertensive medication before pregnancy are often able to discontinue this for the first part of pregnancy because of the physiological fall in blood pressure at this time. Some antihypertensives, such as angiotensin-converting enzyme inhibitors, should be discontinued because of the fetal risk.

If the blood pressure is consistently noted to be >150/100 mmHg, antihypertensive medication will need to be introduced or recommenced. This is to reduce the risk of severe hypertension and the attendant risks of intracerebral haemorrhage, although treatment does not prevent placental abruption or superimposed pre-eclampsia, nor influence perinatal outcome. Preferred antihypertensive agents include methyldopa (centrally acting agent) – which is generally well tolerated, especially if women are forewarned about the common transient side effects of lethargy and postural hypotension – labetolol (alpha- and beta-blocker), and nifedipine (calcium-channel blocker). The aim of antihypertensive medication is to maintain the blood pressure below 160 mmHg systolic and 100–110 mmHg diastolic.

The obstetric management of pre-existing hypertension involves close monitoring for the development of superimposed pre-eclampsia, which may present with elevated blood pressure, new-onset or worsening proteinuria, as well as the development of FGR. Each case must be individually assessed, but early delivery is rarely indicated unless pre-eclampsia develops or the blood pressure is very difficult to control. In general, it is reasonable to await spontaneous labour or attempt vaginal delivery by induction of labour (at around 38 weeks), ensuring the maternal blood pressure is well controlled. Post-natally, the maternal blood pressure will often decrease, but careful observation is required in the first 48 hours because blood pressure tends to increase again on the third or fourth postpartum day. Breastfeeding is encouraged and although some antihypertensive medication may enter the breast milk, the standard antihypertensive medications are not contraindicated in breastfeeding mothers.

Risk factors for developing superimposed pre-eclampsia

- Renal disease
- Maternal age >40 years
- Pre-existing diabetes
- Multiple pregnancy
- Connective tissue disease, e.g. antiphospholipid syndrome
- Coarctation of the aorta
- Blood pressure ≥160/100 mmHg in early pregnancy
- Pre-pregnancy BMI >35
- Previous pre-eclampsia
- Antiphospholipid syndrome

Renal disease

Women with chronic kidney disease are less able to make the renal adaptations necessary for a healthy pregnancy and pregnancy in women with renal disease therefore requires increased maternal and fetal surveillance.

Pre-pregnancy counselling

Pre-pregnancy counselling is recommended in all women with chronic kidney disease and they should be made aware of the risks to the fetus and to their long-term renal function before conception.

Pre-pregnancy counselling discussion should include:

- Safe contraception until pregnancy advised
- Fertility issues if indicated
- Genetic counselling if inherited disorder
- Risks to mother and fetus during pregnancy
- Avoid known teratogens and contraindicated drugs
- Management of antihypertensives
- Low-dose aspirin for most pregnancies

- Need for anticoagulation once pregnant in some conditions
- Need for compliance with strict surveillance
- Likelihood of prolonged admission or early delivery
- Possibility of accelerated decline in maternal renal function
- Need for postpartum follow up.

Chronic kidney disease

Chronic kidney disease (CKD) is classified into five stages based on the level of renal function (Table 12.3). Stages 1 and 2 affect around 3 per cent of women of childbearing age (20–39), and while stages 3–5 affect 1 in 150 women in this age group, pregnancy in these women is less common. Some women are found to have CKD for the first time in their pregnancy, and pregnancy can unmask previously unrecognized renal disease.

Table 12.3 Stages of chronic kidney disease

Stage	Description	Estimated GFR (mL/min/1.73m²)
1	Kidney damage with normal/raised GFR	>90
2	Kidney damage with mildly low GFR	60–89
3	Moderately low GFR	30–59
4	Severely low GFR	15–29
5	Kidney failure	<15 or dialysis

GFR, glomerular filtration rate.

Effect of pregnancy on CKD

Women with CKD stages 1–2 have mild renal dysfunction and usually have an uneventful pregnancy and good renal outcome. Pregnancy with a serum creatinine <110 μmol/L, minimal proteinuria (<1 g/24 hours), and absent or well-controlled hypertension pre-pregnancy has been shown to have little or no adverse effect on long-term maternal renal function. Women with moderate to severe disease (stages 3–5) are at highest risk of complications during pregnancy and of an accelerated decline in their renal function. Pre-existing hypertension and proteinuria greatly increase the risk. If pre-eclampsia develops, maternal renal function often deteriorates further, but any other additional complications, such as postpartum haemorrhage or use of non-steroidal anti-inflammatory drugs, can critically threaten maternal renal function.

Effect of CKD on pregnancy outcome

Pregnancies in mothers with CKD have increased risks of preterm delivery, delivery by Caesarean section (40 per cent) and FGR (increased two-fold). Diastolic blood pressure has been suggested as the greatest risk factor for fetal death, but overall fetal survival is reported at around 95 per cent. The risk of adverse pregnancy outcome correlates with the degree of renal dysfunction (Table 12.4).

Monitoring of patients with CKD during pregnancy

- Blood pressure
- Renal function
  - creatinine

Table 12.4 Estimated effects of renal function on pregnancy outcome and maternal renal function

	Mean pre-pregnancy serum creatinine value		
	<125	125–180	>180
Fetal growth restriction (%)	25	40	65
Preterm delivery (%)	30	60	>90
Pre-eclampsia (%)	22	40	60
Loss of <25% renal function postpartum (%)	0	20	50
End-stage renal failure after 1 year (%)	0	2	35

Data adapted from Williams D, Davison JM. Chronic kidney disease in pregnancy. *BMJ* 2008; 326: 211–5.

- Urine
  - infection
  - proteinuria
- Full blood count
  - haemoglobin
  - ferritin
- Renal ultrasound
- Fetal ultrasound
  - anatomy
  - uterine artery Doppler 20–24 weeks
  - growth.

Dialysis

The incidence of pregnancy on dialysis (stage 5 CKD) is increasing. Dialysis must be adjusted to allow for the physiological changes of pregnancy (plasma volume, fluid retention, electrolytes), and haemodialysis is usually more effective then peritoneal dialysis in achieving this. Complications include preterm delivery, polyhydramnios (30–60 per cent), pre-eclampsia (40–80 per cent) and Caesarean delivery (50 per cent). If conceived on dialysis, 50 per cent of infants survive, but pregnancy before dialysis has a better outcome.

Pregnancy in women with renal transplants

Women with end-stage kidney disease have hypothalamic-gonadal dysfunction and infertility, so conception is rare. Female fertility returns rapidly after renal transplantation and it is estimated that 2–10 per cent of female recipients conceive. Of pregnancies progressing beyond the third trimester, the vast majority (>90 per cent) result in a successful pregnancy outcome. Most transplantation centres advise that conception is safe after the second post-transplantation year, provided the graft is functioning well and no rejection episodes occur in the year before conception.

All pregnancies in transplant recipients are high risk and should be managed by a multidisciplinary team. Lower immunosuppressive steroid dosage, longer time since transplantation and better graft function with absence of chronic rejection, are all associated with better maternal outcomes. Complications of pregnancy in renal transplant patients include high rates of pregnancy-induced hypertension (30–50 per cent), preterm delivery (40–60 per cent), pre-eclampsia

(10–40 per cent) and urinary tract infection (20–40 per cent). Diagnosing pre-eclampsia can be difficult due to the normal rise in blood pressure after 20 weeks and the presence of pre-existing proteinuria. The risk of acute rejection in pregnancy is estimated at 2–10 per cent, and allograft dysfunction may also be difficult to detect during pregnancy. Vaginal delivery is safe, with Caesarean section considered for the usual obstetric indications. From 5 to 15 per cent of women have worse graft function after pregnancy.

Monitoring of renal transplant patients during pregnancy

- Renal function
  - blood pressure
  - creatinine
  - proteinuria
- Drug levels
- Fetal growth
- If renal function declines, exclude
  - obstruction
  - infection
  - rejection.

Predictors of fetal outcome include pre-pregnancy maternal hypertension, diabetes mellitus and maternal drug treatment. Many women have concerns about the immunosuppressive drugs used post-transplantation, and since immunosuppressive medications must be continued throughout pregnancy, the fetus is inevitably exposed to potential fetotoxic and teratogenic agents throughout development. The actual effects of medications on growth and development are difficult to determine and may not be obvious at birth. It is also difficult to assess the relative effects of immunosuppressive agents, since underlying maternal diseases, as well as the concurrent use of other drugs confound interpretation. Prednisolone, azathioprine, cyclosporin and tacrolimus are considered safe.

Gastroenterology

Peptic ulcer disease

Peptic ulceration is less common in pregnancy and pre-existing ulceration tends to improve, probably due to altered oestrogen levels and the improved maternal diet in pregnancy. Complications, such as haemorrhage or perforation, are rare. Treatment with antacids and common anti-ulcer medication (e.g. Ranitidine, Omeprazole) is safe and endoscopy may be performed if indicated by bleeding, epigastric pain or protracted vomiting.

Coeliac disease

Coeliac disease is a gluten-sensitive enteropathy with a prevalence of around 0.3–1 per cent in the general population. It has been estimated that up to 1 in 70 pregnant women are affected by coeliac disease but that many are undiagnosed. Untreated coeliac disease is associated with high rates of spontaneous miscarriage and other adverse pregnancy outcomes such as FGR. There are no specific guidelines for pregnant women with coeliac disease. Standard nutritional advice during pregnancy is appropriate and general guidelines are suitable, in particular advice to take folic acid supplements should be followed. Depending on individual assessment and diet, supplementation with calcium, iron and vitamin B_{12} may also be required.

Inflammatory bowel disease

The majority of patients with inflammatory bowel disease (IBD) are diagnosed during their reproductive years (incidence 5–10 per 100 000), and women with IBD have similar fertility rates to the general population. Pregnancy does not usually alter the course of IBD. However, women with IBD have higher rates of preterm delivery and low birthweight infants, so these pregnancies need to be managed as high-risk pregnancies. Predictors of poor outcome include new-onset IBD, disease activity and previous bowel resection. Overall, there is around a 30 per cent risk of a flare during pregnancy, which increases to 50 per cent if the disease is active at the time of conception. Pregnant women with either ulcerative colitis or Crohn's disease have been shown to have similar rates of disease exacerbation, although flares in the first trimester and postpartum are more common in Crohn's disease. Supplementation with high-dose folic acid (5 mg daily) is recommended and supplemental vitamins D and B_{12} may also be indicated. There is an increased rate of delivery by Caesarean section in IBD. These decisions should be made for the usual obstetric indications, with two exceptions – where there is active perianal disease in Crohn's disease, or where there is an ileoanal pouch.

The use of medication during conception and pregnancy is a cause of concern for many patients with IBD. Methotrexate is contraindicated, but the majority of other medications used to induce or maintain remission, including amniosalicylates and corticosteroids, are considered low risk. The use of azothiaprine and cyclosporin has not been associated with an increase in congenital malformation rates and these drugs are often continued in pregnancy to keep the mother in remission, especially where other drugs have failed. Experience with biological therapy is growing and increasing evidence suggests agents like infliximab are low risk in pregnancy. A relapse of IBD in pregnancy may be treated with aminosalicylates, corticosteroid enemas and high-dose prednisolone (30–60 mg per day with a step-wise reduction).

Pancreatitis

Pancreatitis rarely complicates pregnancy and is not more common in pregnancy. The clinical presentation combines nausea and vomiting with severe epigastric pain, and attacks usually occur in the third trimester of pregnancy. The commonest cause of pancreatitis in pregnancy is gallstones, followed by alcohol, with hypertriglyceridaemia and hyperparathyroidism much rarer causes. Management is supportive, with 10 per cent of women developing significant cardiac, renal and gastrointestinal complications necessitating intensive care.

Liver disease

Viral hepatitis

Viral hepatitis is the commonest cause of jaundice in pregnancy worldwide. Acute viral hepatitis in the first trimester of pregnancy is associated with a higher rate of spontaneous miscarriage. The clinical features of hepatitis are no different to the non-pregnant patient, with the exception of hepatitis E infection and herpes simplex hepatitis. Hepatitis E is more likely to lead to fulminant hepatic failure in pregnancy, and is more common in primagravida and in the third trimester. There is also a significant association with obstetric complications, such as preterm delivery, fetal growth restriction and stillbirth. In underdeveloped countries, 20 per cent of women infected in the third trimester die of fulminant hepatitis. Herpes simplex hepatitis is rare.

While complications are common and associated perinatal mortality high, antiviral agents like acyclovir have dramatically improved outcomes.

The incidence of hepatitis A in pregnancy is around 1 in 1000 and fetal transmission is extremely rare. Acute hepatitis B infection occurs in 1–2 per 1000 pregnancies and 1.5 per cent of pregnant women are chronic carriers. There is no evidence that hepatitis B is any more common in pregnancy. The prevalence of hepatitis C in pregnant women is estimated at 1–2 per cent. Hepatitis C infection is also associated with several adverse pregnancy outcomes, such as preterm rupture of membranes and gestational diabetes, as well as adverse neonatal outcomes, including low birthweight and neonatal unit admission (Table 12.5 and see Chapter 13, Perinatal infections).

Autoimmune hepatitis

Autoimmune hepatitis (chronic active hepatitis) is characterized by progressive hepatic parenchymal destruction, eventually leading to cirrhosis. Its course in pregnancy is variable, with flares reported throughout gestation, and there is a considerable risk of decompensation postpartum. High fetal loss rates (around 20 per cent) have been reported. Immunosuppressive therapy should be continued during pregnancy.

Gallstones

The prevalence of gallstones in pregnancy is around 19 per cent in multiparous women and 8 per cent

in nulliparous women. Acute cholecystitis occurs in around 0.1 per cent of pregnant women. The aetiology of increased biliary sludge and gallstones in pregnancy is multifactorial. Increased oestrogen levels lead to increased cholesterol secretion and supersaturation of bile, and increased progesterone levels cause a decrease in small intestinal motility. Conservative medical management is recommended initially, especially during the first and third trimesters, in which surgical intervention may confer a risk of miscarriage or premature labour, respectively. Medical management involves intravenous fluids, correction of electrolytes, bowel rest, pain management and broad-spectrum antibiotics. However, relapse rates (40–90 per cent) are high during pregnancy and surgical intervention may be warranted, preferentially performed (open or laparoscopic cholecystectomy) in the second trimester.

Primary biliary cirrhosis

Primary biliary cirrhosis (PBC) is an autoimmune disorder characterized by progressive destruction of intrahepatic bile ducts, which ultimately leads to portal hypertension and hepatic failure. PBC is usually associated with reduced fertility and repeated pregnancy loss, with worsening liver function historically reported in pregnancy. More recent series suggest that women maintained on urso-deoxycholic acid tolerate pregnancy well, with no deterioration in liver function, but a risk of flare postpartum is reported.

Table 12.5 Viral hepatitis in pregnancy

	Hepatitis A	Hepatitis B	Hepatitis C	Hepatitis D ('delta')	Hepatitis E	Hepatitis G
Transmission	Faecal-oral	Parenteral Mucosal Sexual	Parenteral Mucosal Sexual	Parenteral	Faecal-oral	Parenteral
Chronic disease	None	2–6% adults	80%	70–80%	None	Rare
Fetal transmission	Rare	20–30%	5–10%	Cases reported	No cases reported	No cases reported
Vaccination	Safe in pregnancy	Safe in pregnancy	None available	HBV safe in pregnancy	None available	None available

HBV, hepatitis B virus.

Cirrhosis

Cirrhosis is not a contraindication to pregnancy, which may be well tolerated if cirrhosis is compensated and without features of portal hypertension. This latter leads to increased risks of maternal complications including variceal haemorrhage, hepatic failure, encephalopathy, jaundice and malnutrition. Bleeding from oesophageal varices has been reported in 25 per cent of pregnant women with cirrhosis, and therefore all pregnant women with cirrhosis should be screened for varices from the second trimester.

Connective tissue disease

Systemic lupus erythematosus

Systemic lupus erythematosus (SLE) is a chronic autoimmune inflammatory disease. It is ten times more common in women, particularly in black and Asian populations, and the incidence is around 1 in 1000 women. It may cause disease in any system, but principally it affects the joints (90 per cent), skin (80 per cent), lungs, nervous system, kidneys and heart. SLE may be diagnosed prenatally or may be suspected for the first time during pregnancy or postpartum, usually as a result of complications. The diagnosis is suggested by the finding of a positive assay for antinuclear antibodies while the presence of antibodies to double-stranded DNA is the most specific for SLE. If 4 of the 11 criteria in the ACR classification system for SLE are present serially or simultaneously, a person is said to have SLE.

American College of Rheumatology (ACR) criteria for classification of SLE

1. Malar rash
2. Discoid rash
3. Photosensitivity
4. Oral ulcers
5. Non-erosive arthritis
6. Pleuritis or pericarditis
7. Renal disorder
8. Neurologic disorder
9. Haematologic disorder
10. Immunologic disorder
11. Positive anti-nuclear antibody

SLE is characterized by periods of disease activity, flares and remissions. Pregnancy increases the risk of flares, but these also become more difficult to diagnose accurately due to coincident pregnancy symptoms. Flares are more common in the late second and third trimesters, and are no more severe than in non-pregnancy. Active disease at the time of conception or new-onset SLE in pregnancy both increase the chance of a flare. SLE is associated with significant risks of miscarriage, fetal death, pre-eclampsia, preterm delivery and FGR. Women with lupus nephritis are at greater risk of these adverse outcomes, although pregnancy does not seem to alter renal function in the long term, and their risk of overall deterioration is higher. Pregnancy outcome is also adversely affected by pre-existing hypertension and the presence of antiphospholipid antibodies.

Differentiation of SLE flare from pre-eclampsia

Pre-eclampsia
- Hypertension
- Proteinuria
- Thrombocytopenia
- Renal impairment

SLE
- Rising anti-DNA titre
- Fall in complement levels
- No increase in serum uric acid
- No abnormal liver function

The term 'antiphospholipid syndrome' (APS) is used to describe the association of anti-cardiolipin antibodies (aCL) and/or lupus anticoagulant (LA) with the typical clinical features of arterial or venous thrombosis, fetal loss after 10 weeks, three or more miscarriages at less than 10 weeks, or delivery before 34 weeks due to intrauterine growth restriction or pre-eclampsia. APS may be primary or found in association with SLE.

Classification criteria for APS

Clinical
- Thrombosis
  - venous
  - arterial

- Pregnancy morbidity
  - fetal death >10 weeks
  - preterm birth <35 weeks due to severe pre-eclampsia or growth restriction
  - three or more unexplained miscarriages <10 weeks
- **Laboratory**
- aCL immunoglobulin (Ig)G and/or IgM
  - medium/high titre
  - two occasions, 8 weeks apart
- LA
  - two occasions, 8 weeks apart

Due to these significant risks, pregnant women with SLE and APS require intensive monitoring for both maternal and fetal indications. The mother should book early to multidisciplinary care and be seen frequently. Baseline renal studies, including a 24-hour urine collection for protein, should be performed. Blood pressure should be monitored closely because of the increased risk of pre-eclampsia. Serial ultrasonography is performed to assess fetal growth, umbilical artery Doppler and liquor volume. If antenatal treatment is required for SLE, steroids, azathioprine, sulphasalazine and hydroxycloroquine may be given safely. Non-steroidal anti-inflammatory drugs should be avoided in the third trimester because of adverse effects on the fetus. In women with APS who have suffered repeated pregnancy loss or severe obstetric complications, the combined use of low-dose aspirin and low-molecular-weight heparin has been shown to reduce the pregnancy loss rate.

Finally, 30 per cent of mothers with SLE also have anti-Ro/LA antibodies, which cross the placenta causing immune damage in the fetus. Several clinical syndromes result, including neonatal lupus and congenital heart block. The risk of neonatal lupus is round 5 per cent, rising to 25 per cent if a previous child was affected, and it manifests as cutaneous lesions 2–3 weeks after birth, disappearing spontaneously without scarring within six months. The risk of congenital heart block is around 2 per cent. It appears *in utero*, is detected at 18–20 weeks, is permanent and difficult to treat and is associated with a 20 per cent rate of perinatal mortality. Of those who survive, over 50 per cent need pacemakers in early infancy. There is a 16 per cent recurrence risk in subsequent pregnancies.

Rheumatoid arthritis

Rheumatoid arthritis (RA) is a chronic inflammatory autoimmune disease affecting primarily the synovial joints. It affects more women than men, and around 1 in 1000 pregnancies is affected. Most women with RA (75 per cent) experience improvement during pregnancy but only 16 per cent enter complete remission from symptoms of the disease. Of those who improve, 90 per cent suffer a flare postpartum. Unlike other connective tissue diseases, no adverse effect of RA on pregnancy is reported, and there is no increase in pregnancy loss rates. The main concern of RA patients is the safety of medication used to control the disease. If paracetamol-based analgesics are insufficient, corticosteroids are preferred to non-steroidal anti-inflammatory drugs, although the latter can be used up to 32 weeks if needed. Azothiaprine and hydroxychloroquine have been used in pregnancy, with no increase in malformation rates reported and no apparent adverse outcomes. Mode of delivery is determined by the usual obstetric indications, except where severe RA limits hip abduction and vaginal delivery is not possible.

Scleroderma

Scleroderma may be either a localized cutaneous form or systemic sclerosis, associated with Raynaud's phenomenon and characterized by progressive fibrosis of skin, oesophagus, lungs, heart and kidneys. No treatment has been shown to influence the course of scleroderma and treatment is usually symptomatic. Women with systemic sclerosis may deteriorate in pregnancy, although it is unclear if this is due to the pregnancy, and those with multi-organ involvement are often advised against pregnancy. The main risks are for those recently diagnosed, with pulmonary hypertension, or with renal disease where rapid deterioration is possible. There are associated adverse fetal outcomes, with increased rates of preterm delivery, pre-eclampsia, growth restriction and perinatal mortality. Finally, venous access, blood pressure monitoring and invasive monitoring may be difficult because of skin and blood vessel involvement.

Endocrinology

Diabetes

Diabetes may complicate a pregnancy either because a woman has pre-existing insulin-dependent diabetes mellitus (IDDM) or non-insulin-dependent diabetes mellitus (NIDDM) before pregnancy or because she develops usually transient impaired glucose tolerance or diabetes during the course of her pregnancy.

Pre-pregnancy counselling

The aim of pre-pregnancy counselling is to achieve the best possible glycaemic control before pregnancy and to educate diabetic women about the implications of pregnancy. Patient information leaflets about pregnancy should make clear the risks of pregnancy in diabetes, and include advice to take high dose (5 mg) folic acid pre-conception and for the first 12 weeks. Hyperglycaemia exerts its teratogenic effects during the period of organogenesis – the first 42 days of pregnancy – often before the pregnancy is medically confirmed. The level of HbA1c in early pregnancy correlates well with the risk of early fetal loss and congenital abnormality. Once HbA1c is >10 per cent, the risk of fetal loss during pregnancy is around 30 per cent, while the risk of congenital malformation is similar. Pre-pregnancy care could significantly reduce the rates of congenital malformation. Therefore, diabetes therapy should be intensified and adequate contraception used until glucose control is good. Targets for therapy pre-pregnancy should be to maintain HbA1c at 6.5 per cent and pre-meal glucose levels of 4–7 mmol/L. Finally, for women with established diabetic nephropathy, the chance of successful pregnancy diminishes sharply as serum creatinine increases (80 per cent chance if 125–180 µmol/L, 75 per cent chance if 180–220 µmol/L and 60 per cent chance if >220 µmol/L). The higher the pre-pregnancy creatinine concentrations, the higher the risk of permanent loss of renal function.

Maternal and fetal complications of diabetes

Congenital abnormality is the most important cause of fetal mortality and morbidity in diabetic pregnancies and is seen two to four times more often than in normal pregnancies, with a three-fold excess of cardiac and neural tube defects. Malformations at present account for 40 per cent of the perinatal mortality associated with diabetic pregnancies. Apart from structural malformations, fetal macrosomia is a major problem associated with traumatic birth, shoulder dystocia and therefore possible hypoxic damage, and still occurs in around one-fifth of diabetic pregnancies. Accelerated growth patterns are typically seen in the late second and third trimesters and are associated with poorly controlled diabetes. Sudden, unexplained, late stillbirths historically occurred in 10–30 per cent of diabetic pregnancies, but are much less common now that the importance of good diabetic control and timely delivery is appreciated. However, this remains a risk in women whose diabetes is poorly controlled and in pregnancies complicated by fetal macrosomia or polyhydramnios.

In general, maternal morbidity in diabetic pregnancies is related to the severity of diabetic-related disease preceding the pregnancy, and those most at risk have pre-existing coronary artery disease. The risk of pre-eclampsia is increased two- to four-fold in women with diabetes, and particularly in those with coexisting microalbuminuria or frank nephropathy. Women with diabetic retinopathy are at risk of progression of the disease and should be kept under careful surveillance (retinal screening at booking, 16–20 weeks and 28 weeks). Other complications include an increased incidence of infection, severe hyperglycaemia or hypoglycaemia, diabetic ketoacidosis and the complications that may arise from the increased operative delivery rate.

Management in pregnancy

Pregnant women with diabetes should be managed in a joint clinic with an obstetrician and physician. Input from a dietician is also important and often a nurse or midwife specialist will act as an adviser to adjust the dose of insulin. Women with pre-existing diabetes should be referred directly to this clinic at booking, and those in whom a diagnosis of gestational diabetes is made at a later stage should also be referred. A plan for the pregnancy should be set out and should include targets for glycaemic control, renal and retinal screening, fetal surveillance and plan for delivery.

The aim of treatment is to maintain blood glucose levels as near normal as possible with a combination of diet and insulin, and control is achieved by matching insulin dose with food intake. Insulin doses will change in pregnancy due to the physiological increase in insulin resistance. Targets for therapy are to maintain HbA1c <6 per cent, with pre-meal glucose levels at 3.5–5.5 mmol/L and 2-hour postprandial levels of 4–6.5 mmol/L. This relative normoglycaemia means that asymptomatic hypoglycaemia can occur more frequently. Therefore, careful self-monitoring of glucose levels by women with diabetes is a critical aspect of care.

Obstetric management is aimed initially at ensuring that the appropriate screening tests are performed, including nuchal translucency scanning, detailed ultrasound assessment for fetal anomalies and fetal echocardiography. Serial growth scans are recommended to detect fetal macrosomia and polyhydramnios, although this is rarely a problem before the third trimester. Any concern for fetal well-being should lead to increased surveillance with Doppler ultrasound and CTG. If antenatal corticosteroids are indicated, an increase of 40 per cent at the time of the first dose and until 24 hours after the second dose will usually prevent loss of control. Timing and mode of delivery should be determined on an individual basis. In general, provided the pregnancy has gone well, management aims to achieve a vaginal delivery between 38 and 39 weeks. However, the development of macrosomia or maternal complications such as pre-eclampsia, together with the rate of failed induction, is such that the Caesarean section rate among diabetic women often is as high as 50 per cent. A sliding scale of insulin and glucose should be commenced in labour, and maternal blood glucose levels maintained at 4–8 mmol/L to reduce risks of neonatal hypoglycaemia. The insulin dose can be halved after delivery.

Effects of pregnancy on diabetes
• Change in eating pattern
• Increase in insulin dose requirements
• Greater importance of tight glucose control
• Increased risk of severe hypoglycaemia
• Risk of deterioration of pre-existing retinopathy
• Risk of deterioration of established nephropathy

Effects of diabetes on pregnancy
• Increased risk of miscarriage
• Risk of congenital malformation
• Risk of macrosomia
• Increased risk of pre-eclampsia
• Increased risk of stillbirth
• Increased risk of infection
• Increased operative delivery rate

Gestational diabetes

Gestational diabetes (GDM) occurs in 2–9 per cent of all pregnancies. Screening for diabetes in pregnancy can be justified to diagnose previously unrecognized cases of pre-existing diabetes and to identify a group of women who are at risk of developing NIDDM later in life. No single screening test has been shown to be perfect in terms of high sensitivity and specificity for gestational diabetes. Urinary glucose is unreliable, and most screening tests now rely on blood glucose estimation, with an oral glucose tolerance test commonly used. The aim of glucose control is to keep fasting levels between 3.5 and 5.5 mmol/L and postprandial levels <7.1 mmol/L, with insulin treatment usually indicated outside these ranges.

GDM is associated with significant rates of maternal and perinatal complications, including macrosomia and its related complications, hypoglycaemia and long-term diabetes. While these risks are well recognized, there has been confusion whether screening and treatment to reduce maternal glucose levels affects outcomes. Recent well-conducted studies suggested that treatment of GDM including dietary advice, blood glucose monitoring and insulin therapy does reduce the rate of serious perinatal outcomes and further reported that maternal hyperglycaemia less severe than that used to define overt diabetes is related to clinically significant problems.

Factors associated with poor pregnancy outcome in diabetes
• Maternal social deprivation
• No folic acid intake pre-pregnancy
• Suboptimal approach of the woman to managing her diabetes
• Suboptimal pre-conception care
• Suboptimal glycaemic control at any stage
• Suboptimal maternity care during pregnancy
• Suboptimal fetal surveillance of big babies

From *Diabetes in pregnancy*, CEMACH, 2007.

Thyroid disease

Thyroid disease is common in women of childbearing age. However, symptoms of thyroid disease, such as heat intolerance, constipation, fatigue, palpitations and weight gain resemble those of normal pregnancy. Physiological changes of pregnancy, including plasma volume expansion, increased thyroid binding globulin production and relative iodine deficiency, also mean that thyroid hormone reference ranges for non-pregnant women are not useful in pregnancy. Free T4 (fT4), free T3 and thyroid stimulating hormone (TSH) should be analysed when assessing thyroid function in pregnancy, and total T3 and T4 not used. There is a fall in TSH and a rise in fT4 concentrations in the first trimester of normal pregnancy, followed by a fall in fT4 concentration with advancing gestation.

Hypothyroidism

Hypothyroidism is found in around 1 per cent of pregnant women. Worldwide, the commonest cause of hypothyroidism is iodine deficiency, but this is rarely seen in the developed world, where autoimmune Hashimoto's thyroiditis is more common. Women diagnosed with hypothyroidism should continue full thyroid replacement during pregnancy and biochemical euthyroidism is the aim. Thyroid function tests should be performed serially in each trimester, or more often if dose adjustments are required. From the fetal perspective, maternal thyroxine levels are most important in the first trimester of pregnancy, where suboptimal replacement therapy is associated with developmental delay and pregnancy loss. Otherwise, hypothyroidism does not seem to influence pregnancy outcome or complications.

Hyperthyroidism

Autoimmune thyrotoxicosis (Graves' disease) affects around 2 per 1000 pregnancies and has usually been diagnosed before pregnancy. Other causes of hyperthyroidism (5 per cent overall) include toxic adenoma, subacute thyroiditis and toxic multinodular goitre. Differentiating symptoms include tremor, eye signs, weight loss and pre-tibial myxoedema. Treatment during pregnancy should be drug therapy, aiming to maintain maternal fT3 and fT4 levels in the high/normal range. Radioactive iodine is contraindicated because it completely obliterates the fetal thyroid gland. Treatment is with carbimazole or propylthiouracil (PTU), but the lowest dose must be used, as high doses cross the placenta and may cause fetal hypothyroidism. Both drugs also cause agranulocytosis. Beta-blockers can be used initially before the antithyroid drugs take effect. Thyroid surgery can be carried out in pregnancy, if indicated due to compression effects, suspicion of malignancy or failed medical therapy.

Disease activity follows the titre of TSH receptor stimulating antibodies, which rises in the first trimester and falls for the remainder of the pregnancy. Uncontrolled thyrotoxicosis is associated with increased risks of miscarriage, preterm delivery and FGR. Thyroid function therefore needs to be closely monitored and many women can reduce their dose of medication, with almost one-third able to stop treatment in pregnancy. Doses usually need to be readjusted postpartum to prevent a relapse. TSH receptor stimulating antibodies cross the placenta and the risk of fetal Graves' disease after 20 weeks is proportional to their level, although still very low overall, as <10 per cent of Graves' disease is associated with high levels of antibodies. Women with positive and rising antibody titres should be serially scanned for signs of fetal thyrotoxicosis. After delivery, thyroid function should be measured using cord blood.

Thyroid storm

A thyroid storm is a life-threatening event that arises in those with underlying thyroid disease, and can be fatal in 20–50 per cent of untreated cases. It is usually the result of either under-treatment or infection, but it may be associated with labour and it can mimic imminent eclampsia. The diagnosis is made on clinical grounds with laboratory confirmation of hyperthyroidism. Features include excessive sweating, pyrexia, tachycardia, atrial fibrillation, hypertension, hyperglycaemia, vomiting, agitation and cardiac failure. Treatment is with PTU and high-dose corticosteroids, while beta-blockers are used to block the peripheral effect of thyroxine and supportive care with rehydration is also required.

Parathyroid disease

Hyperparathyroidism is caused by parathyroid hyperplasia or adenomas, which may be difficult to detect, and leads to hypercalcaemia due to elevated levels of parathyroid hormone (PTH). If diagnosed before pregnancy, the ideal treatment is surgical removal. However, if suspected in pregnancy, parathyroidectomy may still be indicated in severe cases, with mild hyperparathyroidism managed conservatively through hydration and a low calcium diet. The risks to the mother are from hypercalcaemic crises and complications such as acute pancreatitis, while fetal risks include increased rates of miscarriage, intrauterine death, preterm labour and neonatal tetany in untreated cases.

Hypoparathyroidism may be caused by autoimmune disease, but is more commonly a complication of thyroid surgery. It is diagnosed by finding low serum calcium and low PTH levels. Untreated, it is associated with increased risks of second trimester miscarriage and fetal hypocalcaemia, resulting in bone demineralization and neonatal rickets. The aim of treatment is to maintain normocalcaemia through vitamin D and oral calcium supplements, with regular monitoring of calcium and albumin levels during pregnancy.

Pituitary tumours in pregnancy

Hyperprolactinaemia is an important cause of infertility and amenorrhoea, and is most often due to a benign pituitary microadenoma. The diagnosis is confirmed with a combination of measurement of the prolactin level and computed tomography (CT) or magnetic resonance imaging (MRI) of the pituitary fossa. In 80 per cent of cases, it is treated with the dopamine agonists bromocriptine or cabergoline, which cause the tumour to reduce in size. Larger tumours may require surgery or radiotherapy, which is best undertaken before pregnancy.

The pituitary gland enlarges by 50 per cent during pregnancy, but it is rare for microadenomas to cause problems. Serial prolactin levels are unhelpful to monitor tumour growth in pregnancy. Bromocriptine and cabergoline are usually stopped in pregnancy, and visual fields and relevant symptoms, such as frontal headache, are monitored. If there is evidence of tumour growth during pregnancy, bromocriptine or cabergoline should be recommenced, and appropriate neuroimaging arranged. In women with macroadenomas (>1 cm), it is advisable to continue with dopamine agonists because of the risk of the tumour enlarging under oestrogen stimulation.

Adrenal disease

Cushing's syndrome

Cushing's syndrome is rare in pregnancy as most affected women are infertile. It is characterized by increased glucocorticoid production, usually due to hypersecretion of adrenocorticotrophic hormone (ACTH) from a pituitary tumour. However, in pregnancy, adrenal causes (tumours) are more common. Diagnosis is difficult because many of the symptoms – striae, weight gain, weakness, glucose intolerance and hypertension – mimic normal pregnancy changes. If suspected, plasma cortisol levels should be measured (although levels increase in pregnancy) and adrenal imaging with ultrasound, CT or MRI should be used. There is a high incidence of pre-eclampsia, preterm delivery and stillbirth.

Addison's disease

Addison's disease (adrenal insufficiency) is an autoimmune process, associated with clinical symptoms of exhaustion, nausea, hypotension, hypoglycaemia and weight loss. The diagnosis is difficult to make in pregnancy because the cortisol levels, instead of being characteristically decreased, may be in the low–normal range due to the physiological increase in cortisol-binding globulin in pregnancy. Occasionally, the disease may present as a crisis, and treatment consists of glucocorticoid and fluid replacement. In diagnosed and adequately treated patients, the pregnancy usually continues normally. Replacement steroids should be continued in pregnancy and increased at times of stress such as hyperemesis and delivery.

Phaeochromocytoma

Phaeochromocytoma is a rare catecholamine-producing tumour, reported in 1 in 50 000 pregnancies. The tumours arise from the adrenal medulla in 90 per cent of cases. In pregnancy, it may present as a hypertensive crisis and the symptoms may be similar to those of pre-eclampsia. A characteristic feature is paroxysmal hypertension, whereas the other symptoms of headaches, blurred vision, anxiety and convulsions may occur in pre-eclampsia. The diagnosis is confirmed by measurement of catecholamines in a 24-hour urine collection and in plasma, as well as by adrenal imaging. Treatment is by alpha-blockade with prazosin or phenoxybenzamine, but surgical removal is the only cure. Caesarean section is the preferred mode of delivery, as it minimizes the likelihood of sudden increases in catecholamines associated with vaginal delivery. Maternal and perinatal mortality is greatly increased, especially if the diagnosis is not made before pregnancy.

Skin disease

Pre-existing skin disease

Some pre-existing skin conditions, such as eczema or acne, worsen in pregnancy. Atopic eczema is a common pruritic skin condition affecting 1–5 per cent of the general population and causes the commonest pregnancy rash. It can be treated with emollients and bath additives. Hand and nipple eczema are common postpartum. Acne usually improves in pregnancy, but can flare in the third trimester and acne rosacea often worsens. Oral or topical erythromycin can be used, but retinoids are contraindicated. Psoriasis affects 2 per cent of the population and, during pregnancy, it remains unchanged in around 40 per cent of patients, improves in another 40 per cent and worsens in around 15 per cent. Topical steroids can still be used, while methotrexate is contraindicated.

Specific dermatoses of pregnancy

Pemphigoid gestationis

Pemphigoid gestationis (PG) is a rare pruritic autoimmune bullous disorder, with an incidence of around 1 in 60 000 pregnancies. It most commonly presents in the late second or third trimester with lesions beginning on the abdomen 50 per cent of the time and progressing to widespread clustered blisters, sparing the face. Diagnosis is made by the clinical appearance and by direct immunofluorescence. Once established, the disease runs a complex course with exacerbations and remissions, and flares postpartum in 75 per cent of cases. Management aims to relieve pruritus and prevent new blister formation, and is achieved through the use of potent topical steroids and/or oral prednisolone. There is some association with preterm delivery and small for gestational age births, but no increase in pregnancy loss has been reported. PG recurs in most subsequent pregnancies.

Polymorphic eruption of pregnancy

Polymorphic eruption of pregnancy (PEP) is a self-limiting pruritic inflammatory disorder that usually presents in the third trimester and/or immediately postpartum. The estimated incidence is 1 in 160 pregnancies and 75 per cent of affected pregnancies are primagravida. PEP often begins on the lower abdomen involving pregnancy striae, and extends to thighs, buttocks, legs and arms, while sparing the umbilicus and rarely involving face, hands and feet. In 70 per cent of patients the lesions become confluent and widespread, resembling a toxic erythema. Symptomatic treatment is sufficient and pregnancies appear to be otherwise unaffected, with no tendency to recur.

Prurigo of pregnancy

Prurigo of pregnancy is a common pruritic disorder, which occurs in 1 in 300 pregnancies, and presents as excoriated papules on extensor limbs, abdomen and shoulders. It is more common in women with a history of atopy. Prurigo usually starts at around 25–30 weeks of pregnancy and resolves after delivery, with no effect on the mother or baby. Treatment is symptomatic with topical steroids and emollients.

Pruritic folliculitis of pregnancy

Pruritic folliculitis is a pruritic follicular eruption, with papules and pustules that mainly affect the trunk, but can involve the limbs. It is similar in appearance to acne lesions and is sometimes considered a type of hormonally induced acne. Its onset is usually in the second and third trimesters, and it resolves weeks after delivery. Topical steroid treatment is effective.

Key points

- Women with medical conditions that adversely affect pregnancy outcome should be offered pre-pregnancy counselling by appropriately experienced health-care professionals.
- Women with medical problems that preclude safe pregnancy should be offered safe, effective and appropriate contraception.
- Asthma is the commonest chronic disease encountered in pregnancy.
- Pulmonary hypertension is associated with a risk of maternal mortality of up to 50 per cent in pregnancy.
- Women found to be hypertensive in the first half of pregnancy require investigation for possible underlying causes.
- Women with pre-existing hypertension are at increased risk of superimposed pre-eclampsia, FGR and placental abruption.

- Women who become pregnant with serum creatinine values above 125 mol/L have an increased risk of accelerated decline in renal function and poor outcome of pregnancy.
- Pre-existing diabetes increases maternal and fetal obstetric morbidity.
- The incidence of fetal macrosomia in diabetes can be reduced through good blood glucose control.
- The risk of perinatal and maternal morbidity is increased in pregnancies complicated by sickle cell disease.
- The main issue for pregnant women with epilepsy relates to the teratogenic risk of anticonvulsant medication drugs.
- Obstetric cholestasis is associated with an increased risk of term stillbirth.

CASE HISTORY

Mrs M is a 30-year-old woman in her second pregnancy. She has a body mass index of 38. Her first pregnancy was complicated by gestational diabetes, which was detected following screening at 28 weeks gestation. She was poorly compliant with dietary intervention and required insulin treatment from 32 weeks gestation. At 36 weeks, she developed polyhydramnios (amniotic fluid index of 28 cm) and her baby was found to be in a breech position. She subsequently had an elective Caesarean section at 39 weeks gestation, which resulted in the birth of a 4.4 kg male infant.

In this pregnancy, she booked for antenatal care at 18 weeks gestation. Her HbA1c at booking was found to be 9.2 per cent and she was therefore commenced on insulin. An anomaly scan and fetal echocardiography at 22 weeks were normal. Despite weekly attendance at the combined obstetric diabetic clinic, her blood sugar control was poor and serial ultrasound scans from 28 weeks gestation showed fetal growth accelerating beyond the 95th centile. At 36 weeks, she attended complaining of decreased fetal movement. An ultrasound scan showed a singleton fetus with a cephalic presentation and the presence of marked polyhydramnios (AFI 34 cm). A CTG was performed and showed reduced baseline variability with unprovoked decelerations. An urgent Caesarean section was performed and a 4.9 kg male infant was delivered. Within minutes of delivery, the baby was found to have signs of respiratory distress and he was admitted to the neonatal unit. The baby required ventilation for 48 hours. Additionally, the baby became hypoglycaemic within an hour of admission and in total spent 9 days on the neonatal unit while blood glucose levels stabilized and feeding became established.

Mrs M had an oral glucose tolerance 6 weeks following delivery. The 2-hour glucose level was within normal limits.

Additional reading

de Swiet M. *Medical disorders in obstetric practice*. Oxford: Blackwell Science, 2002.

Kaaja RJ, Greer IA. Manifestations of chronic disease during pregnancy. *JAMA* 2005; **294**: 2751–7.

Lombaard H, Pattinson RC. Underlying medical conditions. *Best Practice and Research. Clinical Obstetrics and Gynaecology* 2008; **22**: 847–864.

Taylor R, Davison JM. Type 1 diabetes and pregnancy. *BMJ* 2007; **334**: 742–5.

William D, Davison JM. Chronic kidney disease in pregnancy. *BMJ* 2008; **336**: 211–15.

Williams J, Mozurkewich E, Chilimigras J, Van De Ven C. Critical care in obstetrics: pregnancy-specific conditions. *Best Practice and Research. Clinical Obstetrics and Gynaecology* 2008; **22**: 825–46.

CHAPTER 13

PERINATAL INFECTIONS

Sarah Vause

OVERVIEW

Infectious diseases contracted during pregnancy can have a serious impact on both the mother and the fetus. Some infections cause congenital abnormalities in the fetus (rubella, syphilis, toxoplasmosis, cytomegalovirus, chickenpox). Other infections can be transmitted from mother to baby during pregnancy (parvovirus) or around the time of delivery (human immunodeficiency virus (HIV), hepatitis B, hepatitis C, herpes, group B streptococcus).

For several infectious diseases, screening programmes and effective interventions can improve the outcome for the fetus. For other diseases, early diagnosis and appropriate treatment can be of benefit to both mother and baby.

This chapter will describe some of these infections.

Infections causing congenital abnormalities

Rubella

Infective organism

Rubella virus is a togavirus spread by droplet transmission.

Prevalence

Since the introduction of the measles, mumps and rubella vaccine (MMR), an average of three births affected by congenital rubella a year and four rubella-associated terminations were registered from 1996 to 2000 in the UK. In the 1990s there was reduced uptake of the MMR vaccine for infants due to concern about a possible link with autism. It is too soon to say whether this will eventually lead to an increase in the prevalence of rubella in the community and an increase in incidence of congenital rubella when this cohort of non-immunized infants reach childbearing age.

In England and Wales susceptibility is slightly higher in nulliparous women (2 per cent) than in parous women (1.2 per cent). Certain ethnic groups also appear to have higher susceptibility, such as Asian and black women (5 per cent) and Oriental women (8 per cent), compared with less than 2 per cent in white women, with an overall susceptibility of about 2.5 per cent reported for pregnant women in the UK.

Screening

In the UK, NICE recommendations are that all women should be offered rubella susceptibility screening early in their pregnancy to identify women at risk of contracting rubella infection and to enable vaccination in the post-natal period for the protection of future pregnancies.

This is an unusual antenatal screening test as there is no effective intervention which can be implemented during the index pregnancy to reduce the risk of harm to that fetus, nor does it attempt to identify currently affected pregnancies. The aim of screening for rubella in pregnancy is to identify susceptible women so that postpartum vaccination may protect future pregnancies against rubella infection and its consequences.

For pregnant women who are screened and rubella antibody is not detected, rubella vaccination after pregnancy should be advised. Vaccination during pregnancy is contraindicated because of a theoretical risk that the vaccine itself could be teratogenic, as it is a live vaccine. No cases of congenital rubella syndrome resulting from vaccination during pregnancy have been reported. However, women who are vaccinated postpartum should be advised to use contraception for three months.

Clinical features

Rubella infection is characterized by a febrile rash but may be asymptomatic in the mother in 20–50 per cent of cases.

Features of congenital rubella syndrome can include sensorineural deafness, congenital cataracts, blindness, encephalitis and endocrine problems.

The risk of congenital rubella infection reduces with gestation. If infection of the fetus does occur the defects caused are also less severe with more advanced gestations. Congenital infection in the first 12 weeks of pregnancy among mothers with symptoms is over 80 per cent and reduces to 25 per cent at the end of the second trimester. One hundred per cent of infants infected during the first 11 weeks of pregnancy have rubella defects, whereas primary rubella contracted between 16 and 20 weeks of gestation carries only a minimal risk of deafness. Rubella infection prior to the estimated date of conception or after 20 weeks gestation carries no documented risk to the fetus.

Management

If infection during pregnancy is confirmed, the risk of congenital rubella syndrome should be assessed depending on the gestation when infection occurred. If infection occurred prior to 16 weeks gestation, termination of pregnancy should be offered. If the infection occurs later in pregnancy the woman should be given appropriate information and reassured.

Syphilis

Infective organism

Syphilis is a sexually acquired infection caused by *Treponema pallidum*.

Prevalence

The incidence of infectious syphilis in England and Wales is low, but has increased markedly in the last ten years. The increase has mainly been seen in rates of infection in homosexual men, but part of the increase is due to immigration to the UK from countries where prevalence is higher, for example Eastern Europe.

The prevalence of syphilis in pregnant women has been estimated at approximately 68 per million with regional variation, highest in north-east London. This equates to approximately 50–60 cases per year in the UK.

Clinical features

Primary syphilis may present as a painless genital ulcer 3–6 weeks after the infection is acquired (condylomata lata) (Figure 13.1); however, this may be on the cervix and go unnoticed.

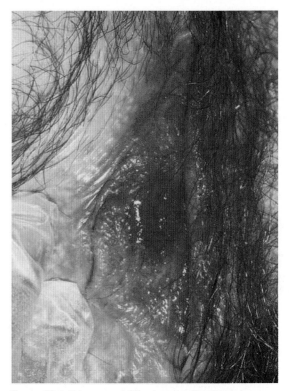

Figure 13.1 Primary syphilitic chancre. (Courtesy of Dr Raymond Maw, Royal Victoria Hospital, Belfast.)

Secondary manifestations occur 6 weeks to six months after infection and present as a maculopapular rash or lesions affecting the mucous membranes. Ultimately, 20 per cent of untreated patients will develop symptomatic cardiovascular tertiary syphilis and 5–10 per cent will develop symptomatic neurosyphilis.

In pregnant women with early untreated (primary or secondary) syphilis, 70–100 per cent of infants will be infected and approximately 25 per cent will be stillborn. Mother-to-child transmission of syphilis in pregnancy is associated with fetal growth restriction (FGR), fetal hydrops, congenital syphilis (which may cause long-term disability), stillbirth, preterm birth and neonatal death. The risk of congenital transmission declines with increasing duration of maternal syphilis prior to pregnancy. Adequate treatment with benzathine penicillin markedly improves the outcome for the fetus.

Screening

Because treatment is so effective, routine antenatal screening for all pregnant women is recommended.

The body's immune response to syphilis is the production of non-specific and specific treponemal antibodies. These can be detected by serological tests. Non-treponemal tests detect non-specific treponemal antibodies and include the Venereal Diseases Research Laboratory (VDRL) and rapid plasma reagin (RPR) tests. Treponemal tests detect specific treponemal antibodies and include enzyme immunoassays (EIA), *T. pallidum* haemagglutination assay (TPHA) and the fluorescent treponemal antibody-absorbed test (FTA-abs). EIA tests that detect immunoglobulin (Ig) G or IgG and IgM are rapidly replacing the VDRL and TPHA combination for syphilis screening in the UK. EIAs are over 98 per cent sensitive and over 99 per cent specific. Non-treponemal tests, on the other hand, may result in false negatives, particularly in very early or late syphilis, in patients with reinfection or those who are HIV positive. The VDRL may be falsely positive in women with lupus. Therefore, positive results should be interpreted with caution and the pregnant woman should be referred for expert assessment and diagnosis in a genitourinary medicine clinic.

None of these serological tests will detect syphilis in its incubation stage, which may last for an average of 25 days.

Management

The initial step is to confirm the diagnosis and to test for any other sexually transmitted diseases. Once a diagnosis of syphilis is confirmed the genitourinary medicine clinic will institute appropriate contact tracing of sexual partners. Older children may also need to be screened for congenital infection.

Parenteral penicillin has a 98 per cent success rate for preventing congenital syphilis. A Jarish–Herxheimer reaction may occur with treatment as a result of release of pro-inflammatory cytokines in response to dying organisms. This presents as a worsening of symptoms, and fever for 12–24 hours after commencement of treatment. It may be associated with uterine contractions and fetal distress. Many clinicians therefore admit women at the time of commencement of treatment for monitoring.

If a woman is not treated during pregnancy her baby should be treated after delivery. An infected baby may be born without signs or symptoms of disease but if not treated immediately, may develop serious problems within a few weeks. Untreated babies often develop developmental delay, have seizures or die.

Toxoplasmosis

Infective organism

Toxoplasma gondii is a protozoan parasite found in cat faeces, soil or uncooked meat. Infection occurs by ingestion of the parasite from undercooked meat or from unwashed hands.

Prevalence

The prevalence varies in different countries. It is 16 per 1000 in France but in the UK it is estimated to be less than two per 1000 pregnancies.

Screening

Only about ten severely affected babies are diagnosed per year in the UK and for this reason the UK National Screening Committee recently reported that screening for toxoplasmosis should not be offered routinely. There is a lack of evidence that antenatal screening and treatment reduces mother-to-child transmission or the complications associated with toxoplasma infection. In the UK women should be advised about appropriate preventative measure such as avoiding eating rare or raw meat, avoiding handling cats and cat litter, and wearing gloves and washing hands when gardening or handling soil.

Even in France where more women acquire infection during pregnancy, and women are screened antenatally, the benefits of such a programme appear to be limited.

Clinical features

The initial infection may be relatively asymptomatic, or may be a glandular fever-like illness. Parasitaemia usually occurs within 3 weeks of infection. Therefore, congenital infection is only a significant risk if the mother acquires the infection during or immediately before pregnancy.

Infection during the first trimester of pregnancy is most likely to cause severe fetal damage (85 per cent), but only 10 per cent of infections are transmitted to the fetus at this gestation. In the third trimester 85 per cent of infections are transmitted, but the risk of fetal damage decreases to around 10 per cent.

Severely infected infants may have ventriculomegaly or microcephaly, chorioretinitis and cerebral calcification. These features may be detected on ultrasound scan. The majority of infected infants are asymptomatic at birth but develop sequelae several years later.

Management

The diagnosis of primary infection with toxoplasmosis during pregnancy is made by the Sabin-Feldman dye test. Enzyme-linked immunosorbant assays are available for IgM antibody. However, IgM may persist for months or even years, so often serial testing for rising titres is necessary. If suspicion of congenital toxoplasmosis has arisen because of an abnormal ultrasound scan of the fetus, an amniocentesis can be performed. Polymerase chain reaction (PCR) analysis of amniotic fluid is highly accurate for the identification of *T. gondii*.

Spiramycin treatment can be used in pregnancy (a 3-week course of 2–3 g per day). This reduces the incidence of transplacental infection but has not been shown to definitively reduce the incidence of clinical congenital disease.

If toxoplasmosis is found to be the cause of abnormalities detected on ultrasound scan of the fetus, then termination of pregnancy can be offered.

Cytomegalovirus

Infective organism

Cytomegalovirus (CMV) is a DNA herpes virus. It is transmitted by respiratory droplet transmission and is excreted in the urine.

Prevalence

It is a common virus in the UK and about 60 per cent of women are already immune when they become pregnant and, consequently, approximately 40 per cent are susceptible to infection. The incidence of infection in pregnancy is estimated to be around 1–2 per cent of pregnancies. Of those infected, approximately 30 per cent will transmit the viral infection to the fetus and of these approximately 30 per cent of the fetuses will be affected by the virus.

Clinical features

Primary infection often produces no symptoms or mild non-specific flu-like symptoms in the mother.

The diagnosis is often made after abnormalities are seen in the fetus on ultrasound scan. The main features seen in an affected fetus are FGR, microcephaly, ventriculomegaly, ascites or hydrops.

Some fetuses which are infected may not show any features on ultrasound, but may later be found to have neurological damage such as blindness, deafness or developmental delay. The neonate can also be anaemic and thrombocytopenic, with hepatosplenomegaly, jaundice and a purpural rash.

Management

A serological diagnosis can be made by demonstrating the development of CMV antibodies in a seronegative woman, who initially develops CMV IgM antibody, and subsequently IgG antibody. Virology labs usually keep the initial sample taken at booking, so if infection is suspected a sample taken at the time of presentation can be compared with the initial booking sample to determine whether seroconversion has occurred. Since IgM can be secreted for several months, it is not sufficient to simply demonstrate IgM in a sample at the time of presentation; it has to be a new finding in a woman who was negative for IgM at the time of booking.

If there is a suspicion that the fetus may be infected, amniotic fluid can be tested for the virus by PCR. Since the virus is excreted in fetal urine it can be found in amniotic fluid.

If abnormalities are detected on ultrasound and these are felt to be due to congenital CMV infection, termination of pregnancy should be offered. A much more difficult situation is when CMV infection is known to have occurred, but the fetus appears normal on ultrasound, as there is approximately a 20 per cent chance of neurological abnormality in the fetus.

Like other herpes viruses, CMV has the capacity to establish latency and be reactivated. After infection the virus is excreted for weeks or months by adults and for years by infants. It persists in the lymphocytes throughout life and can be transmitted by blood transfusion or transplantation. Reactivation occurs intermittently, with shedding in the genital urinary or respiratory tract. Reactivation during pregnancy very rarely causes congenital CMV infection.

Chickenpox

Infective organism

Chickenpox is caused by the varicella zoster virus (VZV), a herpes virus which is transmitted by droplet spread.

Prevalence

In the UK 90 per cent of adults are immune to chickenpox. However, contact with chickenpox is common in pregnancy and approximately one in 200 women will contract chickenpox during their pregnancy.

Clinical features

Non-immune pregnant women are more vulnerable to chickenpox and may develop a serious pneumonia, hepatitis or encephalitis. It can occasionally be fatal with the mortality rate being approximately five times higher in pregnant women than in non-pregnant adults. Pneumonia occurs in about 10 per cent of women with chickenpox and seems more severe at later gestations. It may also cause the fetal varicella syndrome (FVS) or varicella infection of the newborn.

Management

Women should be asked whether they have had chickenpox at the initial booking visit. If they have not had chickenpox, they should be advised to avoid contact with it during pregnancy, and if they accidentally come into contact with it should advise their doctor or midwife about the exposure as soon as possible.

When contact occurs with chickenpox, a careful history must be taken to confirm the significance of the contact (length of exposure and closeness of contact) and the susceptibility of the patient. Significant contact is defined as being in the same room as someone for 15 minutes or more, or face-to-face contact.

Testing for immunity

If a women reports that she has been in contact with chickenpox, she should have a blood test for confirmation of VZV immunity, by testing for VZV IgG. This can usually be performed within 24–48 hours and the virology laboratory may be able to use serum stored from booking antenatal bloods. At least 80–90 per cent of women tested will have VZ IgG and can be reassured.

Management of the non-immune woman exposed to chickenpox

If the pregnant woman is not immune to VZV and she has had a significant exposure, she should be given varicella zoster immunoglobulin (VZIG) as soon as possible. VZIG is effective when given up to 10 days after contact and may prevent or attenuate the disease. Women who have had exposure to chickenpox (regardless of whether or not they have received VZIG) should be asked to notify their doctor or midwife early if a rash develops.

Management of chickenpox in pregnancy

Women with chickenpox should avoid contact with susceptible individuals; that is, other pregnant women and neonates, until the lesions have crusted over. This is usually about 5 days after the onset of the rash. Symptomatic treatment and hygiene is advised to prevent secondary bacterial infection of the lesions.

The UK Advisory Group on Chickenpox recommends that oral aciclovir 800 mg five times per day for 7 days be prescribed for pregnant women with chickenpox if they present within 24 hours of the onset of the rash and if they are more than 20 weeks gestation. Aciclovir should be used cautiously before 20 weeks gestation. VZIG has no therapeutic benefit once chickenpox has developed. If the woman smokes cigarettes, has chronic lung disease, is taking corticosteroids or is in the latter half of pregnancy, a hospital assessment should be considered, even in the absence of complications.

Women hospitalized with varicella should be nursed in isolation from babies or potentially susceptible pregnant women or non-immune staff. Delivery during the viraemic period may be extremely hazardous. The maternal risks are bleeding, thrombocytopenia, disseminated intravascular coagulopathy and hepatitis. There is a high risk of varicella infection of the newborn with significant morbidity and mortality. Supportive treatment and intravenous aciclovir is therefore desirable, allowing resolution of the rash and transfer of protective antibodies from the mother to the fetus. However, delivery may be required in women to facilitate assisted ventilation in cases where varicella pneumonia is complicated by respiratory failure.

The fetus

Spontaneous miscarriage does not appear to be increased if chickenpox occurs in the first trimester.

FVS is characterized by one or more of the following:

- skin scarring in a dermatomal distribution;
- eye defects (microphthalmia, chorioretinitis, cataracts);
- hypoplasia of the limbs;
- neurological abnormalities (microcephaly, cortical atrophy, developmental delay and dysfunction of bowel and bladder sphincters).

This only occurs in a minority of infected fetuses (approximately 1 per cent). FVS has been reported to complicate maternal chickenpox that occurs as early as 3 weeks and up to 28 weeks of gestation. The risk appears to be lower in the first trimester (0.55 per cent). No case of FVS has been reported when maternal infection has occurred after 28 weeks.

If the mother has contracted chickenpox during pregnancy, referral to a fetal medicine specialist should be considered at 16–20 weeks or 5 weeks after infection for discussion and detailed ultrasound examination, when findings such as limb deformity, microcephaly, hydrocephalus, soft-tissue calcification and fetal growth restriction can be detected. A time lag of at least 5 weeks after the primary infection is advised as it takes several weeks for these features to manifest.

Maternal infection around the time of delivery

If maternal infection occurs at term, there is a significant risk of varicella of the newborn. Elective delivery should normally be avoided until 5–7 days after the onset of maternal rash to allow for the passive transfer of antibodies from mother to child. Neonatal ophthalmic examination should be organized after birth.

If birth occurs within the 7-day period following the onset of the maternal rash, or if the mother develops the chickenpox rash within the 7-day period after birth, the neonate should be given VZIG. The infant should be monitored for signs of infection until 28 days after the onset of maternal infection.

Neonatal infection should be treated with aciclovir following discussion with a neonatologist and virologist. VZIG is of no benefit once neonatal chickenpox has developed.

Contact with shingles

Following the primary infection, the virus remains dormant in sensory nerve root ganglia but can be reactivated to cause a vesicular erythematous skin rash in a dermatomal distribution known as herpes zoster or shingles. The risk of a pregnant woman acquiring infection from an individual with herpes zoster in non-exposed sites (for example, thoracolumbar) is remote.

Other congenital infections associated with pregnancy loss and preterm birth

Parvovirus

Infective organism

Parvovirus is a relatively common infection in pregnancy, and is spread by droplet infection.

Incidence

Fifty per cent of women at childbearing age are immune to PVB19 infection and therefore 50 per cent are susceptible to infection during pregnancy. It occurs most commonly in those pregnant women who work with young children, for example teachers. In some years the incidence of parvovirus is higher than others.

Clinical features

In adults, symptoms are a mild flu-like illness. In children it may cause a characteristic rash (slapped cheek syndrome). In the fetus it can cause an aplastic anaemia. The anaemic fetus may then become hydropic due to high output cardiac failure and liver congestion. This is the most common presentation during pregnancy and is seen on ultrasound scan. If a fetus is hydropic, the velocity of blood flow in the fetal middle cerebral artery can be measured. If the velocity is high, it is suggestive of anaemia, and parvovirus would be one of several differential diagnoses.

Management

The diagnosis is made by demonstrating seroconversion of the mother, who develops IgM antibodies to parvovirus, having previously tested negative. Viral DNA amplifications using PCR in maternal and fetal serum or amniotic fluid, is the most sensitive and accurate diagnostic test.

A hydropic fetus may recover spontaneously as the mother and fetus recover from the virus, or may require treatment by *in utero* transfusion.

Infection in the first 20 weeks of pregnancy can lead to hydrops fetalis and intrauterine death, as treatment by intrauterine transfusion is not possible at early gestations. Prior to 20 weeks the fetal loss rate is approximately 10 per cent.

If the anaemia is treated by *in utero* transfusion, the fetus can make a complete recovery. Parvovirus does not cause neurological damage, and if the fetus survives the anaemia, there can be a completely normal outcome. After 20 weeks gestation the fetal loss rate is estimated to be approximately 1 per cent.

Listeria

Infective organism

Listeria monocytogenes is an aerobic and facultatively anaerobic motile Gram-positive bacillus. It has an unusual life cycle with obligate intracellular replication. People with reduced cell-mediated immunity, e.g. pregnant women and the elderly, are therefore most at risk.

Incidence

The incidence of listeria infection in pregnant women is estimated at 12 per 100 000 compared to 0.7 per 100 000 in the general population. Contaminated food is the usual source of infection. Usual sources include unpasteurized milk, ripened soft cheeses and pâté. It is therefore recommended that pregnant women should be offered information on how to reduce the risk of listeriosis by dietary modification. Listeria is not transmitted in hot cooked foods and does not multiply in the freezer; however, it survives and multiplies at refrigerator temperatures and hence can be transmitted in chilled foods, e.g. milk, soft cheese, prawns and pâté.

Clinical features

Pregnant women with listeriosis most commonly suffer from a flu-like illness with fever and general malaise. About a third of women may be asymptomatic. Transmission to the fetus may either occur via the ascending route through the cervix, or transplacentally secondary to maternal bacteraemia. Approximately 20 per cent of affected pregnancies result in miscarriage or stillbirth. Premature delivery may occur in over 50 per cent. Neonates may have respiratory distress, fever, sepsis or neurological

symptoms and the overall neonatal mortality rate has been estimated at 38 per cent.

Management

The diagnosis of listeria depends on clinical suspicion and isolation of the organism from blood, vaginal swabs or the placenta. Meconium staining of the amniotic fluid in a preterm fetus may increase clinical suspicion for listeriosis.

For women with listeriosis during pregnancy, intravenous antibiotic treatment (ampicillin 2 g given every 6 hours) is indicated.

Malaria

Infective organisms

Although malaria can be caused by five species of malarial parasite (*Plasmodium falciparum*, *P. vivax*, *P. ovale*, *P. malariae* and *P. knowlesi*) the species which carries the worst prognosis for the mother and fetus, and the organism of greatest importance on a worldwide scale, is *P. falciparum*. This is a protozoan parasite transmitted by the female anopheline mosquito.

Incidence

Incidence varies depending on geographical location, but is endemic in sub-Saharan Africa, South Asia and some parts of South America. It is estimated that one billion people worldwide carry parasites at any time, and 0.5–3 million people per year die from malaria. Pregnant women have an increased risk of malarial infection compared to their non-pregnant adult counterparts. The incidence of parasitaemia has been found to be higher in primiparous women (66 per cent) than multiparous women (21–29 per cent).

In endemic areas where many women are semi-immune, malarial parasites may often be found in large numbers sequestrated in the placenta, even when blood films are negative. This may lead to the diagnosis being missed, unless a high index of suspicion is maintained.

Clinical features

Maternal effects include a cyclical spiking pyrexia, which may be associated with miscarriage and preterm labour. Severe anaemia may develop rapidly, but many women from endemic areas may also have other risk factors for severe anaemia. Hypoglycaemia is common and may be severe in pregnancy. Pulmonary oedema, due to abnormal capillary permeability, results in high mortality (approximately 50 per cent). Haemolysis causes jaundice and renal failure.

Fetal effects include premature delivery and low birthweight (<2500 g). Placental sequestration of parasites is associated with abnormal uteroplacental Doppler waveforms and is also implicated in the higher rate of transmission of HIV. Coinfection with HIV is common in many of the areas where malaria is endemic and both the vertical transmission of malaria and HIV to the fetus seem to be more common if the two infections coexist.

Management

If malaria is suspected, prompt symptomatic and supportive treatment with appropriate antimalarial therapy is important. The choice of antimalarial will vary, depending on local patterns of disease and drug resistance, and expert advice should be sought. In endemic areas preventative strategies include the use of insecticide-treated bed nets and intermittent preventative treatment during pregnancy.

If women from non-endemic areas are planning to travel to endemic areas they should only do this if absolutely necessary during their pregnancy. Insecticide sprays, mosquito nets, appropriate clothing to reduce the risk of mosquito bites and drug prophylaxis can all be used. Expert advice on which antimalarial is appropriate for the area is important. The risks of teratogenicity must be balanced against the serious risk of contracting malaria in pregnancy.

Infections acquired around the time of delivery with serious neonatal consequences

Herpes

Infective organism

Herpes simplex virus (HSV) is a double-stranded DNA virus. There are two viral types, HSV-1 and HSV-2. The majority of orolabial infections are caused by HSV-1. These infections are usually acquired during childhood through direct physical contact such as kissing. Genital herpes is a sexually transmitted infection and is most commonly caused by HSV-2. However, there is an increasing prevalence of genital HSV-1 infections in many countries, including the UK, USA and Scandinavia.

Incidence

Genital herpes is the most common ulcerative sexually transmitted infection in the UK. Neonatal herpes is a viral infection with a high morbidity and mortality which is most commonly acquired at or near the time of delivery due to contact with infected secretions. It is rare, with an incidence of 1 in 60 000 live births.

Clinical features

Genital herpes presents as ulcerative lesions on the vulva, vagina or cervix. The woman may give a history of this being a recurrent problem, in which case the lesion is often less florid. A primary infection may be associated with systemic symptoms and may cause urinary retention.

Neonatal herpes may be caused by HSV-1 or HSV-2, as either viral type can cause genital herpes. Almost all cases of neonatal herpes occur as a result of direct contact with infected maternal secretions, although cases of post-natal transmission have been described.

Neonatal herpes is classified into three subgroups: disease localized to skin, eye and/mouth, local central nervous system disease (encephalitis alone) and disseminated infection with multiple organ involvement (Table 13.1).

Factors influencing transmission include the type of maternal infection (primary or recurrent), the presence of transplacental maternal neutralizing antibodies, the duration of rupture of membranes before delivery, the use of fetal scalp electrodes and the mode of delivery. The risks are greatest when a woman acquires a new infection (primary genital herpes) in the third trimester, particularly within 6 weeks of

Table 13.1 Classification of neonatal herpes

	Death (in treated babies) %	Neurological morbidity %
Localized to skin, eye and/ mouth	Rare	<2
Local CNS disease	6	70
Disseminated infection	30	17

CNS, central nervous system.

delivery, as viral shedding may persist and the baby is likely to be born before the development of protective maternal antibodies. Very rarely, congenital herpes may occur as a result of transplacental intrauterine infection.

Management

Symptomatic genital herpes infections are confirmed by direct detection of HSV. A swab for viral detection should be used. Any woman with suspected first-episode genital herpes should be referred to a genitourinary physician, who will confirm the diagnosis by viral culture or PCR, advise on management and arrange a screen for other sexually transmitted infections. The use of aciclovir is associated with a reduction in the duration and severity of symptoms and a decrease in the duration of viral shedding.

It may be difficult to distinguish clinically between recurrent and primary genital HSV infections, as many first episode HSV infections are not true primary infections (Figure 13.2). Advice of a GUM consultant should be sought, as recommendations

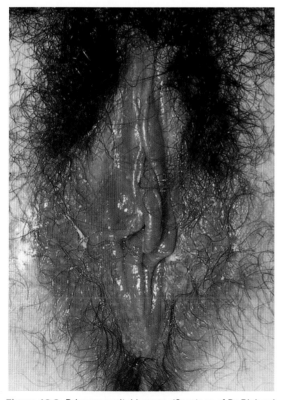

Figure 13.2 Primary genital herpes. (Courtesy of Dr Richard Lau, St Georges's Hospital, London.)

about the mode of delivery depend on whether the woman has a primary or recurrent infection.

Primary infections

Caesarean section should be recommended to all women presenting with primary episode genital herpes lesions at the time of delivery, or within 6 weeks of the expected date of delivery. The rationale for elective Caesarean section in the prevention of neonatal herpes is to reduce exposure of the fetus to HSV in genital secretions.

For women who develop primary genital herpes lesions within 6 weeks of delivery and who opt for a vaginal birth, rupture of membranes should be avoided and invasive procedures such as fetal scalp electrodes, or fetal scalp pH measurement should not be used. Intravenous aciclovir given intrapartum to the mother and subsequently to the neonate may be considered. The neonatologist should be informed and may advise acyclovir treatment of the baby.

Recurrent episodes

A recurrent episode of genital herpes occurring during the antenatal period is not an indication for delivery by Caesarean section.

Women presenting with recurrent genital herpes lesions at the onset of labour should be advised that the risk to the baby of neonatal herpes is very small (1–3 per cent). Although Caesarean section is not routinely recommended for women with recurrent genital herpes lesions at the onset of labour, the mode of delivery should be discussed with the woman and individualized according to the clinical circumstances and the woman's preferences.

Some women feel that they would not wish to accept the small risk of neonatal herpes infection associated with active recurrent genital herpes at the time of delivery and would opt for Caesarean delivery if HSV lesions were detected at the onset of labour. For these women, daily suppressive aciclovir given from 36 weeks of gestation until delivery may reduce the likelihood of active HSV lesions at term.

Women with recurrent genital herpes lesions and confirmed rupture of membranes at term should be advised to have delivery expedited by the appropriate means. Invasive procedures in labour should be avoided for women with recurrent genital herpes lesions. The neonatologist should be informed of babies born to mothers with recurrent genital herpes lesions at the time of labour.

Group B streptococcus

Infective organism

Group B streptococcus (GBS) (*Streptococcus agalactiae*) is a Gram-positive coccus frequently found as a vaginal commensal. It can cause sepsis in the neonate and transmission can occur from the time the membranes are ruptured until delivery.

Prevalence

GBS is recognized as the most frequent cause of severe early-onset (less than 7 days of age) infection in newborn infants. Approximately 25 per cent of women in the UK carry GBS as a commensal in the vagina. The incidence of early-onset GBS disease in the UK is 0.5 per 1000 births.

   The mortality from early-onset GBS disease in the UK is 6 per cent in term infants and 18 per cent in preterm infants. Even when treated appropriately, some infants will still die of early-onset disease, particularly when the disease is well established prior to birth.

Screening

Universal screening is carried out in the USA but this practice has not been adopted in the UK. The incidence of early-onset GBS disease in the UK in the absence of systematic screening or widespread intrapartum antibiotic prophylaxis is similar to that seen in the USA after universal screening and intrapartum antibiotic prophylaxis, despite comparable vaginal carriage rates.

   The RCOG green-top guidelines review current evidence relating to GBS and conclude that 'Routine screening (either bacteriological or risk based) for antenatal GBS carriage is not recommended.'

Clinical features

The mother will not have symptoms as GBS is a common vaginal commensal.

   An infected neonate may demonstrate signs of neonatal sepsis including sudden collapse, tachypnoea, nasal flaring, poor tone, jaundice, etc.

Management

Antenatal

If GBS is detected incidentally, antenatal treatment is not recommended as it does not reduce the likelihood of GBS colonization at the time of delivery.

Intrapartum antibiotic prophylaxis

It is during labour that infection of the fetus/neonate occurs. Antibiotics given in labour are estimated to be 60–80 per cent effective in reducing early-onset neonatal GBS infection. The difficulty is knowing which women require treatment.

   Different approaches are used for screening, to determine which women should receive intrapartum antibiotics.

Risk factor-based prophylaxis

Approximately 15 per cent of all UK pregnancies have one or more of the following risk factors:

- intrapartum fever
- prolonged rupture of membranes (PROM) greater than 18 hours
- prematurity less than 37 weeks
- previous infant with GBS.

Using this strategy, 25 per cent of women will receive intrapartum antibiotics with 50–69 per cent reduction in early-onset GBS infection in the neonate.

   To prevent one neonatal death 5882 women need to be treated.

Bacteriological screening using vaginal and rectal swabs

All women would need to have vaginal and rectal swabs at 35–37 weeks gestation. Twenty-seven per cent of women will receive intrapartum antibiotics, with 86 per cent reduction in early-onset GBS infection in the neonate. In the UK, at least 24 000 women would need to be screened and at least 7000 colonized women treated with antibiotics to prevent one neonatal death.

Vaginal and rectal swabs and risk factor screening in combination

Three per cent of women would receive intrapartum antibiotics with a 51 per cent reduction in early-onset GBS infection in the neonate.

   The RCOG therefore recommends that intrapartum antibiotic prophylaxis is discussed with women with the following risk factors, and that the argument for using prophylaxis is stronger if more than one risk factor is present; furthermore, if the women has had a previous baby with neonatal GBS or if GBS bacteruria is detected, as this is associated with a higher risk of neonatal disease.

- Intrapartum fever (>38°)
- Prolonged rupture of membranes (PROM) >18 hours
- Prematurity <37 weeks
- Previous infant with GBS
- Incidental detection of GBS in current pregnancy
- GBS bacteruria.

It is recommended that intravenous penicillin 3 g be given as soon as possible after the onset of labour and 1.5 g 4-hourly until delivery. Clindamycin 900 mg should be given intravenously 8-hourly to those allergic to penicillin.

There is no good evidence to support the administration of intrapartum antibiotic prophylaxis to women in whom GBS carriage was detected in a previous pregnancy.

If chorioamnionitis is suspected, broad-spectrum antibiotic therapy including an agent active against GBS should replace GBS-specific antibiotic prophylaxis.

Women undergoing planned Caesarean delivery in the absence of labour or membrane rupture do not require antibiotic prophylaxis for GBS, regardless of GBS colonization status. The risk of neonatal GBS disease is extremely low in this circumstance.

The neonate

Many infants with early-onset GBS disease have symptoms at or soon after birth. Neonatal sepsis can progress rapidly to death. Whether they received intrapartum antibiotics or not, any newborn infant with clinical signs compatible with infection should be treated promptly with broad-spectrum antibiotics, which provide cover against early-onset GBS disease and other common pathogens. Blood cultures should always be obtained before antibiotic treatment is commenced, and CSF cultures should be considered. Randomized controlled trials have not provided a sufficient evidence base for clear treatment recommendations in well, newborn infants whose mothers had risk factors for GBS. Some clinicians will recommend treatment of the infants, while others will prefer to observe them because the balance of risks and benefits of treatment is uncertain. Each hospital will have its own guideline.

Chlamydia

Infective organism

Chlamydia trachomatis is an obligate intracellular organism.

Prevalence

Chlamydia is the most common sexually transmitted organism in the UK and USA. Between one in 8–10 men and women who are sexually active and under 25 years old screen positive for Chlamydia. In the UK an opportunistic chlamydia screening programme for under 25 year olds has been initiated. Whilst it is not a routine antenatal screening test in the UK, NICE recommends that all women booking for antenatal care, who are younger than 25 years, are informed of the National Screening Programme.

Clinical features

During pregnancy chlamydia is frequently asymptomatic in the pregnant woman. Infection with chlamydia is associated with preterm rupture of membranes, preterm delivery and low birthweight. Transmission to the fetus occurs at the time of delivery and can cause conjunctivitis and pneumonia.

Management

Treatment with azithromycin or erythromycin is recommended. Tetracyclines such as doxycycline should be avoided if possible during pregnancy. Appropriate contact tracing can be arranged via a genitourinary medicine clinic.

Gonorrhoea

Infective organism

Neisseria gonorrhoeae is a Gram-negative diplococcus.

Prevalence

The prevalence of gonorrhoea in pregnancy varies with the population studied. In the UK it is the second most common bacterial sexually transmitted disease.

Clinical features

Gonococcal infection in women is frequently asymptomatic, or women may present with a mucopurulent discharge or dysuria. Rarely, disseminated gonorrhoea may cause low grade fever, a rash and polyarthritis. There is an increased risk of coinfection with chlamydia, and an increased risk of preterm rupture of membranes and preterm birth. Transmission to the fetus occurs at the time of delivery and can cause opthalmia neonatorum.

Management

Bacteriological swabs should be taken and specific swabs/testing for concomitant infection with chlamydia should also be undertaken. Cephalosporins are effective against gonococcus, but empirical treatment for chlamydia should also be considered. Appropriate contact tracing can be arranged via a genitourinary medicine clinic.

Perinatal infections causing long-term disease

HIV

Infective organism

The HIV virus is an RNA retrovirus transmitted through sexual contact, blood and blood products, shared needles for i.v. drug users, vertical (mother-to-child) transmission which mainly occurs in the late third trimester, during labour or delivery or breastfeeding.

Prevalence

The prevalence of HIV infection in pregnant women in London in 2001 was about one in 286 (0.35 per cent), a 22 per cent increase from the year 2000 (one in 349 or 0.29 per cent). Elsewhere in England, the prevalence of HIV infection is reported to be around one in 2256 (0.044 per cent). Most of the pregnant women with HIV in the UK have acquired their infection through heterosexual exposure. Many of the women are of black African ethnicity and were probably infected in sub-Saharan Africa before immigrating to the UK.

Screening

Routine antenatal screening has increased detection rates and new treatments have increased life expectancy.

In the UK, all pregnant women should be offered screening for HIV early in pregnancy because appropriate antenatal interventions can reduce maternal-to-child transmission of HIV infection from 25 to 30 per cent to less than 2 per cent. Care needs to be taken to ensure that the woman understands the reasons for screening, and that appropriate interventions would be of benefit to her baby. She should also consider the consequences of a positive result prior to embarking on screening, but be reassured about confidentiality and support, should this be the case. A positive HIV antibody test result should be given to the woman in person by an appropriately trained health professional; this may be a specialist nurse, midwife, HIV physician or obstetrician. The issue of disclosure of the HIV diagnosis to her partner should be handled with sensitivity and she should be reassured that her confidentiality will be respected.

Some women remain at risk of becoming infected with HIV during their pregnancy. These women should be offered repeat testing during pregnancy. Rapid HIV tests should be offered to women who present for labour unbooked.

Clinical features

Infection with HIV begins with an asymptomatic stage with gradual compromise of immune function eventually leading to acquired immunodeficiency syndrome (AIDS). The time between HIV infection and development of AIDS ranges from a few months to as long as 17 years in untreated patients.

Management

The principal risks of mother-to-child (vertical) transmission are related to maternal plasma viral load, obstetric factors and infant feeding (Table 13.2).

Interventions to reduce the risk of HIV transmission can reduce the risk of vertical transmission from 25 to 30 per cent to less than 2 per cent:

* anti-retroviral therapy, given antenatally and intrapartum to the mother and to the neonate for the first 4–6 weeks of life
* delivery by elective Caesarean section
* avoidance of breastfeeding.

The implementation of these three interventions combined is associated with a vertical transmission rate of less than 2 per cent.

All women who are HIV positive should be advised to take antiretroviral therapy during pregnancy and at delivery. The optimal regimen is determined by an

Table 13.2 Risk factors for vertical transmission of HIV

Increased risk of transmission	Reduced risk of transmission
Advanced maternal HIV disease	
High maternal plasma viral load	Low or undetectable viral counts at time of delivery
Low CD4 lymphocyte counts	
	Antiretroviral therapy
	Delivery by Caesarean section
Prolonged rupture of membranes	
Chorioamnionitis	
Preterm delivery	
Obstetric interventions such as FBS or fetal scalp electrodes	
Coexisting viral infections e.g. herpes, hepatitis C	
Breastfeeding doubles transmission rate	Exclusive formula feeding

FBS, fetal blood sampling.

HIV physician on a case-by-case basis. The decision to start, modify or stop antiretroviral therapy should be undertaken by an HIV physician. The choice of treatment and the gestation at which it is commenced will depend on whether the woman needs treatment for her own health or simply to prevent vertical transmission. It also depends on her viral load, viral resistance and whether the woman agrees to delivery by lower segment Caesarean section.

Women who do not require HIV treatment for their own health require antiretroviral therapy to prevent mother-to-child transmission. For these women antiretroviral therapy is usually commenced in the second trimester and should be continued intrapartum. A maternal sample for plasma viral load should be taken at delivery. Antiretroviral therapy is usually discontinued soon after delivery but the precise time of discontinuation should be discussed with the HIV physician.

An elective vaginal delivery is an option for women taking triple drug antiretroviral therapy who have a viral load below 50 copies/mL at the time of delivery. Women who opt for a planned vaginal delivery should have their membranes left intact for as long as possible. Use of fetal scalp electrodes and fetal blood sampling should be avoided. A Caesarean delivery is recommended if a woman is taking azidothymidine monotherapy, or if viral load is above 50 copies/mL at the time of delivery.

A Caesarean delivery should be recommended for women with hepatitis C coinfection as the risk of transmission is higher.

Lactic acidosis is a recognized complication of certain highly active antiretroviral therapy (HAART) regimens and may mimic the symptoms and signs of pre-eclampsia. Presentation with symptoms or signs of pre-eclampsia, cholestasis or other signs of liver dysfunction during pregnancy may indicate drug toxicity and early liaison with HIV physicians should be sought. Where this condition is suspected, liver function tests and blood lactate should be monitored. The presenting symptoms of lactic acidosis are often non-specific but may include gastrointestinal disturbance, fatigue, fever and breathlessness.

Management of infants

The cord should be clamped as early as possible after delivery and the baby should be bathed immediately after the birth.

In the UK, where safe infant feeding alternatives are available, all women who are HIV positive should be advised not to breastfeed their babies as this increases the risk of mother-to-child transmission.

All infants born to women who are HIV positive should be treated with antiretroviral therapy from birth. Zidovudine is usually administered orally to the neonate for 4–6 weeks, unless the mother started antiretroviral therapy late in pregnancy. HAART may be considered for neonates of mothers who started antiretroviral therapy late in pregnancy.

Maternal antibodies crossing the placenta are detectable in most neonates of mother who are HIV positive. This means that neonates test positive for HIV antibodies. For this reason, direct viral amplification by PCR is used for the diagnosis of infant infections. Typically, tests are carried out at birth, then at 3 weeks, 6 weeks and six months.

Hepatitis B

Infective organism

The hepatitis B virus (HBV) is a DNA virus that is transmitted mainly in blood, but also in other body fluids such as saliva, semen and vaginal fluid. Drug users who share needles are at high risk. In some areas in the world, e.g. China, chronic hepatitis B is prevalent and vertical transmission is very common.

Prevalence

Two billion people worldwide are infected with HBV. More than 350 million have chronic (lifelong) infections.

In the UK, approximately one in 1000 people are thought to have the virus. The prevalence of hepatitis B surface antigen (HBsAg) in pregnant women in the UK has been found to range from 0.5 to 1 per cent. There is wide variation in prevalence among different ethnic groups, and oriental women in particular appear to have a higher prevalence of HBsAg.

Screening

Serological screening for HBV should be offered to pregnant women so that effective post-natal intervention can be offered to infected women to decrease the risk of mother-to-child transmission.

As many as 85 per cent of babies born to mothers who are positive for the hepatitis e antigen (eAg) will become HBsAg carriers and subsequently become chronic carriers, compared with 31 per cent of babies who are born to mothers who are eAg negative. It has been estimated that chronic carriers of HBsAg are 22 times more likely to die from hepatocellular carcinoma or cirrhosis than non-carriers.

Mother-to-child transmission of the HBV is approximately 95 per cent preventable through administration of vaccine and immunoglobulin to the baby at birth. To prevent mother-to-child transmission, all pregnant women who are carriers of HBV need to be identified. Because of the high proportion of cases of mother-to-child transmission that can be prevented through vaccination and immunization, the UK National Screening Committee recommends that all pregnant women be screened for HBV.

Clinical features

Hepatitis B is a virus that infects the liver, but many people with hepatitis B viral infection have no symptoms. The HBV has an incubation period of 6 weeks to six months.

Management

Women who screen positive for hepatitis B should be referred to a hepatologist for ongoing monitoring for the long-term consequences of chronic infection, for example hepatocellular carcinoma.

To prevent vertical transmission of hepatitis B, a combination of hepatitis B immunoglobulin and hepatitis B vaccine may be given. Virology laboratories will usually advise on the appropriate regime. The combined treatment provides better therapy than either alone. The passive immunoglobulin provides immediate protection against any virus transmitted to the baby from contact with blood during delivery, and should be given immediately after delivery. The active vaccine provides ongoing protection from subsequent exposure in the household. The active vaccine is given in three doses: at birth, at one month and at six months of age.

Hepatitis C

Infective organism

The hepatitis C virus (HCV) is an RNA virus. Acquisition of the virus occurs predominantly through infected blood products and injection of drugs. It can also occur with tattooing and body piercing. Mother-to-child transmission can occur due to contact with infected maternal blood around the time of delivery, and the risk is higher in those coinfected with HIV. Sexual transmission is extremely rare.

Prevalence

In the UK the overall antenatal prevalence has been estimated to be around 1 per cent, with regional variation. The risk of mother-to-child transmission is estimated to lie between 3 and 5 per cent and it is estimated that 70 births each year are infected with HCV as a result of mother-to-child transmission in the UK. The risk of mother-to-child transmission of HCV increases with increasing maternal viral load.

Screening

Current recommendations are that pregnant women should not be offered routine screening for HCV. This is because there is a lack of evidence-based effective interventions for the treatment of HCV in pregnancy, and a lack of evidence about which interventions reduce vertical transmission of HCV from mother to child.

Clinical features

HCV is a major public health concern due to its long-term consequences on health. It is one of the major causes of liver cirrhosis, hepatocellular carcinoma and liver failure. Following initial infection, only 20 per cent of women will have hepatic symptoms, 80 per cent being asymptomatic. The majority of pregnant women with hepatitis C will not have reached the phase of having the chronic disease, and may well be unaware that they are infected.

Management

Testing for HCV in the UK involves detection of anti-HCV antibodies in serum with subsequent confirmatory testing by PCR for the virus, if a positive result is obtained. Upon confirmation of a positive test, a woman should be offered post-test counselling and referral to a hepatologist for management and treatment of her infection.

In non-pregnant adults, interferon and ribavirin can be used to treat hepatitis C infection, but these are contraindicated in pregnancy.

There is no strong evidence regarding mode of delivery in women with hepatitis C. Consensus groups therefore do not recommend elective Caesarean section for all women with hepatitis C, although it is recommended if the woman is also HIV positive.

Key points

- Infectious diseases contracted during pregnancy can have a serious impact on both the mother and the fetus.
- Infections can cause congenital abnormalities in the fetus (rubella, syphilis, toxoplasmosis, cytomegalovirus, chickenpox). Some infections can be transmitted from mother to baby during pregnancy and affect the fetus *in utero* (parvovirus, syphilis).
- Some infections can be transmitted to the fetus around the time of delivery, and appropriate obstetric management can reduce the risk of transmission (HIV, hepatitis B, hepatitis C, herpes, group B streptococcus).
- For some infections screening programmes and effective interventions can improve the outcome for the mother and baby.

New developments

- In recent years a non-invasive method has been developed to diagnose and monitor fetal anaemia. This is done by using Doppler ultrasound to measure the velocity of blood flow in the fetal middle cerebral artery. Faster flow is indicative of fetal anaemia. This has improved the diagnosis and management of fetuses infected with parvovirus, as the main effect of this infection is anaemia.
- Antiretroviral HIV therapies have been developed and research has focused on which therapies are more appropriate for different groups of women.
- Hepatitis B vaccination programmes are being extended worldwide. In some countries such as Taiwan, this has already resulted in lower transmission rates and a reduction in childhood hepatocellular carcinoma.
- Further research is needed into the treatment of hepatitis C in pregnancy with antiviral agents, and into the most appropriate mode of delivery in women with hepatitis C. The development of a hepatitis C vaccination would confer long-term health benefits.

CASE HISTORY

Ms B is a 30-year-old shop assistant. This is her first pregnancy and she attends for a routine anomaly scan at 20 weeks gestation. She has no family history or past medical history of note and has been well throughout her pregnancy.

On the ultrasound scan the fetus is seen to be small, approximately 18 weeks size. The ventricles in the brain measure 12 mm (the upper limit of normal is 10 mm).

There is a small amount of fetal ascites and some fetal skin oedema.

What are the possible causes?

These ultrasound findings could be due to congenital infection, chromosomal abnormality in the fetus or genetic disorders. Various infections could cause these ultrasound abnormalities including syphilis, rubella, CMV and toxoplasmosis.

continued ➤

What would you do next?

The first steps would be to take a careful history for symptoms suggestive of a viral illness or contact with illness.

The results of her routine screening blood tests taken at the booking visit should be checked. (These showed that she was immune to rubella and tested negative for syphilis.)

The virology lab should be asked whether they had retained the original sample and this should be checked for toxoplasmosis and cytomegalovirus antibodies. (She did not have any antibodies to these on her initial sample.) A further sample should be taken to be tested for toxoplasmosis and cytomegalovirus antibodies to see whether antibodies had developed. This would suggest recent infection.

She should be offered an amniocentesis to exclude chromosomal abnormalities. The amniotic fluid should also be tested for toxoplasma and CMV.

Results

The initial booking blood sample did not have any antibodies for CMV. The sample sent on the day of her anomaly scan had CMV IgM, suggesting a recent infection. The PCR on the amniotic fluid showed that it contained CMV.

These results together with the ultrasound findings confirm a diagnosis of congenital CMV infection.

What would you do next?

The results should be explained to Ms B. The likelihood of a very poor prognosis for the baby should be explained and termination of pregnancy offered. Throughout this she would need support and compassion. It should also be explained to her that since she would now be immune to CMV this would not happen again in a future pregnancy.

CHAPTER 14

LABOUR

Alec McEwan

OVERVIEW

Labour can be defined as the process by which regular painful contractions bring about effacement and dilatation of the cervix and descent of the presenting part, ultimately leading to expulsion of the fetus and the placenta from the mother. This gross oversimplification hides a multitude of medical, social, cultural and ethical variables which combine together in a complex interplay and mean that labour and delivery can often have a long-lasting physical and emotional impact, which may be positive or negative. A doctor or midwife who manages labour must be aware of the normal anatomy and physiology of the mother and fetus, what distinguishes an abnormal from a normal labour, and when it is appropriate to intervene.

Introduction

Approximately 600 000 women give birth in the United Kingdom each year. Labour and delivery are both a physical and emotional challenge for the mother and represent a potentially hazardous journey for the fetus. There is a complex interaction between the 'powers' of the uterus (the contractions), the 'passages' of the birth canal (the bony pelvis and the soft tissues of the pelvic floor and perineum) and the 'passenger' (the fetus) which means that no two labours are ever quite the same. Contractions are necessary to promote dilatation of the uterine cervix and descent of the fetus, however during each one, the placenta is temporarily deprived of blood flow, and consequently the fetus of its oxygen supply.

Labour brings great joy and happiness to the majority of families, but maternal and fetal outcomes are not always good, and are frequently suboptimal. Maternal death is rare in the Western world, but remains frequent in many countries that have less developed healthcare systems. Complications of labour account for a significant proportion of maternal deaths in these countries, where childbirth is often unattended. This must not be confused with 'natural childbirth', a term used to describe a form of care in labour that utilizes minimal technology and natural methods of pain relief. Women have widely different expectations of labour and delivery, influenced by previous experiences, friends and family, social, religious and cultural factors, the media and healthcare professionals. In the Western world, the expectation is usually that the outcome will be 'normal' and this is one reason why rates of litigation are so high following supposed intrapartum mismanagement. Maternal choice remains a high priority for policymakers, and also most midwives and obstetricians. Where a woman should give birth, who should care for her in labour, how she might deliver and with what kind of pain relief, are all key issues that are decided by a multitude of factors, including maternal choice. Natural childbirth may be sought by women who perceive that birth in the Western world has been 'hijacked' by modern medicine and modern doctors. Conversely, there is now a small but significant minority of women who have the opposite philosophy: they have opted to avoid labour altogether and to elect for planned Caesarean section. Although this remains a contentious issue, many women have an increasing expectation that mode of delivery should be a matter of choice. The average Caesarean section rate in the UK is approximately 21 per cent, including both emergency and elective Caesarean sections. Although this is recognized by most as being too high, the reason for the steady rise in Caesarean births and the ideal rate are unclear. Undoubtedly, maternal choice is an important factor. How far maternal wishes should be followed remains a matter of debate. Healthcare professionals have a duty to provide good quality evidence to pregnant women to help them in their decision-making. Conflict should be avoided and a degree of compromise is often required to optimize outcomes.

Before exploring the process of labour in detail, an understanding of the anatomy of the female pelvis and the fetus is crucial if the mechanisms of labour are to be understood.

Fetal and maternal anatomy relevant to labour

The pelvis

The pelvic brim or inlet

The pelvic brim is the inlet of the pelvis and is bounded in front by the symphysis pubis (the joint separating the two pubic bones), on each side by the upper margin of the pubic bone, the ileopectineal line and the ala of the sacrum, and posteriorly by the promontory of the sacrum (Figure 14.1). The normal transverse diameter in this plane is 13.5 cm and is wider than the anterior–posterior (AP) diameter,

which is normally 11 cm (Figure 14.2). The angle of the inlet is normally 60° to the horizontal in the erect position, but in Afro-Caribbean women this angle may be as much as 90° (Figure 14.3). This increased angle may delay the head entering the pelvis during labour.

The pelvic mid-cavity

The pelvic mid-cavity can be described as an area bounded in front by the middle of the symphysis pubis,

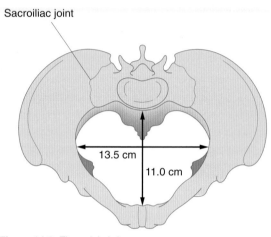
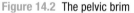

Figure 14.2 The pelvic brim

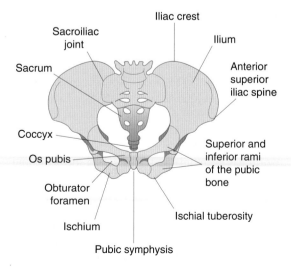

Figure 14.1 The bony pelvis

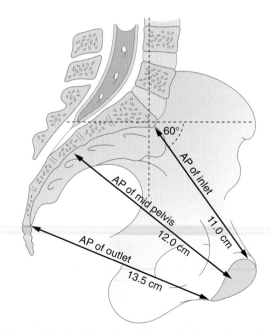

Figure 14.3 Sagittal section of the pelvis demonstrating the anterior–posterior (AP) diameters of the inlet and outlet

on each side by the pubic bone, the obturator fascia and the inner aspect of the ischial bone and spines, and posteriorly by the junction of the second and third sections of the sacrum. The cavity is almost round, as the transverse and anterior diameters are similar at 12 cm. The ischial spines are palpable vaginally and are used as landmarks to assess the descent of the head on vaginal examination (station). They are also used as landmarks for providing an anaesthetic block to the pudendal nerve. The pudendal nerve passes behind and below the ischial spine on each side. The pelvic axis describes an imaginary curved line, a path that the centre of the fetal head must take during its passage through the pelvis.

The pelvic outlet

The pelvic outlet is bounded in front by the lower margin of the symphysis pubis, on each side by the descending ramus of the pubic bone, the ischial tuberosity and the sacrotuberous ligament, and posteriorly by the last piece of the sacrum. The AP diameter of the pelvic outlet is 13.5 cm and the transverse diameter is 11 cm (Figure 14.4). Therefore, the transverse is the widest diameter at the inlet, but at the outlet it is the AP. Recognizing this is crucial to the understanding of the mechanism of labour.

The pelvic measurements given here are obviously average values and relate to bony points. Maternal stature, previous pelvic fractures and metabolic bone disease, such as rickets, may all be associated with measurements less than these population means. Furthermore, as the pelvic ligaments at the pubic ramus and the sacroiliac joints loosen towards the end of the third trimester, the pelvis often becomes more flexible and these diameters may increase during labour. It is now uncommon to perform x-rays or computed tomography (CT) scans of the pelvis to measure the pelvis because they have, on the whole,

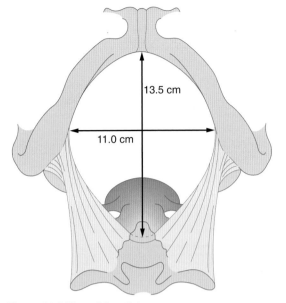

Figure 14.4 The pelvic outlet

proven to be of minimal clinical use in predicting the outcome of labour.

A variety of pelvic shapes has been described, and these may contribute to difficulties encountered in labour. The gynaecoid pelvis is the most favourable for labour, and the most common (Figure 14.5). Other pelvic shapes are shown in Figures 14.6 to 14.8. An android-type pelvis is said to predispose to deep transverse arrest (see Figure 14.22) and the anthropoid shape encourages an occipito-posterior (OP) position (see below). A platypelloid pelvis also is associated with an increased risk of obstructed labour.

The pelvic floor

This is formed by the two levator ani muscles which, with their fascia, form a musculofascial gutter during the second stage of labour (Figure 14.9).

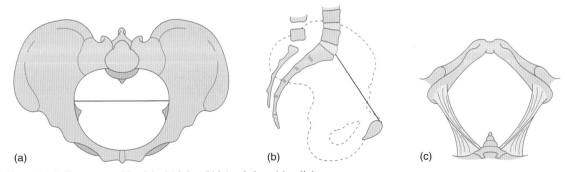

(a)   (b)   (c)

Figure 14.5 The gynaecoid pelvis: (a) brim, (b) lateral view, (c) outlet

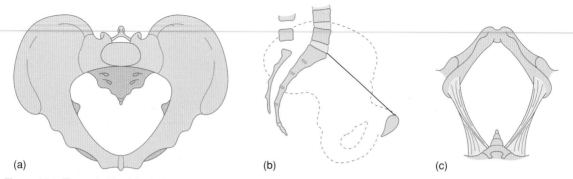

Figure 14.6 The android pelvis: (a) brim, (b) lateral view, (c) outlet

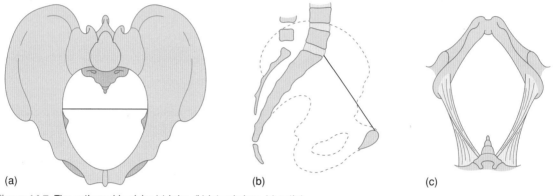

Figure 14.7 The anthropoid pelvis: (a) brim, (b) lateral view, (c) outlet

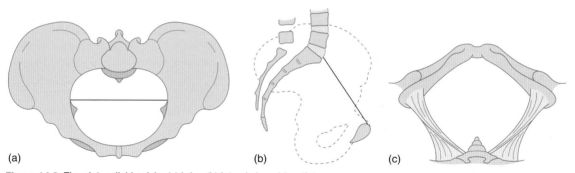

Figure 14.8 The platypelloid pelvis: (a) brim, (b) lateral view, (c) outlet

The perineum

The final obstacle to be negotiated by the fetus during labour is the perineum. The perineal body is a condensation of fibrous and muscular tissue lying between the vagina and the anus (Figure 14.10). It receives attachments of the posterior ends of the bulbo-cavernous muscles, the medial ends of the superficial and deep transverse perineal muscles, and the anterior fibres of the external anal sphincter. It is always involved in a second-degree perineal tear and an episiotomy.

The fetal skull

The bones, sutures and fontanelles

The fetal skull is made up of the vault, the face and the base. The sutures are the lines formed where the individual bony plates of the skull meet one another.

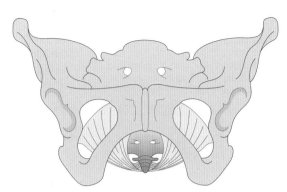

Figure 14.9 The musculofascial gutter of the levator sling

At the time of labour, the sutures joining the bones of the vault are soft, unossified membranes, whereas the sutures of the face and the skull base are firmly united (Figure 14.11).

The vault of the skull is formed by the parietal bones and parts of the occipital, frontal and temporal bones. Between these bones there are four membranous sutures: the sagittal, frontal, coronal and lambdoidal sutures.

Fontanelles are the junctions of the various sutures. The anterior fontanelle, or bregma (diamond shaped), is at the junction of the sagittal, frontal and coronal sutures. The posterior fontanelle (triangular shaped) lies at the junction of the sagittal suture and the lambdoidal sutures between the two parietal bones and the occipital bone. The fact that these sutures are not united is important for labour. It allows these bones to move together and even to overlap. The parietal bones usually tend to slide over the frontal and occipital bones. Furthermore, the bones themselves are compressible. Together, these characteristics of the fetal skull allow a process called 'moulding' to occur, which effectively reduces the diameters of the fetal skull and encourages progress through the bony pelvis, without harming the underlying brain (Figure 14.12). However, severe moulding can be a sign of cephalopelvic disproportion (see below under Cephalopelvic disproportion).

The area of the fetal skull bounded by the two parietal eminences and the anterior and posterior fontanelles is termed the 'vertex'.

The diameters of the skull

The fetal head is ovoid in shape. The attitude of the fetal head refers to the degree of flexion and extension at the upper cervical spine. Different longitudinal diameters are presented to the pelvis in labour

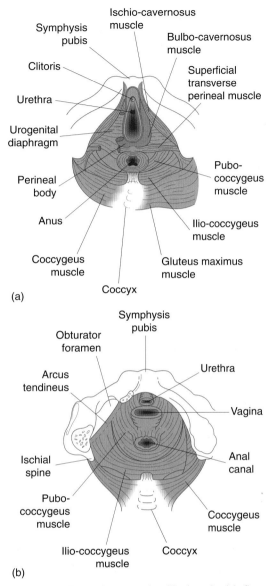

Figure 14.10 The perineum, perineal body and pelvic floor from below, showing superficial (a) and deeper (b) views. The pelvic floor muscles are made up of the levator ani (pubo-coccygeus and ilio-coccygeus)

depending on the attitude of the fetal head (Figures 14.13 and 14.14).

The longitudinal diameter that presents in a well-flexed fetal head (vertex presentation) is the suboccipito-bregmatic diameter. This is usually 9.5 cm and is measured from the suboccipital region to the centre of the anterior fontanelle (bregma). The longitudinal diameter that presents in a less well-flexed head, such as is found in the OP position, is

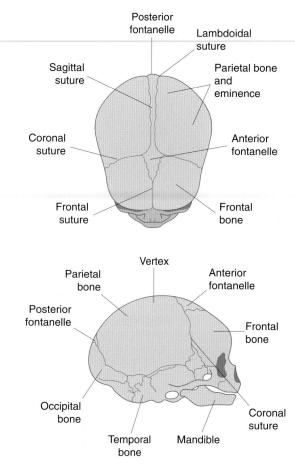

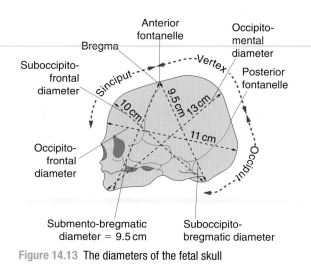

Figure 14.13 The diameters of the fetal skull

the suboccipito-frontal diameter, and is measured from the suboccipital region to the prominence of the forehead. It measures 10 cm.

With further extension of the head, the occipito-frontal diameter presents. This is measured from the root of the nose to the posterior fontanelle and is 11.5 cm. The greatest longitudinal diameter that may present is the mento-vertical, which is taken from the chin to the furthest point of the vertex and measures 13 cm. This is known as a brow presentation and it is usually too large to pass through the normal pelvis.

Extension of the fetal head beyond this point results in a smaller diameter. The submento-bregmatic diameter is measured from below the chin to the anterior fontanelle and is 9.5 cm. This is clinically a face presentation.

Figure 14.11 The fetal skull from superior and lateral views

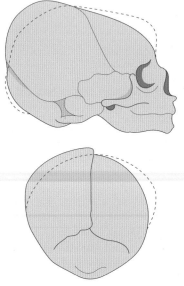

Figure 14.12 A schematic representation of moulding of the fetal skull

Key points

The female pelvis and fetal skull

- The pelvic inlet is wider in the transverse than in the AP diameter.
- The pelvic outlet is wider in the AP than in the transverse diameter.
- Pelvic measurements may widen during labour due to pelvic ligament laxity.
- The soft tissues of the pelvic floor and perineum have a vital role to play in labour.
- Moulding may reduce the absolute measurements of the fetal skull during labour.
- The degree of flexion of the fetal skull at the cervical spine (the attitude) determines the diameter of the fetal skull presenting to the pelvis.

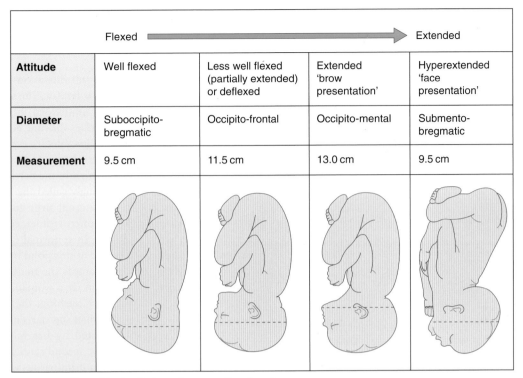

	Flexed ⟶ Extended			
Attitude	Well flexed	Less well flexed (partially extended) or deflexed	Extended 'brow presentation'	Hyperextended 'face presentation'
Diameter	Suboccipito-bregmatic	Occipito-frontal	Occipito-mental	Submento-bregmatic
Measurement	9.5 cm	11.5 cm	13.0 cm	9.5 cm

Figure 14.14 The effect of fetal attitude on the presenting diameter

The process of labour

The onset of labour

The onset of labour can be defined as regular contractions bringing about progressive cervical change. Therefore, a diagnosis of labour is usually made in retrospect. Loss of a 'show' (a blood-stained plug of mucus passed from the cervix) or spontaneous rupture of the membranes (SROM) does not define the onset of labour, although they may occur at the same time. Labour can be well established before either of these events occur, and both may precede labour by many days. Although much is understood about the physiology of labour in humans, the initiating biological event is still unclear (see below under Understanding the physiology of labour). It is certainly true however that the uterine body and cervix undergo a number of changes in preparation for labour which start a number of weeks before its onset.

The stages of labour

Labour can be divided into three stages. The definitions of these stages rely predominantly on anatomical criteria, and in certain situations this may be a disadvantage, as labour is essentially a physiological process. In normal labour, the division into three stages is of little clinical significance. The important events in normal labour are the diagnosis of labour and the maternal urge to push, which usually corresponds with full dilatation of the cervix and the baby's head resting on the perineum. Defining the three stages of labour becomes more relevant if the labour does not progress normally. Because the definition of a normal labour can only be made retrospectively, there is difficulty in defining exactly when a normal labour becomes abnormal. Indeed, this definition will be different depending on the gestation, the previous obstetric record and the onset of labour. The average duration of first labours is approximately 8 hours, and that of subsequent labours 5 hours. First labours rarely last more than 18 hours, and second and subsequent labours not usually more than 12 hours.

The stages of labour are as follows.

First stage

This describes the time from the diagnosis of labour to full dilatation of the cervix (10 cm) (Figure 14.15).

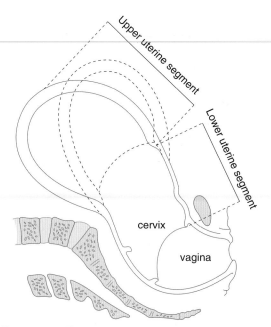

Figure 14.15 The thick upper segment and the thin lower segment of the uterus at the end of the first stage of labour. The dotted lines indicate the position assumed by the uterus during contraction

The first stage of labour can be divided into two phases. The 'latent phase' is the time between the onset of labour and 3–4 cm dilatation. During this time, the cervix becomes 'fully effaced'. Effacement is a process by which the cervix shortens in length as it becomes included into the lower segment of the uterus. The process of effacement may begin during the weeks preceding the onset of labour, but will be complete by the end of the latent phase. The cervical os cannot usually begin to dilate until effacement is complete. Effacement and dilatation should be thought of as consecutive events in the nulliparous woman, but may occur simultaneously in the multiparous woman. Dilatation is expressed in centimetres between 0 and 10. The duration of the latent phase is variable, and time limits are arbitrary. However, it usually lasts between 3 and 8 hours, being shorter in multiparous women.

The second phase of the first stage of labour is called the 'active phase' and describes the time between the end of the latent phase (3–4 cm dilatation) and full dilatation (10 cm). It is also variable in length, usually lasting between 2 and 6 hours. Again, it is usually shorter in multiparous women. Cervical dilatation during the active phase usually occurs at 1 cm/hour or more in a normal labour (again, an arbitrary value), but is only considered abnormal if it occurs at less than 2 cm/hour.

Second stage

This describes the time from full dilatation of the cervix to delivery of the fetus or fetuses. The second stage of labour may also be subdivided into two phases. The passive phase describes the time between full dilatation and the onset of involuntary expulsive contractions. There is no maternal urge to push and the fetal head is still relatively high in the pelvis. The second phase is rather confusingly called the 'active second stage'. There is a maternal urge to push because the fetal head is low (often visible), causing a reflex need to 'bear down'. In a normal labour, second stage is often diagnosed at this point because the maternal urge to push prompts the midwife to perform a vaginal examination. If a woman never reaches a point of involuntary pushing, the active second stage is said to begin when she starts making voluntary active efforts directed by her midwife. Conventionally, a normal active second stage should last no longer than 2 hours in a primiparous woman and 1 hour in those who have delivered vaginally before. Again, these definitions are largely arbitrary, but there is evidence that a second stage of labour lasting more than 3 hours is associated with increased maternal and fetal morbidity.

Use of epidural anaesthesia may influence the length and the management of the second stage of labour.

Third stage

This is the time from delivery of the fetus or fetuses until delivery of the placenta(e). The placenta is usually delivered within a few minutes of the birth of the baby. A third stage lasting more than 30 minutes should be considered abnormal, unless the woman has opted for 'physiological management' (see below under Third stage under Management of normal labour) in which case it is reasonable to extend this definition to 60 minutes.

The duration of labour

More than any other objective measurement, the duration of labour determines the impact of childbirth, particularly on mothers but also on babies, and also on those who care for both of them. The morale of most women starts to deteriorate after 6 hours in labour, and after 12 hours the rate of deterioration significantly accelerates. There is a greater incidence of fetal hypoxia and need for operative delivery associated with longer labours. Shorter labours will also mean that personal attention for each woman in labour is a realistic possibility. An early artificial rupture of membranes (ARM) does shorten the length of labour, but does not necessarily alter the outcome.

It is difficult to define prolonged labour, but it would be reasonable to suggest that labour lasting longer than 12 hours in nulliparous women and 8 hours in multiparous women should be regarded as prolonged.

The mechanism of labour

This refers to the series of changes in position and attitude that the fetus undergoes during its passage through the birth canal. It is described here for the vertex presentation and the gynaecoid pelvis. The relation of the fetal head and body to the maternal pelvis changes as the fetus descends through the pelvis. This is essential so that the optimal diameters of the fetal skull are present at each stage of the descent.

Engagement

The head normally enters the pelvis in the transverse position or some minor variant of this, so taking advantage of the widest diameter. Engagement is said to have occurred when the widest part of the presenting part has passed successfully through the inlet. Engagement has occurred in the vast majority of nulliparous women prior to labour, but not so for the majority of multiparous women.

The number of fifths of the fetal head palpable abdominally is often used to describe whether engagement has taken place. If more than two-fifths of the fetal head is palpable abdominally, the head is not yet engaged.

Descent

Descent of the fetal head is needed before flexion, internal rotation and extension can occur (Figure 14.16). During the first stage and first phase of the second stage of labour, descent of the fetus is secondary to uterine action. In the active phase of the second stage of labour, descent of the fetus is helped by voluntary use of abdominal musculature and the Valsalva manoeuvre ('pushing').

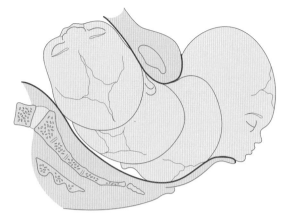

Figure 14.16 Descent and flexion of the head followed by internal rotation and ending in birth of the head by extension

Flexion

The fetal head may not always be completely flexed when it enters the pelvis. As the head descends into the narrower mid-cavity, flexion should occur. This passive movement occurs, in part, due to the surrounding structures and is important in minimizing the presenting diameter of the fetal head.

Internal rotation

If the head is well flexed, the occiput will be the leading point and on reaching the sloping gutter of the levator ani muscles, it will be encouraged to rotate anteriorly so that the sagittal suture now lies in the AP diameter of the pelvic outlet (i.e. the widest diameter). If the fetus has engaged in the OP position, internal rotation can occur from an OP position to an occipito-anterior (OA) position. This long internal rotation may explain the increased duration of labour associated with this malposition. Alternatively, an OP position may persist, resulting in a 'face to pubes' delivery. More often, the persistent OP position is associated with extension of the fetal head and a resulting increase in the diameter presented to the pelvic outlet. This may lead to obstructed labour and the need for instrumental delivery or even Caesarean section.

Extension

Following completion of internal rotation, the occiput is underneath the symphysis pubis and the bregma is near the lower border of the sacrum. The soft tissues of the perineum still offer resistance, and may be traumatized in the process. The well-flexed head now extends and the occiput escapes from underneath the symphysis pubis and distends the vulva. This is known as 'crowning' of the head. The head extends further and the occiput underneath the symphysis pubis acts as a fulcrum point as the bregma, face and chin appear in succession over the posterior vaginal opening and perineal body. This extension and movement minimize soft-tissue trauma by utilizing the smallest diameters of the head for the birth.

Restitution

When the head is delivering, the occiput is directly anterior. As soon as it escapes from the vulva, the head aligns itself with the shoulders, which have entered the pelvis in the oblique position. The slight rotation of the occiput through one-eighth of the circle is called 'restitution'.

External rotation

In order to be delivered, the shoulders have to rotate into the direct AP plane (remember the widest diameter at the outlet). When this occurs, the occiput rotates through a further one-eighth of a circle to the transverse position. This is called external rotation (Figure 14.17).

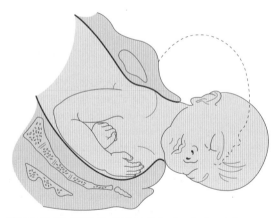

Figure 14.17 External rotation of the head after delivery as the anterior shoulder rotates forward to pass under the subpubic arch

Delivery of the shoulders and fetal body

When restitution and external rotation have occurred, the shoulders will be in the AP position. The anterior shoulder is under the symphysis pubis and delivers first, and the posterior shoulder delivers subsequently. Although this process may occur without assistance, lateral traction is often exerted by gently pulling the fetal head in a downward direction

to help release the anterior shoulder from beneath the pubic symphysis.

Normally the rest of the fetal body is delivered easily, with the posterior shoulder guided over the perineum by traction in the opposite direction, so sweeping the baby on to the maternal abdomen.

Understanding the physiology of labour

The mechanism responsible for initiating human parturition is still unknown and is somewhat different from that in all other animal models that have been studied. There are, however, certain processes that seem to be of particular importance.

The onset of labour occurs when those factors which inhibit contractions and maintain a closed cervix diminish and are succeeded by the actions of factors which do the opposite. Both mother and fetus make contributions toward this.

The myometrium

Myometrial cells contain filaments of actin and myosin, which interact and bring about contraction in response to an increase in intracellular calcium. Prostaglandins and oxytocin increase intracellular free calcium ions, whereas beta-adrenergic compounds and calcium-channel blockers do the opposite. Separation of the actin and myosin filaments brings about relaxation of the myocyte, however, unlike in any other muscle cell of the body, this actin–myosin interaction occurs along the full length of the filaments so that a degree of shortening occurs with each successive interaction. This progressive shortening of the uterine smooth muscle cells is called retraction and occurs in the cells of the upper part of the uterus. The result of this retraction process is the development of the thicker, actively contracting 'upper segment'. At the same time, the lower segment of the uterus becomes thinner and more stretched. Eventually, this results in the cervix being taken up into the lower segment of the uterus so forming a continuum with the lower uterine segment (see Figure 14.15). The cervix effaces and then dilates, and the fetus descends in response to this directional force.

It is essential that the myocytes of the uterus contract together in a coordinated fashion. Individual myometrial cells are laid down in a mesh of collagen. There is cell-to-cell communication by means of gap junctions, which facilitate the passage of various products of metabolism and electrical current between cells. These gap junctions are absent for most of the pregnancy but appear in significant numbers at term. Gap junctions increase in size and number with the progress of labour and allow greater coordination of myocyte activity. Prostaglandins stimulate their formation, while beta-adrenergic compounds possibly do the opposite. A uterine pacemaker from which contractions originate probably does exist but has not been demonstrated histologically.

Uterine contractions are involuntary in nature and there is relatively minimal extrauterine neuronal control. The frequency of contractions may vary during labour and with parity. Throughout the majority of labour, they occur at intervals of 2–4 minutes. Their duration also varies during labour, from 30 to 60 seconds, or occasionally longer. The intensity or amplitude of the intrauterine pressure generated with each contraction averages between 30 and 60 mmHg.

The cervix

The cervix contains muscle cells and fibroblasts separated by a 'ground substance' made up of extracellular matrix molecules. Interactions between collagen, fibronectin and dermatan sulphate (a proteoglycan) during the earlier stages of pregnancy keep the cervix rigid and closed. Contractions at this point do not bring about effacement or dilatation. Under the influence of prostaglandins, and other humoral mediators, there is an increase in proteolytic activity and reduction in collagen and elastin. Interleukins bring about a pro-inflammatory change with a significant invasion by neutrophils. Dermatan sulphate is replaced by the more hydrophilic hyaluronic acid, which results in an increase in water content of the cervix. This causes cervical softening or 'ripening', so that contractions, when they begin, can bring about the processes of effacement and dilatation.

Hormonal factors

Progesterone maintains uterine quiescence by suppressing prostaglandin production, inhibiting communication between myometrial cells and preventing oxytocin release. Oestrogen opposes the action of progesterone. Prior to labour, there is a reduction in progesterone receptors and an increase in the concentration of oestrogen relative to the progesterone. Prostaglandin synthesis by the chorion and the decidua is enhanced, leading to an increase in calcium influx into the myometrial cells. This change in the hormonal milieu also increases gap junction formation between individual myometrial cells, creating a functional syncytium, which is necessary for coordinated uterine activity. The production of corticotrophin-releasing hormone (CRH) by the placenta increases in concentration towards term and potentiates the action of prostaglandins and oxytocin on myometrial contractility. The fetal pituitary secretes oxytocin and the fetal adrenal gland produces cortisol, which stimulates the conversion of progesterone to oestrogen.

Which of these hormonal steps initiates labour is unclear. As labour becomes established, the output of oxytocin increases through the Fergusson reflex. Pressure from the fetal presenting part against the cervix is relayed via a reflex arc involving the spinal cord and results in increased oxytocin release from the maternal posterior pituitary.

Place of birth

The most recent recommendation from the National Institute for Health and Clinical Excellence (NICE) (see Clinical Guideline 55) is that women should be offered the choice of planning birth at home, in a midwife-led unit, or in an obstetric unit. Currently, less than 5 per cent of women deliver at home in most areas of the UK. Not all women have access to a midwifery-run unit. Some of these units are based within a hospital environment, and some are stand-alone. The evidence base guiding women on the outcomes of birth in the different settings is poor and full of bias. The chances of a normal birth at home, or in a midwifery unit, are higher than in an obstetric unit, but these women self-select and are more likely to be multiparous and without complicating factors. Use of epidural pain relief is restricted to consultant-led hospital labour wards, and this is known to increase the chances of delivery by forceps or ventouse. There is simply too little information to state conclusively where it is safest to give birth, from a maternal or fetal perspective. All women should be informed, however, that unexpected emergencies can occur in labour and that the outcome from these may be better in a hospital setting. It should also be made clear that the need for transfer into hospital, during labour, is possible from home or a midwifery-run unit. Women with issues which increase the chances of problems occurring during labour should be recommended to deliver in an obstetric unit and NICE have published a list of obstetric, fetal and medical factors to help guide midwives and obstetricians when they are counselling women. Also, a variety of indications are listed for intrapartum transfer into an obstetric unit, including high maternal pyrexia in labour, delay in labour, concerns regarding fetal well-being, hypertension, retained placenta and complicated perineal trauma requiring suturing.

Management of normal labour

Women are told to contact their local labour suite or their community midwife if they think their waters may have broken (rupture of membranes) or when their contractions are occurring every 5 minutes or more. It is important to recognize that women have very different thresholds for seeking advice and reassurance. The need for pain relief may result in admission to hospital before either of these two criteria is reached. Whether at home or in hospital, the attending midwife will then make an assessment of the situation based on the history and on clinical examination.

History

The following are important points to note in the admission history:

- Details of previous births and the size of previous babies (the uneventful birth of normal or large babies is encouraging). A previous Caesarean section, for example, is an adverse feature, especially if it was performed because of a mechanical problem.
- The frequency, duration and perception of strength of the contractions and when they began.
- Whether the membranes have ruptured and, if so, the colour and amount of amniotic fluid lost.
- The presence of abnormal vaginal discharge or bleeding.
- The recent activity of the fetus.
- Any medical issues of note that may influence the labour and delivery, e.g. pregnancy-induced hypertension, fetal growth restriction.

- Does she have any special requirements, e.g. an interpreter, or particular emotional/psychological needs?
- What are her expectations of the labour and delivery? Has she made a birth plan? What did she hope to use for pain relief?

General examination

It is important to recognize women who have a raised body mass index, as this may complicate the management of labour. The temperature, pulse and blood pressure must be recorded and a sample of urine tested for protein, blood, ketones, glucose and nitrates.

Abdominal examination

After the initial inspection for scars indicating previous surgery, it is important to determine the lie of the fetus (longitudinal, transverse or oblique) and the nature of the presenting part (cephalic or breech). If it is a cephalic presentation, the degree of engagement must be determined. A head that remains high and unengaged is a poor prognostic sign for successful delivery. If there is any doubt as to the presentation or if the head is high (five-fifths palpable), an ultrasound scan will determine the presenting part or the reason for the high head (e.g. OP position, deflexed head, placenta praevia, fibroid, etc.) An attempt to estimate the size of the fetus should be made.

Abdominal examination also includes an assessment of the contractions; this takes time (at least 10 minutes) and is done by palpating the uterus directly, not by looking at the tocograph, which provides information only on the frequency and duration of contractions, not the strength.

Vaginal examination

A full explanation of the purpose and technique of vaginal examination is given to the woman and her consent must be obtained. Many women find vaginal examinations extremely distressing and every effort should be made to maintain the woman's dignity and privacy. The index and middle fingers are passed to the top of the vagina and the cervix. The cervix is examined for dilatation, effacement and application to the presenting part. The dilatation is estimated digitally in centimetres. When no cervix can be felt, this means the cervix is fully dilated (10 cm). The length of the cervix should be recorded. The cervix at 36 weeks is about 3 cm long. It gradually shortens by the process of effacement. In early labour, it may still be uneffaced. At about 4 cm of dilatation, the cervix should be fully effaced. Providing the cervix is at least 4 cm dilated, it should be possible to determine both the position and the station of the presenting part.

In a normal labour, the vertex will be presenting and the position can be determined by locating the occiput. The occiput is identified by feeling for the triangular posterior fontanelle. Failure to feel the posterior fontanelle may be because the head is deflexed, the occiput is posterior or there is so much caput that the sutures cannot be felt. All of these indicate the possibility of a prolonged labour. Normally, the occiput will be transverse (OT position) or anterior (OA). Relating the lowest part of the head to the ischial spines will give an estimation of the station. This vaginal assessment of station should always be taken together with assessment of the degree of engagement by abdominal palpation. If the head is at or below the ischial spines (0 to +1 or more) and the occiput is anterior (OA), the outlook is favourable for vaginal delivery.

The condition of the membranes should also be noted. If they have ruptured, the colour and amount of fluid draining should be noted. Copious amounts of clear fluid are a good prognostic feature; scanty, heavily blood-stained or meconium-stained fluid is a warning sign for fetal compromise.

Women who are found not to be in established labour should be offered appropriate analgesia and support. Most can safely go home, to return when the contractions increase in strength and frequency.

The admission history and examination act as an initial screen for abnormal labour and increased maternal/fetal risk. If all features are normal and reassuring, the woman will remain under midwifery care. If there are risk factors identified, medical involvement in the form of the on-call obstetric team may be appropriate.

Women in labour should have their pulse measured hourly and their temperature and blood pressure every 4 hours. The frequency of contractions should be recorded every 30 minutes and a vaginal examination performed every 4 hours (unless other factors suggest it needs to be repeated on a different time-frame). It should be noted when the woman voids urine, and this should be tested for ketones and protein. Once the second stage is reached, the blood pressure and pulse should be performed hourly, and vaginal examinations offered every hour also.

Fetal assessment in labour

A healthy term fetus is usually able to withstand the rigours of a normal labour. However, with each contraction, placental blood flow and oxygen transfer are temporarily interrupted and a fetus that is already compromised before labour will become increasingly so. Insufficient oxygen delivery to the fetus causes a switch to anaerobic metabolism and results in the generation of lactic acid and hydrogen ions. In excess, these saturate the buffering systems of the fetus and cause a metabolic acidosis which, in the extreme, can cause neuronal damage and permanent neurological injury, even intrapartum fetal death. Hypoxia and acidosis cause a characteristic change in the fetal heart rate pattern, which can be detected by ausculatation and the cardiotocograph (CTG). Meconium is often passed by a healthy fetus at or after term as a result of maturation of gastrointestinal physiology; in this scenario, it is usually thin and a very dark green or brown colour. However, it may also be expelled from a fetus exposed to marked intrauterine hypoxia or acidosis; in this scenario, it is often thicker and much brighter green in colour.

Fetal assessment in labour takes four forms:

1. observation of the colour of the liquor – fresh meconium staining and heavy bleeding are markers of potential fetal compromise
2. intermittent auscultation of the fetal heart using a Pinard stethoscope or a hand-held Doppler ultrasound,
3. continuous external fetal monitoring (EFM) using CTG,
4. fetal scalp blood sampling (FBS).

The fetal heart rate (FHR) should be auscultated with a Pinard stethoscope, or by using a hand-held Doppler device, early on in the initial assessment. It should be listened to for at least a minute, immediately after a contraction. This should be repeated every 15 minutes during first stage, and at least every 5 minutes in second stage. The practice of performing an 'admission cardiotocograph' on all women is no longer recommended, however a CTG should be performed if there are issues which might complicate labour and delivery. Most of these women will also be advised to have continuous electronic fetal monitoring (EFM) throughout labour, using the CTG. This may negatively impact on their mobility. Women who begin labour with intermittent auscultation may be advised to change to continuous EFM if any of the following events occur during their labour:

- significant meconium staining to the liquor;
- abnormal fetal heart rate detected by intermittent auscultation;
- maternal pyrexia;
- fresh vaginal bleeding;
- augmentation of contractions with oxytocin;
- at the request of the woman.

The quality of a CTG recording is sometimes poor because of fetal position or maternal obesity. A fetal scalp electrode may overcome this problem. It is fixed into the skin of the fetal scalp and picks up the fetal heart rate directly. It rarely causes any harm to the fetus but requires a certain degree of cervical dilatation to be fitted, and for the membranes to be ruptured if they have remained intact.

The interpretation of the fetal heart rate pattern on a CTG is discussed in Chapter 6, Antenatal imaging and assessment of fetal well-being. In brief,

features of a normal fetal heart rate pattern include a baseline rate of between 110 and 160 bpm (beats per minute), a baseline variability of between 5 and 25 bpm, and the absence of decelerations. Interpreting the CTG in labour is somewhat different to that of an antenatal CTG, particularly in second stage. The absence of accelerations is of uncertain significance during labour, and the presence of simple variable decelerations, or early decelerations, later on in labour is extremely common and not usually a sign of significant fetal compromise.

Each feature of the CTG (baseline rate, variability, decelerations and accelerations) should be assessed each time a CTG is reviewed. Each feature can be described as 'reassuring', 'non-reassuring' or 'abnormal' according to certain strict nationally agreed definitions outlined in the NICE guideline on intrapartum management. If all four features are reassuring then the CTG is considered 'normal' (see Figure 14.18). If one feature is non-reassuring (and the other three are reassuring) then the CTG is described as 'suspicious'. If there are two or more non-reassuring features, or any abnormal features, then the CTG is 'pathological'. Any reversible causes must be considered and addressed and further assessment of the fetus made with fetal blood sampling. If this is not possible or safe then the baby should be delivered without delay.

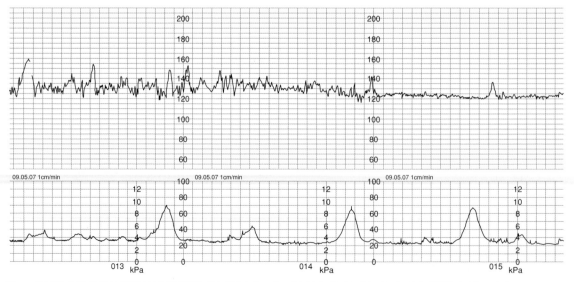

Figure 14.18 A normal cardiotocograph (CTG), showing a baseline fetal heart rate of approximately 120 bpm, frequent accelerations, baseline variability of 10–15 bpm and no decelerations. The uterus is contracting approximately once every 5 minutes

Unfortunately, the CTG can be difficult to interpret and it carries a significant false-positive rate, i.e. it often raises the possibility of fetal compromise when in truth the fetus is still in good condition. In order that the use of the CTG does not lead to unnecessary intervention, a fetal blood sampling may be performed during labour to measure fetal pH and base excess directly (see below under Management of possible fetal compromise). Often, these results are normal even when the CTG is abnormal.

The use of electronic fetal monitors, only introduced in the 1970s, has been controversial and their value in 'low-risk' labours is doubtful. Education and training are crucial in the proper use of all equipment. Unfortunately, these devices were introduced before CTG recordings and their outcomes were fully understood. There is little doubt that babies' lives have been saved by the use of electronic fetal monitors, but they have also contributed to the rise in the Caesarean section and instrumental delivery rates and they lead to reduced mobility in labour and increased parental anxiety. This remains a challenge.

The partogram

The introduction of a graphic record of labour in the form of a partogram has been an important development. This record allows an instant visual assessment of the rate of cervical dilatation and comparison with an expected norm, according to the parity of the woman, so that slow progress can be recognized early and appropriate actions taken to correct it where possible. Other key observations are entered on to the chart, including the frequency and strength of contractions, the descent of the head in fifths palpable, the amount and colour of the amniotic fluid draining, and basic observations of maternal well-being, such as blood pressure, pulse rate and temperature (Figure 14.19).

A line can be drawn on the partogram at the end of the latent phase demonstrating progress of 1 cm dilatation per hour. Another line ('the action line') can be drawn parallel and 4 hours to the right of it. If the plot of actual cervical dilatation reaches the action line, indicating slow progress, then consideration should be given to a number of different measures which aim to improve progress (see below). Progress can also be considered slow if the cervix dilates at less than 1 cm every 2 hours.

Management during first stage

Key management principles of first stage of labour

- The first stage of labour is timed from the diagnosis of onset of labour to full dilatation of the cervix.
- Provision of continuity of care and emotional support to the mother.
- Observation of the progress of labour with timely intervention if it becomes abnormal.
- Monitoring of fetal well-being.
- Adequate and appropriate pain relief consistent with the woman's wishes.
- Adequate hydration to prevent ketosis.

Women who are in the latent phase of labour should be encouraged to mobilize and should be managed away from the labour suite where possible. Indeed, they may well go home, to return later when the contractions are stronger or more frequent. Encouragement and reassurance are extremely important. Intervention during this phase is best avoided unless there are identified risk factors. Simple analgesics are preferred over nitrous oxide and epidurals. There is no reason to restrict eating and drinking, although lighter foods and clear fluids may be better tolerated. Vaginal examinations are usually performed every 4 hours to determine when the active phase has been reached (approximately 4 cm dilatation and full effacement). Thereafter, the timing of examinations should be decided by the midwife. Four-hourly is standard practice, however, this frequency may be increased if the midwife thinks that progress is unusually slow or fast. The lower limit of normal progress is 1 cm dilatation every 2 hours once the active phase has been reached. Descent of the presenting part through the pelvis is another crucial component of progress and should be recorded at each vaginal examination. Full dilatation may be reached, but if descent is inadequate, vaginal delivery will not occur.

During the first stage, the membranes may be intact, may have ruptured spontaneously or may have been ruptured artificially. Generally speaking, if the membranes are intact, it is not necessary to rupture them if the progress of labour is satisfactory.

Maternal and fetal observations are carried out as described previously, and recorded on the partogram. Women should receive one-to-one care (i.e. from

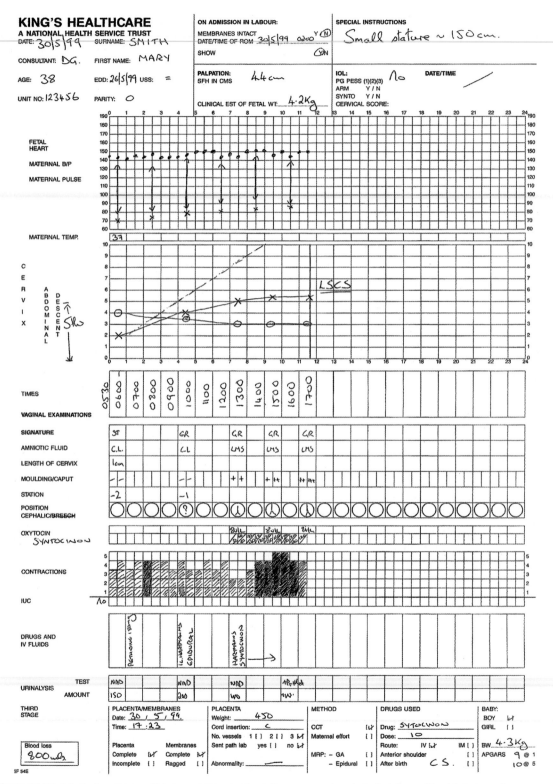

Figure 14.19 A typical partogram. This is a partogram of a nulliparous woman of short stature with a big baby and an augmented labour. The labour culminates in an emergency Caesarean section for cephalopelvic disproportion

a dedicated midwife) and should not be left alone for any significant period of time once labour has established. They should be able to choose birth partners themselves and should be able to adopt whatever positions they find most comfortable. Mobility during labour is encouraged and it is likely that standing upright encourages progress. Unfortunately, many women adopt a supine position, especially if there is a need for continuous EFM (i.e. the CTG). Women may drink during established labour and those who are becoming dehydrated may benefit from intravenous fluids to prevent ketosis, which can impair uterine contractility. Light diet is acceptable if they have no obvious risk factors for needing a general anaesthetic and if they have not had pethidine or diamorphine for pain relief. Shaving and enemas are unnecessary and antacids need only be given to women with risk factors for complications, or to those who have had opioid analgesia. A variety of methods of pain relief are available, depending on the location of the birth, and these are discussed below under Pain relief in labour.

'Active management of labour' was a collection of interventions which was routinely recommended to nulliparous women to maximize the chances of a normal birth. It included one-to-one midwifery care, 2-hourly vaginal examinations and early artificial rupture of membranes and use of oxytocin augmentation if progress fell more than 2 hours behind the schedule of 1 cm dilatation per hour. A variety of studies failed to show any obvious benefit of active management, except that derived from one-to-one care, the only component now recommended for all women in normal labour.

Second stage

If the labour has been normal, the first sign of the second phase of the second stage is likely to be an urge to push experienced by the mother. Full dilatation of the cervix should be confirmed by a vaginal examination if the head is not visible. The woman will get an expulsive reflex with each contraction, and will generally take a deep breath, hold it, and strain down (the Valsalva manoeuvre). Women will be guided by their own urge to push, however, the midwife has an important role to play, with advice, support and reassurance if progress is poor. Women should be discouraged from lying supine, or semi-supine, and should adopt any other position that they

find comfortable. Lying in the left lateral position and squatting are particularly effective options. There is insufficient good quality evidence to either support or discourage water-birth. Maternal and fetal surveillance intensifies in second stage, as described previously. The development of fetal acidaemia may accelerate, and maternal exhaustion and ketosis increase in line with the duration of active pushing. Use of regional analgesia may interfere with the normal urge to push, and second stage is more often diagnosed on a routine scheduled vaginal examination. Pushing is usually delayed for at least an hour if an epidural is *in situ* (the 'passive stage'), however, the baby should be delivered within 4 hours of reaching full dilatation.

Descent and delivery of the head

The progress of the descent of the head can be judged by watching the perineum. At first, there is a slight general bulge as the woman strains. When the head stretches the perineum, the anus will begin to open, and soon after this the baby's head will be seen at the vulva at the height of each contraction. Between contractions, the elastic tone of the perineal muscles will push the head back into the pelvic cavity. The perineal body and vulval outlet will become more and more stretched, until eventually the head is low enough to pass forwards under the subpubic arch. When the head no longer recedes between contractions (crowning), this indicates that it has passed through the pelvic floor, and delivery is imminent. Vaginal and perineal tears are common consequences of vaginal birth, particularly during first deliveries. The 'hands-on' approach has been very popular. As crowning occurs, the hands of the accoucheur are used to flex the fetal head and guard the perineum. The belief is that controlling the speed of delivery of the fetal head will limit maternal damage, however, there is little evidence to support this practice over the alternative 'hands-off' approach. Once the head has crowned, the woman should be discouraged from bearing down by telling her to take rapid, shallow breaths ('panting'). An episiotomy is a surgical cut, performed with scissors, which extends from the vaginal fourchette in a mediolateral direction, usually to the right, through the perineum and incorporating the lower vaginal wall (see Chapter 15, Operative intervention in obstetrics). It is performed during instrumental birth (ventouse or forceps), or to hasten delivery if there is suspected fetal compromise. It will only assist the birth if the head has passed through the pelvic floor, so should not be performed too early. It does not help prevent more severe perineal injury and its routine use in normal spontaneous labour was abandoned some time ago. Effective analgesia is required, and this will usually be with infiltration of local anaesthetic if the woman does not have an epidural.

Delivery of the shoulders and rest of the body

Once the fetal head is born, a check is made to see whether the cord is wound tightly around the neck, thereby making delivery of the body difficult. If this is the case, the cord may need to be clamped and divided before delivery of the rest of the body. With the next contraction, there is external rotation of the head and the shoulders can be delivered. To aid delivery of the shoulders, the head should be pulled gently downwards and forwards until the anterior shoulder appears beneath the pubis. The head is then lifted gradually until the posterior shoulder appears over the perineum and the baby is then swept upwards to deliver the body and legs. If the infant is large and traction is necessary to deliver the body, it should be applied to the shoulders only, and not to the head. Shoulder dystocia (difficulty in delivering the shoulders) is discussed in Chapter 16, Obstetric emergencies.

Immediate care of the neonate

After the infant is born, it lies between the mother's legs or is delivered directly on to the maternal upper abdomen. The baby will usually take its first breath within seconds. There is no need for immediate clamping of the cord, and indeed about 80 mL of blood will be transferred from the placenta to the baby before cord pulsations cease, reducing the chances of neonatal anaemia and iron deficiency. The baby's head should be kept dependent to allow mucus in the respiratory tract to drain, and oropharyngeal suction should only be applied if really necessary. After clamping and cutting the cord, the baby should have an Apgar score calculated at 1 minute of age (see Chapter 19, Neonatology) which is then repeated at 5 minutes. Immediate skin-to-skin contact between mother and baby will help bonding, and promote the further release of oxytocin, which will encourage uterine contractions. The baby should be dried and covered with a warm blanket or towel, maintaining this contact. Initiation of breastfeeding should be encouraged within the first hour of life, and routine newborn measurements of head circumference, birthweight and temperature are usually performed soon after this hour has elapsed. Before being taken from the delivery room, the first dose of vitamin K should be given (if parental consent has been given) and the infant should have a general examination for abnormalities and a wrist label attached for identification.

Third stage

This is timed from the delivery of the baby to the expulsion of the placenta and membranes. This normally takes between 5 and 10 minutes.

Separation of the placenta occurs because of the reduction of volume of the uterus due to uterine contraction and the retraction (shortening) of the lattice-like arrangement of the myometrial muscle fibres. A cleavage plane develops within the decidua basalis and the separated placenta lies free in the lower segment of the uterine cavity. Signs of separation are:

- lengthening of the cord protruding from the vulva;
- a small gush of blood from the placental bed, which normally stops quickly due to a retraction of the myometrial fibres;
- rising of the uterine fundus to above the umbilicus (Figure 14.20);
- the fundus becomes hard and globular compared to the broad, softer fundus prior to separation.

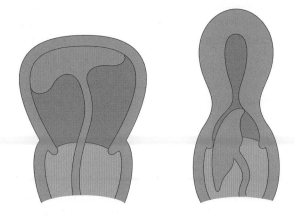

Figure 14.20 Signs of separation and descent of the placenta. After separation, the uterine upper segment rises up and feels more rounded

Management of the third stage can be described as 'active' or 'physiological'. Modern active management of the third stage is a package of care which includes the following:

- intramuscular injection of 10 IU of oxytocin, given as the anterior shoulder of the baby is delivered, or immediately after delivery of the baby;
- early clamping and cutting of the umbilical cord;
- controlled cord traction (see Figure 14.21).

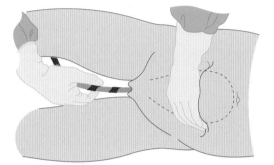

Figure 14.21 Delivering the placenta by controlled cord traction

Active management of the third stage should be recommended to all women because high quality evidence shows that it reduces the incidence of postpartum haemorrhage from 15 to 5 per cent. When the signs of placental separation are recognized, controlled cord traction is used to expedite delivery of the placenta. When a contraction is felt, the left hand should be moved suprapubically and the fundus elevated with the palm facing towards the mother. At the same time, the right hand should grasp the cord and exert steady traction so that the placenta separates and is delivered gently, care being taken to peel off all the membranes, usually with a twisting motion. Uterine inversion is a rare complication which may occur if the uterus is not adequately controlled with the left hand and excessive traction is exerted on the cord in the absence of a uterine contraction (see Chapter 16, Obstetric emergencies).

In approximately 2 per cent of cases, the placenta will not be expelled by this method. If no bleeding occurs, a further attempt at controlled cord traction should be made after 10 minutes. If this fails, the placenta is 'retained' and will require manual removal under general or regional anaesthesia in the operating theatre. Direct injection of oxytocin into the umbilical vein may bring about delivery of the placenta while preparations are being made for theatre.

Physiological management of the third stage is where the placenta is delivered by maternal effort, and no uterotonic drugs are given to assist this process. It is associated with heavier bleeding, but women who are not at undue risk of postpartum haemorrhage should be supported if they choose this option. In the event of haemorrhage, or if the placenta remains undelivered after 60 minutes of physiological management, active management should be recommended.

After completion of the third stage, the placenta should be inspected for missing cotyledons or a succenturiate lobe. If these are suspected, manual removal of the placenta (possibly under ultrasound guidance) should be arranged, because in this situation the risk of postpartum haemorrhage is high.

Finally, the vulva of the mother should be inspected for any tears or lacerations. Minor tears do not require suturing, but tears extending into the perineal muscles (or, indeed, an episiotomy) will require careful repair (see Chapter 15, Operative intervention in obstetrics).

Key points

The key features of normal labour are:
- spontaneous onset,
- single cephalic presentation,
- 37–42 weeks gestation,
- no artificial interventions,
- unassisted spontaneous vaginal delivery,
- dilatation of at least 1 cm every 2 hours in the active phase of first stage,
- an active second stage of no more than 2 hours in a primiparous woman, and no more than 60 minutes in multiparous women,
- a third stage lasting no more than 30 minutes with active management.

Pain relief in labour

The provision of analgesia in childbirth varies between cultures. Some women and their carers believe that there is an advantage in avoiding analgesia, whereas other women will use all methods on offer to limit their pain. Professionals who are knowledgeable about labour and are sympathetic to the labouring woman should give advice regarding pain relief in labour. The method of pain relief is to some extent dependent on the previous obstetric record of the woman, the course of labour and also the estimated length of labour. Just as one woman's labour can be made into an unhappy experience by unsolicited and unnecessary analgesia, pain relief that is inadequate, or offered too late, can ruin another's. It should be remembered that the final decision rests with the woman, although there are certain circumstances in which particular forms of analgesia are contraindicated and should not be offered.

Non-pharmacological methods

One-to-one care in labour from a midwife or effective birth partner has been shown to reduce the need for analgesia. Relaxation and breathing exercises may help the woman to manage her pain. Prolonged hyperventilation can make the woman dizzy and can cause alkalosis. Homeopathy, acupuncture and hypnosis are sometimes employed, but their use has not been associated with a significant reduction in pain scores or with a reduced need for conventional methods of analgesia, and they are probably not widely applicable.

Relaxation in warm water during the first stage of labour often leads to a sense of well-being and allows women to cope much better with the pain. The temperature of the water should not exceed 37.5ºC. Clearly, a woman in labour cannot use an opiate or have an epidural sited while in water. Transcutaneous electrical nerve stimulation (TENS) works on the principle of blocking pain fibres in the posterior ganglia of the spinal cord by stimulation of small afferent fibres (the 'gate' theory). It has been shown to be ineffective in reducing pain scores or the need for other forms of analgesia and should no longer be offered to women in established labour. It does not have any adverse effects, but is often disappointing. It may still be of use in the latent phase of labour.

Pharmacological methods

Opiates, such as pethidine and diamorphine, are still used in most obstetric units and indeed can be administered by midwives without the involvement of the medical staff. This may be one of the reasons for their popularity. They should be available in all birth settings but they provide only limited pain relief during labour and furthermore may have significant side effects including:

- nausea and vomiting (they should always been given with an anti-emetic);
- maternal drowsiness and sedation;
- delayed gastric emptying (increasing the risks if general anaesthesia is subsequently required);
- short-term respiratory depression of the baby;
- possible interference with breastfeeding.

Opiates tend to be given as intramuscular injections, however, an alternative is a subcutaneous or intravenous infusion by a patient-controlled analgesic device (PCA). This allows the woman, by pressing a dispenser button, to determine the level of analgesia that she requires. If a very short-acting opiate is used, the opiate doses can be timed with the contractions. This method of pain relief is particularly popular among women who cannot have an epidural and find non-pharmacological options insufficient.

Inhalational analgesia

Nitrous oxide (NO) in the form of Entonox (an equal mixture of NO and oxygen) is used on most labour wards. It has a quick onset, a short duration of effect, and is more effective than pethidine. It may cause light-headedness and nausea. It is not suitable for prolonged use from early labour because hyperventilation may result in hypocapnoea, dizziness and ultimately tetany and fetal hypoxia. It is most suitable later on in labour or while awaiting epidural analgesia.

Epidural analgesia

Epidural (extradural) analgesia is the most reliable means of providing effective analgesia in labour. Failure to provide an epidural is one of the most frequent causes of anxiety and disappointment among labouring women. The epidural service must be well organized to be effective, and fortunately resources are now in place so that a significant delay in the placement of an epidural is unusual.

Indications

The decision to have an epidural sited should be a combined one between the woman, her midwife, the obstetric team and the anaesthetist. The woman must be informed about the risks and benefits and the final decision in most cases rests with the woman unless there is a definite contraindication. It is important to warn the woman that she may temporarily lose sensation and movement in her legs, and that intravenous access and a more intensive level of maternal and fetal monitoring will be necessary, for example with continuous electronic fetal monitoring (the CTG). The effect of epidural analgesia on labour and the operative delivery rate has been a controversial issue. The evidence is now clear that epidural analgesia does not increase Caesarean section rates. However, second stage is longer and there is a greater chance of instrumental delivery, which may be lessened by a more liberal use of oxytocin infusions during second stage in primiparous women with an epidural. In certain clinical situations, an epidural in the second stage of labour may assist a vaginal delivery by relaxing the woman and allowing time for the head to descend and rotate.

The main indication is for effective pain relief. There are other maternal and fetal conditions for which epidural analgesia would be advantageous in labour. These are:

- prolonged labour,
- maternal hypertensive disorders,
- multiple gestation,
- certain maternal medical conditions,
- a high risk of operative intervention.

The main contraindications are:

- coagulation disorders,
- local or systemic sepsis,
- hypovolaemia,
- insufficient numbers of trained staff (both anaesthetic and midwifery).

An epidural will limit mobility and for this reason is not ideal for women in early labour. However, women in severe pain, even in the latent phase of labour, should not be denied regional anaesthesia. Neither is advanced cervical dilatation necessarily a contraindication to an epidural. It is more important to assess the rate of progress, the anticipated length of time to delivery and the type of delivery expected.

Complications of regional analgesia

- Accidental dural puncture during the search for the epidural space should occur in no more than 1 per cent of cases. The needle used for an epidural is wider bore than that used for a spinal. If the subarachnoid space is accidentally reached with an epidural needle, there is a risk that the hole left afterwards in the dura will be large enough to allow the leakage of cerebrospinal fluid. This results in a 'spinal headache'. This is characteristically experienced on the top of the head and is relieved by lying flat and exacerbated by sitting upright. If the headache is severe or persistent, a blood patch may be necessary. This involves injecting a small volume of the woman's blood into the epidural space at the level of the accidental dural puncture. The resulting blood clot is thought to block off the leak of cerebrospinal fluid.

- Accidental total spinal anaesthesia (injection of epidural doses of local anaesthetic into the subarachnoid space) causes severe hypotension, respiratory failure, unconsciousness and death if not recognized and treated immediately. The mother requires intubation, ventilation and circulatory support. Hypotension must be treated with intravenous fluids, vasopressors and left uterine displacement, although urgent delivery of the baby may be required to overcome aorto-caval compression and so permit maternal resuscitation.

- Spinal haematomata and neurological complications are rare, and are usually associated with other factors such as bleeding disorders.

- Drug toxicity can occur with accidental placement of a catheter within a blood vessel. This is normally noticed by aspiration prior to injection.

- Bladder dysfunction can occur if the bladder is allowed to overfill because the woman is unaware of the need to micturate, particularly after the birth while the spinal or epidural is wearing off. Over-distension of the detrusor muscle of the bladder can permanently damage it and leave long-term voiding problems. To avoid this, catheterization of the bladder should be carried out during labour if the woman does not void significant volumes of urine spontaneously.

- Backache during and after pregnancy is not uncommon. There is now good evidence that epidural analgesia does not cause backache.

- Hypotension is now an uncommon complication of epidural anaesthesia, but can still occur with an epidural although more commonly with a spinal. It can usually be rectified easily with fluid boluses, but may need vasopressors. Occasionally, maternal hypotension will lead to fetal compromise (see below).

- Short-term respiratory depression of the baby is possible because all modern epidural solutions contain opioids which reach the maternal circulation and may cross the placenta.

Technique

After detailed discussion, the woman's back is cleansed and local anaesthetic is used to infiltrate the skin. The woman may be in an extreme left lateral position, or sat up but leaning over. Flexion at the upper spine and at the hips helps to open up the spaces between the vertebral bodies of the lumbar spine. Aseptic technique is used. The epidural catheter is normally inserted at the L2–L3, L3–L4 or L4–L5 interspace and should come to lie in the epidural space, which contains blood vessels, nerve roots and fat (Figure 14.22). The catheter is aspirated to check for position and, if no blood or cerebrospinal fluid is obtained, a 'test dose' is given to confirm the catheter position (Figure 14.23). This test dose is a small volume of dilute local anaesthetic that would not be expected to have any clinical effect. If indeed it has no obvious effect on sensation in the lower limbs, the catheter is correctly sited. If, however, there is a sensory block, leg weakness and peripheral vasodilatation, the catheter has been inserted too far and into the subarachnoid (spinal) space. Inserting the normal dose of local anaesthetic into the spinal space by accident would risk complete motor and respiratory paralysis. If none of these signs is observed 5 minutes after injection of the test dose, a loading dose can be administered. The epidural solution is usually a mixture of low-concentration local anaesthetic (e.g. 0.0625–0.1 per cent bupivacaine) with an opioid such as fentanyl. Combining the opioid with the local anaesthetic reduces the amount of local anaesthetic required and this reduces the motor blockade and peripheral autonomic effects of the epidural (e.g. hypotension).

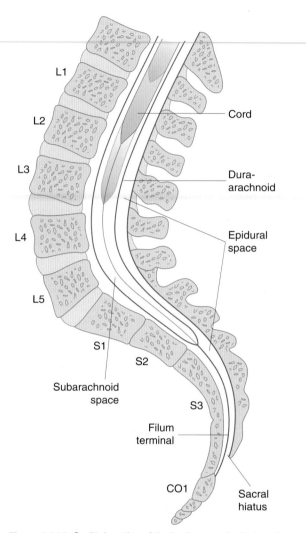

Figure 14.22 Sagittal section of the lumbo-sacral spinal cord

After the loading dose is given, the mother should be kept in the right or left lateral position, and her blood pressure should be measured every 5 minutes for 15 minutes. A fall in blood pressure may result from the vasodilatation caused by blocking of the sympathetic tone to peripheral blood vessels. This hypotension is usually short lived, but may cause a fetal bradycardia due to redirection of maternal blood away from the uterus. It should be treated with intravenous fluids and, if necessary, vasoconstrictors such as ephedrine. The mother should never lie supine, as aorto-caval compression can reduce maternal cardiac output and so compromise placental perfusion. Hourly assessment of the level of the sensory block using a cold spray is critical in the detection of a block

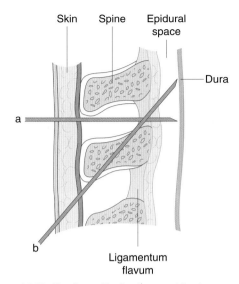

Skin   Spine   Epidural space

Dura

a

b

Ligamentum flavum

Figure 14.23 Needle positioning for an epidural anaesthetic. Midline (a) and paramedian (b) approaches

which is creeping too high and risking respiratory compromise. Regional analgesia can be maintained throughout labour with either intermittent boluses or continuous infusions. Patient-controlled epidural analgesia is an option. Women should be encouraged to move around and adopt whichever upright position suits them best. Full mobility is unlikely.

Reducing the rate of an epidural infusion in the second stage may increase the maternal awareness to push, but care should be taken that the analgesic effect is not compromised. Regional anaesthesia should be continued until after completion of the third stage of labour, including repair of any perineal injury.

Spinal anaesthesia

A spinal block is considered more effective than that obtained by an epidural, and is of faster onset. A fine-gauge atraumatic spinal needle is passed through the epidural space, through the dura and into the subarachnoid space, which contains the cerebrospinal fluid. A small volume of local anaesthetic is injected, after which the spinal needle is withdrawn. This may be used as the anaesthetic for Caesarean sections, trial of instrumental deliveries (in theatre), manual removal of retained placentae and the repair of difficult perineal and vaginal tears. Spinals are not used for routine analgesia in labour.

Combined spinal–epidural (CSE) analgesia has gained in popularity. This technique has the advantage of producing a rapid onset of pain relief and the provision of prolonged analgesia. Because the initiating spinal dose is relatively low, this is a viable option for pain relief in labour.

CASE HISTORY

Mrs W is a 32-year-old para 1 (previous normal vaginal delivery at term), with no medical or obstetric history of note, who realized she was pregnant at approximately 6 weeks gestation. She made an appointment with a local community midwife who confirmed the pregnancy and took a detailed history. In the absence of risk factors, she was booked under midwifery care. The midwife discussed the options for the place of birth and the woman chose the local obstetric unit because she had elected to have an epidural in her previous labour and thought she would like the option once again. A dating scan, organized by the midwife, agreed with the menstrual estimated delivery date (EDD), and screening tests in the second trimester were all reassuring. Regular visits through the second and third trimesters did not reveal any new problems.

At 39 weeks gestation, after a week of increasingly uncomfortable but irregular uterine tightenings, Mrs W experienced a 'show'. Her contractions remained irregular for a further 24 hours. Finally, they began to come frequently and, when they reached every 5 minutes, she phoned her midwife, who recommended assessment at the local maternity unit. Mrs W called her own

parents, who came to look after her first child, and she and her husband drove to the hospital.

On admission, the midwife took a history and performed an abdominal examination. The head was well engaged and the contractions were coming every 3 minutes. Maternal observations were normal on admission, as was the fetal heart rate when auscultated with a Pinard stethoscope. A vaginal examination showed the membranes to be intact and the cervix to be fully effaced and 4 cm dilated. The vertex was found to be 1 cm above the spines. Mrs W therefore remained under the care of the midwives and the on-call medical staff were not involved.

She remained mobile and continued to drink while in labour, but did not want anything to eat. She spent some time in the bath, as this helped her cope with the pain of the contractions. The midwife listened regularly to the fetal heart, during and after contractions, later choosing to use a hand-held Doppler device. The fetal heart rate remained steady and of a normal rate. Maternal observations also remained normal. Three hours later, her membranes ruptured spontaneously and the liquor was clear. Permission was given for an internal examination and Mrs W was found to be 9 cm dilated.

continued ≫

She was finding the contractions much more painful but, with support and reassurance from her partner and the midwife, did not require anything more than nitrous oxide for analgesia.

One hour later, she was aware of a strong urge to 'bear down' and began involuntarily pushing. The midwife confirmed second stage with another vaginal examination and the pushing continued. Mrs W was encouraged to remain upright, but chose to lie in a supine position on the bed. She later found the left lateral position ideal for pushing, as suggested by the midwife. The fetal heart was listened to during and after each and every contraction during the second stage. Twenty minutes later, the maternal anus began

to dilate slightly and the vertex became visible soon after. Three further contractions later, the head had delivered. The rest of the body came with the fourth. The midwife delivered the baby on to the maternal abdomen and clamped and cut the cord a few minutes later. An intramuscular injection of Syntocinon (oxytocin) was given by a second midwife as the baby was born, and the placenta delivered 5 minutes later, aided by controlled cord traction. She had sustained no perineal damage and the placenta appeared complete. The first breastfeed was established and vitamin K was given to the baby. A check by the paediatrician suggested all was well and Mrs W left hospital 7 hours later with her husband and new baby.

Abnormal labour

Labour becomes abnormal when there is poor progress (as evidenced by a delay in cervical dilatation or descent of the presenting part) and/or the fetus shows signs of compromise. Also, if there is a fetal malpresentation, a multiple gestation, a uterine scar, or if labour has been induced, labour cannot be considered normal.

Poor progress in labour

Poor progress in the first stage of labour

Poor progress in labour has been defined already as cervical dilatation of less than 2 cm in 4 hours, usually associated with failure of descent and rotation of the fetal head.

Progress in labour is dependent on three variables:

1. the powers, i.e. the efficiency of uterine contractions,
2. the passenger, i.e. the fetus (with particular respect to its size, presentation and position),
3. the passages, i.e. the uterus, cervix and bony pelvis.

Abnormalities in one or more of these factors can slow the normal progress of labour. Plotting the findings of serial vaginal examinations on the partogram will help to highlight poor progress during the first stage of labour.

Dysfunctional uterine activity

This is the most common cause of poor progress in labour. It is more common in primigravidae and perhaps in older women and is characterized by weak and infrequent contractions. The assessment of uterine contractions is most commonly carried out by clinical examination and by using external uterine tocography. However, this can only provide information about the frequency and perhaps duration of contractions. Intrauterine pressure catheters are available and these do give a more accurate measurement of the pressure being generated by the contractions, but they are rarely necessary. A frequency of four to five contractions per 10 minutes is usually considered ideal. Fewer contractions than this does not necessarily mean progress will be slow, but more frequent examinations may be indicated to detect poor progress earlier. Women should be offered hydration, good pain relief and emotional support. When poor progress in labour is suspected it is usual to recommend repeat vaginal examination 2, rather than 4, hours after the last. If delay is confirmed, the woman should be offered artificial rupture of membranes (ARM) and, if there is still poor progress in a further 2 hours, advice should be sought from an obstetrician regarding the use of an oxytocin infusion to augment the contractions. The infusion is commenced at a slow rate initially, and increased carefully every 30 minutes, according to a well-defined protocol. Continuous EFM is necessary as excessively frequent and augmented contractions may cause fetal compromise (see Figure 14.38). Women should be offered an epidural before oxytocin is started, and they need to be aware that although ARM and oxytocin will bring forward the time of birth somewhat, they will not influence the mode of delivery, or other outcomes.

Multiparous women are less likely to experience poor progress in labour secondary to dysfunctional uterine activity. Extreme caution must be exercised when making this diagnosis in a multiparous woman where an alternative explanation, such as malposition or malpresentation, is more likely. An obstetrician must be closely involved in the assessment of such a woman and the decision to augment with oxytocin must be considered very carefully indeed. Excessive uterine contractions in a truly obstructed labour may result in uterine rupture in a multiparous woman, a complication which is extremely rare in primiparous women. Augmentation with oxytocin is contraindicated if there are concerns regarding the condition of the fetus.

If progress fails to occur despite 4–6 hours of augmentation with oxytocin, a Caesarean section will usually be recommended.

Cephalopelvic disproportion

Cephalopelvic disproportion (CPD) implies anatomical disproportion between the fetal head and maternal pelvis. It can be due to a large head, small pelvis or a combination of the two. Women of small stature (<1.60 m) with a large baby in their first pregnancy are likely candidates to develop this problem. The pelvis may be unusually small because of previous fracture or metabolic bone disease. Rarely, a fetal anomaly will contribute to CPD. Obstructive hydrocephalus may cause macrocephaly, and fetal thyroid and neck tumours may cause extension at the fetal neck. Relative CPD is more common and occurs with malposition of the fetal head. The occipito-posterior position is associated with deflexion of the fetal head and presents a larger skull diameter to the maternal pelvis (Figures 14.14 and 14.24).

Cephalopelvic disproportion is suspected in labour if:

- progress is slow or actually arrests despite efficient uterine contractions;
- the fetal head is not engaged;
- vaginal examination shows severe moulding and caput formation;
- the head is poorly applied to the cervix.

Oxytocin can be given carefully to a primigravida with mild to moderate CPD as long as the CTG is reactive. Relative disproportion may be overcome if the malposition is corrected (i.e. conversion to a flexed OA position). Oxytocin must never be used in a multiparous woman where CPD is suspected.

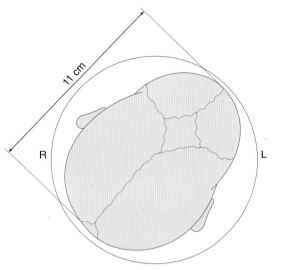

Figure 14.24 Vaginal palpation of the head in the right occipito-posterior position. The circle represents the pelvic cavity, with a diameter of 12 cm. The head is poorly flexed so that the anterior fontanelle is easily felt

Malpresentations

Vital to good progress in labour is the tight application of the fetal presenting part on to the cervix. Face presentations (Figures 14.25 and 14.26) may apply themselves poorly to the cervix and the resulting progress in labour may be poor, although vaginal birth is still possible. Brow presentations are associated with the mento-vertical diameter, which is simply too large

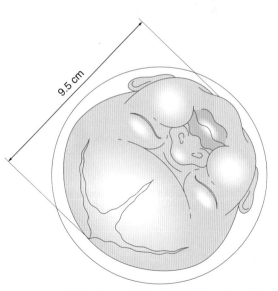

Figure 14.25 Vaginal examination in the left mento-anterior position. The circle represents the pelvic cavity, with a diameter of 12 cm

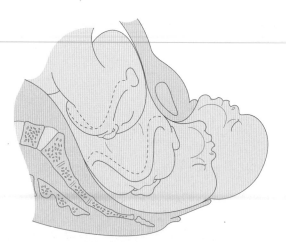

Figure 14.26 The mechanism of labour with a face presentation. The head descends with increasing extension. The chin reaches the pelvic floor and undergoes forward rotation. The head is born by flexion

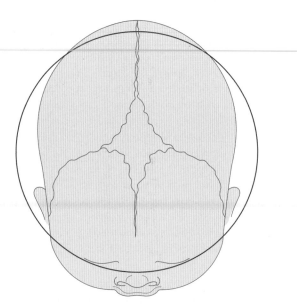

Figure 14.28 Vaginal examination with brow presentation. The circle represents the pelvic cavity, with a diameter of 12 cm. The mento-vertical diameter of 13 cm is too large to permit engagement of the head

to fit through the bony pelvis unless flexion occurs or hyperextension to a face presentation (Figures 14.27 and 14.28). Brow presentation therefore often manifests as poor progress in first stage, often in a multiparous woman. Shoulder presentations cannot deliver vaginally and once again poor progress will

occur. Malpresentations are more common in women of high parity and some carry a risk of uterine rupture if the labour is allowed to continue.

Abnormalities of the birth canal (the 'passages')

The bony pelvis may cause delay in the progress of labour as discussed above (CPD). Abnormalities of the uterus and cervix can also delay labour. Unsuspected fibroids in the lower uterine segment can prevent descent of the fetal head. Delay can also be caused by 'cervical dystocia', a term used to describe a non-compliant cervix which effaces but fails to dilate because of severe scarring, usually as a result of a previous cone biopsy. Caesarean section may be necessary. It is rare for the soft tissues of the pelvic floor to cause significant delay in labour.

Poor progress in the second stage of labour

Birth of the baby is expected to take place within 3 hours of the start of the active second stage (pushing) in nulliparous women, and 2 hours in parous women. Delay is diagnosed if delivery is not imminent after 2 hours of pushing in a nulliparous labour (1 hour for a parous woman). The causes of second-stage delay can again be classified as abnormalities of the powers, the passenger and the passages. Secondary uterine inertia is a common cause of second stage delay, and

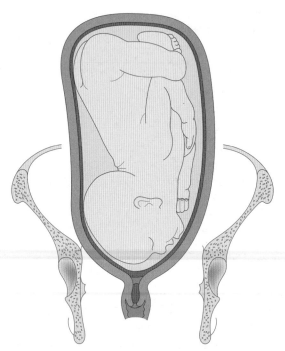

Figure 14.27 Brow presentation. The head is above the brim and not engaged. The mento-vertical diameter of the head is trying to engage in the transverse diameter at the brim

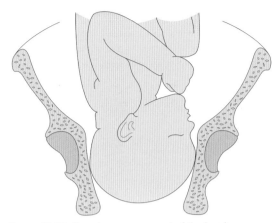

Figure 14.29 Deep transverse arrest of the head

prevents internal rotation of the fetal head. This may result in the arrest of the descent of the fetal head at the level of the ischial spines in the transverse position, a condition called deep transverse arrest (Figure 14.29).

Instrumental birth should be considered for prolonged second stage (see Chapter 15, Operative intervention in obstetrics). This may be safely performed in the labour room, or may be more safely carried out in theatre with easy recourse to Caesarean delivery if the attempt is unsuccessful, or if an attempt is deemed unwise when the woman is examined with the benefits of effective anaesthesia.

may be exacerbated by epidural analgesia. Having achieved full dilatation, the uterine contractions become weak and ineffectual and this is sometimes associated with maternal dehydration and ketosis. If no mechanical problem is anticipated, the treatment is with rehydration and intravenous oxytocin, if the woman is primiparous. Delay can also occur because of a persistent OP position of the fetal head. In this situation, the head will either have to undergo a long rotation to OA or be delivered in the OP position, i.e. face to pubes. By the time delay in second stage in labour has been diagnosed, NICE recommend that oxytocin should not be started. Inefficient uterine activity therefore needs to be corrected proactively at the beginning of the second stage.

Delay in the second stage can also occur because of a narrow mid-pelvis (android pelvis), which

Risk factors for poor progress in labour
• Small woman
• Big baby
• Dysfunctional uterine activity
• Malpresentation
• Malposition
• Early membrane rupture
• Soft-tissue/pelvic malformation

Patterns of abnormal progress in labour

The use of a partogram to plot the progress of labour improves the detection of poor progress. Indeed, three patterns of abnormal labour are commonly described (Figure 14.30).

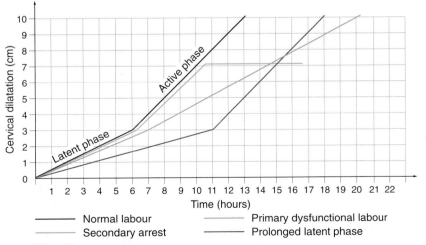

Figure 14.30 Abnormalities of the partogram

Prolonged latent phase occurs when the latent phase is longer than the arbitrary time limits discussed previously. It is more common in primiparous women and probably results from a delay in the chemical processes that occur within the cervix which soften it and allow effacement. Prolonged latent phase can be extremely frustrating and tiring for the woman. However, intervention in the form of ARM or oxytocin infusion will increase the likelihood of poor progress later in the labour and the need for Caesarean birth. It is best managed away from the labour suite with simple analgesics, mobilization and reassurance. 'Primary dysfunctional labour' is the term used to describe poor progress in the active phase of labour (<2 cm cervical dilatation/4 hours) and is also more common in primiparous women. It is most commonly caused by inefficient uterine contractions, but can also result from CPD and malposition of the fetus. Secondary arrest occurs when progress in the active phase of first stage is initially good but then slows, or stops altogether, typically after 7 cm dilatation. Although inefficient uterine contractions may be the cause, fetal malpositions, malpresentations and CPD feature more commonly than in primary dysfunctional labour.

Key points

Poor progress in labour
- There are different patterns of poor progress in labour.
- Inefficient uterine activity is the most common cause of poor progress in labour.
- Fetal malposition, malpresentation and true CPD are other causes of poor progress, and may occur in isolation or in combination with inefficient uterine contractions.
- ARM is a simple intervention which may shorten labour, but does not influence the overall outcome.
- The use of oxytocin is relatively safe in nulliparous women.
- Use of oxytocin augmentation in multiparous women is less safe because of the greater risk of uterine hyperstimulation, fetal compromise and uterine rupture in the face of obstruction.
- Oxytocin does not have a significant impact on the mode of delivery, but does shorten the length of labour.

Fetal compromise in labour

Concern for the well-being of the fetus is one of the most common reasons for medical intervention during labour. The fetus may already be compromised before labour, and the reduction in placental blood flow associated with contractions may uncover this and ultimately lead to fetal hypoxia and eventually acidosis. Fetal compromise may present as fresh meconium staining to the amniotic fluid, or an abnormal CTG. However, neither of these findings confirms fetal hypoxia or acidosis. Meconium can be passed for benign reasons, such as fetal maturity, and it is well recognized that the abnormal CTG carries a very high false-positive rate for the diagnosis of fetal compromise. Intervention for 'presumed fetal compromise' is therefore more accurate than 'fetal distress'. In many cases, babies delivered by Caesarean section or instrumental birth for presumed fetal compromise are found to be in good condition.

Risk factors for fetal compromise in labour

- Placental insufficiency – intrauterine growth restriction (IUGR) and pre-eclampsia
- Prematurity
- Postmaturity
- Multiple pregnancy
- Prolonged labour
- Augmentation with oxytocin
- Uterine hyperstimulation
- Precipitate labour
- Intrapartum abruption
- Cord prolapse
- Uterine rupture/dehiscence
- Maternal diabetes
- Cholestasis of pregnancy
- Maternal pyrexia
- Chorioamnionitis
- Oligohydramnios

Recognition of fetal compromise

Meconium staining of the amniotic fluid is considered significant when it is either thick or tenacious, dark green, bright green or black. Any particulate meconium should also be of concern. Thin and light meconium is more likely to represent fetal gut maturity than fetal compromise. However, when any meconium is seen in the liquor, consideration should be given to starting continuous EFM with the CTG and this is mandatory if the meconium is thick and dark. Another reason for commencing the CTG is if a change in the heart rate is noted with intermittent auscultation, particularly fetal tachycardia, bradycardia or fetal heart rate decelerations. The CTG may have already been running throughout the labour because of underlying risk factors which predate the labour.

Interpretation of the CTG is a skilled business, and there is significant inter-observer variability. There are national guidelines, which should be used to classify the CTG as 'normal', 'suspicious' or 'pathological'. Interpretation of the CTG is discussed in more detail in Chapter 6, Antenatal imaging and assessment of fetal well-being. Examples are given in Figures 14.31–14.36.

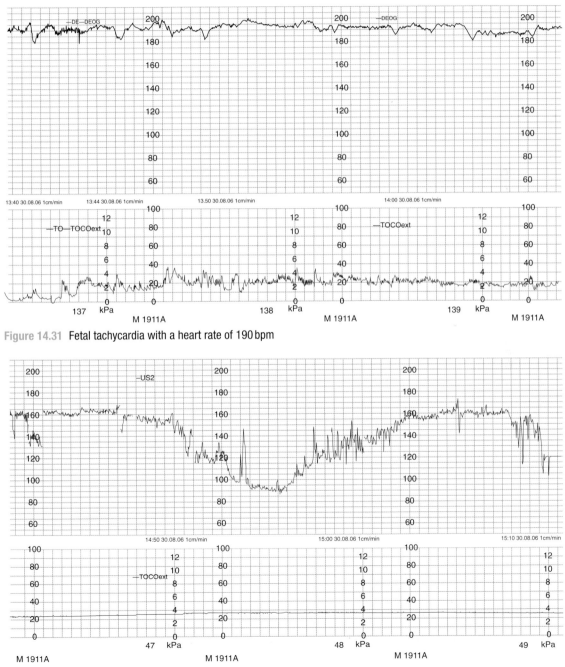

Figure 14.31 Fetal tachycardia with a heart rate of 190 bpm

Figure 14.32 Fetal bradycardia to a heart rate of 90 bpm, lasting approximately 11 minutes

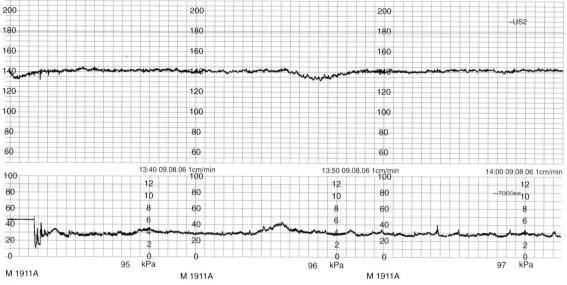

Figure 14.33 Loss of baseline variability (<5 bpm), with a fetal heart rate of 140 bpm

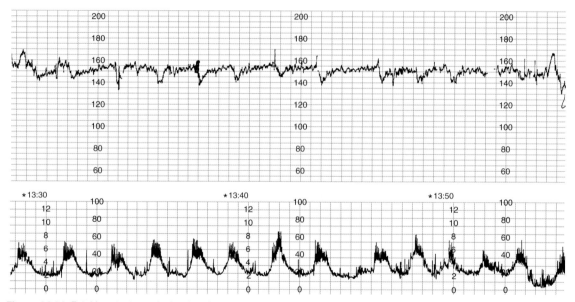

Figure 14.34 Fetal heart rate: early decelerations

CTG signs suggestive of fetal compromise

- Fetal tachycardia (>160 bpm, or a steady rise over the course of the labour)
- Loss of baseline variability (<5 bpm)
- Recurrent late decelerations
- Persistent variable decelerations
- Fetal bradycardia (<100 bpm for more than 3 minutes)

Management of possible fetal compromise

A number of resuscitative manoeuvres should be considered when a CTG is classified as 'suspicious'. It is reasonable to continue observation of the CTG and more complex intervention is not required. If a CTG becomes 'pathological', these reversible factors should also be considered, but it is also important to carry out an immediate vaginal examination to exclude malpresentation and cord prolapse and to assess the

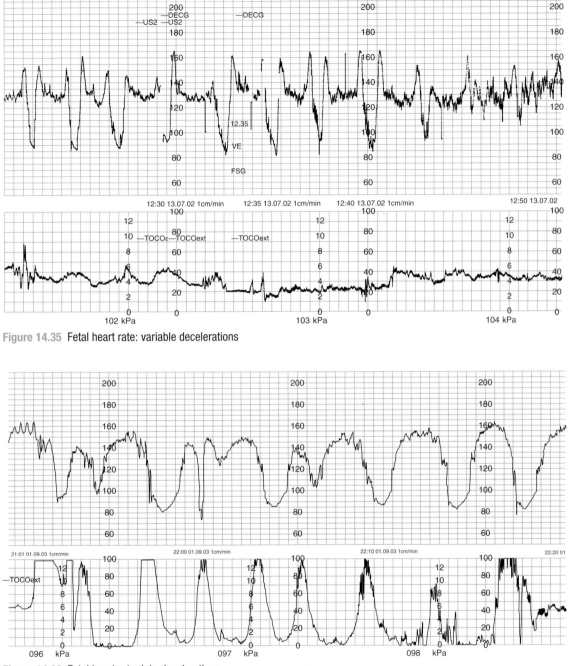

Figure 14.35 Fetal heart rate: variable decelerations

Figure 14.36 Fetal heart rate: late decelerations

progress of the labour. If the cervix is fully dilated, it may be possible to deliver the baby vaginally using the forceps or ventouse. Alternatively, if the cervix is not fully dilated, a fetal blood sampling can be considered. This is usually only possible when the cervix is dilated 3 cm or more. A normal result will permit labour to continue, although it may need to be repeated every 30–60 minutes if the CTG abnormalities persist or worsen. An abnormal result mandates immediate delivery, by Caesarean section if the cervix is not fully dilated. An instrumental delivery may be possible if the cervix is fully dilated.

Resuscitating the fetus in labour

- Maternal dehydration and ketosis can be corrected with intravenous fluids.
- Maternal hypotension secondary to an epidural can be reversed by a fluid bolus, although a vasoconstrictor such as ephedrine is occasionally necessary.
- Uterine hyperstimulation from excess oxytocin can be treated by turning off the infusion temporarily and using tocolytic drugs, such as terbutaline.
- Venocaval compression and reduced uterine blood flow can be eased by turning the woman into a left lateral position.

Fresh, thick meconium in the presence of a reassuring CTG is still a cause for concern, and although the labour should be allowed to continue, the threshold for intervention will be lowered and a paediatrician should be present at delivery.

Fetal blood sampling

- Explanation is given and consent obtained from the woman. She is asked to lie in the left lateral position.
- An amnioscope is inserted into the vagina and its distal end is placed at right angles on to the fetal head. The scalp is cleaned and a small cut is made using a blade with a guard. The resulting blood is collected into a microtube. The amount of blood required is approximately 0.25 mL.
- A normal pH value is above 7.25. A pH below 7.20 is confirmation of fetal compromise. Values between 7.20 and 7.25 are 'borderline'.
- The base deficit can also be useful in interpretation of the fetal scalp pH. A base excess of more than −10 demonstrates a significant metabolic acidosis, with increasing risk of fetal neurological injury beyond this level.
- More than one fetal scalp sample may be necessary over the course of the labour. A downward trend in the fetal scalp pH values is to be expected and should be assessed together with how the labour is progressing.
- If an abnormal CTG persists in labour, then, despite normal values, fetal scalp sampling should be repeated every 60 minutes, or sooner if the CTG deteriorates. If the result is borderline, it should be repeated no more than 30 minutes later.

Mrs S is a 30-year-old gravida 2 para 1. She is 153 cm tall. Her previous baby weighed 3.2 kg at term and was delivered by forceps after a prolonged second stage. The father of this second baby is a new partner.

She has been admitted in spontaneous labour 10 days past her due date. Her hand-held records show concern from her midwife that this is a significantly larger baby than last time. Indeed, a scan at 36 weeks gestation placed the abdominal and head circumference measurements on the 97th centiles. A subsequent glucose tolerance test was normal.

Despite good progress in the earlier part of the labour, dilatation has arrested at 7 cm. On examination, the head is found to be 3/5 palpable per abdomen; the position is left occipito-transverse and the contractions are poor. There is meconium-stained amniotic fluid.

What risks do Mrs S and her baby face?

The large fetal size and the short maternal stature raise the possibility of CPD. The previous need for a forceps delivery of only an average-size baby may indicate small pelvic diameters. There is a risk of obstructed labour, poor progress and the need for a Caesarean section. The meconium may simply be a sign of fetal maturity, but it may also indicate a degree of fetal compromise. At the very least, it poses the risk of meconium aspiration at delivery.

What care should Mrs S receive?

She should be informed of the concerns and provided with adequate pain relief. Fetal monitoring with a continuous CTG should begin (fortunately, this proves to be reassuring). There is no need for an FBS at this point.

She should then be assessed by an obstetric consultant or an experienced registrar, who must make a diagnosis as to the cause of this secondary arrest in first stage. Has the delay in labour occurred simply because of poor uterine contractions? Is there CPD, exacerbated by fetal malposition?

If there is no caput or moulding, and the contractions do indeed prove to be poor and infrequent, any maternal dehydration should be corrected and a cautious trial of oxytocin can be considered. However, this woman has significant risk factors for CPD, and augmenting the labour with oxytocin risks uterine rupture if the labour is truly obstructed. An alternative option is to offer a Caesarean section at this point, or reassess 2 hours later without augmentation.

What subsequent assessment should be undertaken?

If oxytocin is used, a repeat examination should be performed by the same doctor 2 hours later. If the augmentation has been unsuccessful and the cervix is no further dilated, a Caesarean section is indicated. Even if full dilatation is reached, a vaginal delivery cannot be guaranteed. The obstetrician must be confident that the head has descended appropriately, without the development of excessive moulding or caput.

Labour in special circumstances

Women with a uterine scar

Some women will have a pre-existing uterine scar, usually because of a previous Caesarean section. Approximately 20 per cent of all deliveries in developed countries are by Caesarean section and 99 per cent are performed through the lower segment of the uterus because blood loss is less, healing is better and the risk of subsequent rupture is lower than that following an upper segment or 'classical' Caesarean section. There are still a few indications for upper segment Caesarean section and it is important that these women are counselled appropriately. It is estimated that uterine rupture or dehiscence (partial rupture) occurs in approximately 1 in 200 women who labour spontaneously with a pre-existing lower segment uterine scar. The risk is two to three times higher than this in women with a previous upper segment incision.

Signs of uterine rupture include severe lower abdominal pain, vaginal bleeding, haematuria, cessation of contractions, maternal tachycardia and fetal compromise (often a bradycardia, see Figure 14.32). Uterine rupture carries serious maternal risks (shock, need for blood transfusion and operative repair, possibly a hysterectomy) and also serious fetal risks (including hypoxia, permanent neurological injury and intrapartum death).

Rupture of the uterus is particularly likely to occur:

- late in the first stage of labour,
- with induced or accelerated labour,
- in association with a large baby.

Labour after a previous Caesarean section is known as 'vaginal birth after Caesarean' (VBAC). Approximately 70–80 per cent of women who attempt a VBAC will give birth vaginally and the remainder will need repeat Caesarean delivery. The chances of a successful vaginal birth depend on a number of factors, including a previous history of vaginal birth, size of the baby and the original indication for the first Caesarean.

Relative contraindications to VBAC include:

- two or more previous Caesarean section scars,
- the need for induction of labour (IOL)

- a previous labour progress and outcome suggestive of CPD.

A previous classical Caesarean section is an absolute contraindication to attempting vaginal birth.

If a woman with a previous history of a Caesarean section delivery is admitted in labour, intense surveillance is required to identify early signs of uterine rupture. Continuous CTG monitoring is strongly recommended and there should be a low threshold for urgent delivery by repeat Caesarean section.

Some women will have scars on the uterus as a result of a previous myomectomy. In general, there is minimal danger of rupture of a myomectomy scar unless the uterine cavity was extensively opened during the procedure.

Malpresentations

Breech presentation

The antenatal management of breech presentation and the mechanics of the delivery are discussed in Chapter 8, Antenatal obstetric complications. For this discussion, it is sufficient to list some of the complications of a breech labour, which include the following:

- Increased risk of prolapsed cord: this is particularly so with footling breech presentations, and to a lesser extent with the flexed breech. This can cause rapid and severe hypoxia in the fetus (see Chapter 16, Obstetric emergencies).
- Increased risk of CTG abnormalities: cord compression is common during a breech vaginal delivery.
- Mechanical difficulties with the delivery of the shoulders and/or after-coming head: damage to the visceral organs or the brachial plexus can occur if traction is exerted on the breech. Delay in the delivery of the head may occur with the larger fetus, leading to prolonged compression of the umbilical cord and asphyxia. An uncontrolled rapid delivery of the head may occur with a smaller fetus and this predisposes to tentorial tears and intracranial bleeding.

The majority of persistent breech presentations recognized antenatally are delivered by Caesarean section to avoid these risks. Although this is evidence based, and it is probably safer for breech babies to be delivered this way, the most frequent cause of harm in breech labours is the failure to recognize and respond to CTG abnormalities, rather than mechanical problems at the very end of the labour. There is still a place for the vaginal delivery of a breech presentation. Maternal choice and the failure to detect breech presentation until very late in labour will mean that there will continue to be a need for obstetricians to be expert in the skills of breech vaginal delivery.

Poor progress in a breech labour is taken by most to be an indication for Caesarean section. However, a few would support the use of augmentation with oxytocin if contractions are infrequent.

Face presentation

This malpresentation occurs in about 1:500 labours and is due to complete extension of the fetal head (Figure 14.14). In the majority of cases, the cause for the extension is unknown, although it is frequently attributed to excessive tone of the extensor muscles of the fetal neck. Rarely, extension may be due to a fetal anomaly such as a thyroid tumour. The presenting diameter is the submento-bregmatic, which measures 9.5 cm, and is approximately the same in dimension as the suboccipito-bregmatic (vertex) presentation. Despite this, engagement of the fetal head is late and progress in labour is frequently slow, possibly because the facial bones do not mould. It is diagnosed in labour by palpating the nose, mouth and eyes on vaginal examination (Figure 14.25). If progress in labour is excellent, and the chin remains mento-anterior, vaginal delivery is possible, the head being delivered by flexion (Figure 14.26). If the chin is posterior (mento-posterior position), delivery is impossible, as extension over the perineum cannot occur. In this circumstance, Caesarean section is performed. Oxytocin should not be used, and if there is any concern about fetal condition, Caesarean section should be carried out. Forceps delivery is permitted for low mento-anterior face presentations.

Brow presentation

This arises when there is less extreme extension of the fetal neck than that with a face presentation. It can be considered a midway position between vertex and face. It is the least common malpresentation, occurring in 1:2000 labours. The causes of this are similar to those of face presentation, although some brow presentations arise as a result of exaggerated extension associated with OP position. The presenting diameter is the mento-vertical (measuring 13.5 cm) (Figures 14.14 and 14.27). This is incompatible with a vaginal delivery. It is diagnosed in labour by palpating the anterior fontanelle, supra-orbital ridges and nose on vaginal examination (Figure 14.28). If this presentation persists, delivery will only be achieved by Caesarean section.

Shoulder presentation

This is reported as occurring in 1:300 pregnancies at term, but few of these women will go into labour. Shoulder presentation occurs as the result of a transverse or oblique lie of the fetus and the causes of this abnormal presentation include placenta praevia, high parity, pelvic tumour and uterine anomaly (see Chapter 8, Antenatal obstetric complications). Delivery should be by Caesarean section. Delay in making the diagnosis risks cord prolapse and uterine rupture.

Multiple gestations

About 1:80 pregnancies at term are multi-fetal. High-order multiples, such as triplets and quadruplets, are now invariably delivered by Caesarean section, because of the difficulties in monitoring more than two fetuses and the elevated risks of fetal compromise. The second twin is at greater risk of sustaining intrapartum injury than the presenting twin, or a singleton. Currently, the evidence base does not strongly support recommending elective Caesarean delivery for all twins and this is the subject of a large on-going multinational randomized controlled trial. Nevertheless, elective (i.e. planned) Caesarean section is frequently performed in twin pregnancies for a variety of justifiable reasons.

Indications for elective Caesarean section in twin pregnancy

- Malpresentation of the first twin
- Second twin larger than the first
- Evidence of IUGR in one or both twins
- Monoamniotic twins
- Placenta praevia
- Maternal request

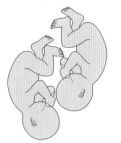
Cephalic/Cephalic (60%)

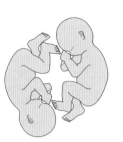
Cephalic/Breech (20%)

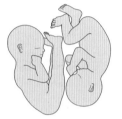
Breech/Cephalic (10%)

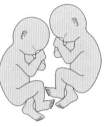
Breech/Breech (10%)

Figure 14.37 The four most common patterns of fetal presentation in a twin pregnancy

In 70–80 per cent of twin gestations the presenting twin is cephalic, with the majority of the remainder being breech (see Figure 14.37). Essentially, the lie and the presentation of the second twin are not crucially important. However, planned Caesarean section will usually be performed if the first twin presents by the breech, and certainly if it is transverse.

The mechanics of the delivery of twins is discussed in greater detail in Chapter 9, Twins and higher multiple gestations. Suffice to say that CTG abnormalities, fetal compromise, malpresentations, cord prolapse, need for emergency Caesarean section and postpartum haemorrhage all occur more commonly than in singleton labours.

Key points

Labour

- Most labours are uncomplicated and the outcomes are good.
- Labour can be a hazardous journey for the baby.
- Abnormalities of the uterine contractions (the 'powers'), the fetus (the 'passenger') and the pelvis and lower genital tract (the 'passages') can cause abnormal labour.
- The term 'fetal distress' is unhelpful and often misleading. If there are concerns regarding fetal well-being in labour,

---

the term 'presumed fetal compromise' should be used instead.
- Augmentation of labour with oxytocin will often correct poor uterine contractions and may help to resolve fetal malposition.
- Augmentation of labour with oxytocin can be dangerous in multiparous women, in those with a uterine scar, and in cases of malpresentation.

Induction of labour

Induction of labour is the planned initiation of labour prior to its spontaneous onset. Approximately one in five deliveries in the United Kingdom occur following induction of labour. The reasons for IOL are listed below. Broadly speaking, an IOL is performed when the risks to the fetus and/or the mother of the pregnancy continuing outweigh those of bringing the pregnancy to an end. It should only be performed if there is a reasonable chance of success and if the risks of the process to the mother and/or fetus are acceptable. If either of these is not the case, a planned Caesarean section should be performed instead.

Common indications for induction of labour

- Prolonged pregnancy
- Fetal growth restriction
- Pre-eclampsia and other maternal hypertensive disorders
- Deteriorating maternal illnesses
- Prelabour rupture of membranes
- Unexplained antepartum haemorrhage
- Diabetes mellitus
- Twin pregnancy continuing beyond 38 weeks
- Intrahepatic cholestasis of pregnancy
- Maternal iso-immunization against red cell antigens
- 'Social' reasons

The most common reason for IOL is prolonged pregnancy (previously described as 'post-term' or 'post-dates'). There is evidence that pregnancies extending beyond 42 weeks gestation are associated with a higher risk of stillbirth, fetal compromise in labour, meconium aspiration and mechanical problems at delivery. Because of this, women are usually recommended IOL between 41 and 42 weeks gestation. Induction for prolonged pregnancy does not increase the rate of Caesarean section. The evidence is good quality, and the recommendation a strong one, however 300–400 pregnancies need to be induced to prevent the one perinatal death which would have occurred if the pregnancies had been managed expectantly beyond 42 weeks gestation. Women who choose not to be induced for this reason are offered more intensive serial fetal monitoring (see Chapter 8, Antenatal obstetric complications).

Prelabour rupture of membranes (PROM) is another common indication for IOL. It is not uncommon for the membranes to rupture and the subsequent onset of labour to be significantly delayed. The longer the time delay between membrane rupture and the delivery of the baby, the greater the risk of ascending infection (chorioamnionitis) and neonatal infectious morbidity. At term (beyond 37 weeks), good quality evidence supports IOL approximately 24 hours following membrane rupture. This policy, endorsed in the NICE guideline on IOL, reduces rates of chorioamnionitis, endometritis and admissions to the neonatal unit. The evidence is less clear at present when PROM occurs preterm. Before 34 weeks, some other additional indication is needed to justify IOL if the membranes rupture (e.g. maternal infection, fetal compromise, growth restriction). Between 34 and 37 weeks, in an otherwise straightforward pregnancy, the risks and benefits of IOL need to be assessed on an individual basis.

Pre-eclampsia and other maternal hypertensive disorders often indicate earlier delivery. Pre-eclampsia at term is normally managed with IOL, however at very preterm gestations (<34 weeks), or where there is rapid deterioration or significant fetal compromise, Caesarean delivery may be a better option. Maternal diabetes, twin gestation and intrahepatic cholestasis of pregnancy are all common reasons for IOL at 38 weeks gestation, and sometimes earlier. The evidence base could be better, and a number of randomized controlled trials are underway to address these issues.

Suspected fetal macrosomia, in the absence of maternal diabetes, and isolated oligohydramnios at term are not evidence-based indications for IOL. Indeed, a number of trials have demonstrated an increased risk of Caesarean section, without improved perinatal morbidity and mortality, when IOL is performed because of concerns regarding large fetal size.

'Social' induction of labour is controversial and is performed to satisfy the domestic and organizational needs of the woman and her family. It is mostly discouraged, and there must be careful counselling as to the potential risks involved. These are determined essentially by the parity and the cervical condition. If the situation is favourable for vaginal birth, with higher parity and a favourable cervix (see below under The Bishop score), 'soft' indications are more acceptable. In any circumstance, an induced labour cannot be considered 'normal' and should be carefully supervised.

There are a number of absolute contraindications to IOL, including placenta praevia and severe fetal compromise. Deteriorating maternal condition with major antepartum haemorrhage, pre-eclampsia or cardiac disease may favour Caesarean delivery. Breech presentation is a relative contraindication to IOL, and women with a previous history of caesarean birth need to be informed of the greater risk of uterine rupture. Preterm gestation is not an absolute contraindication, but induction at <34 weeks is associated with a much higher risk of failure and the need for subsequent Caesarean section.

The Bishop score

As the time of spontaneous labour approaches, the cervix becomes softer, shortened, moves forward and starts to dilate. This reflects the natural preparation for labour. If labour is induced before this process is nearly complete, the induction process will tend to take longer. Bishop produced a scoring system (Table 14.1) to quantify how far this process had progressed prior to the IOL. High scores (a 'favourable' cervix) are associated with an easier, shorter induction that is less likely to fail. Low scores (an 'unfavourable' cervix) point to a longer IOL that is more likely to fail and result in Caesarean section.

Methods

Induction of labour was traditionally performed by artificial rupture of membranes. In the mid-1950s, synthetic oxytocin (Syntocinon) became available and was then used as an intravenous adjunct after rupture of the membranes. In unfavourable cases, it was often unsuccessful and sometimes it was impossible to rupture the membranes. In the late 1960s, prostaglandin became available. Various routes and various preparations have been used,

Table 14.1 Modified Bishop score

Score	0	1	2	3
Dilatation of cervix (cm)	0	1 or 2	3 or 4	5 or more
Consistency of cervix	Firm	Medium	Soft	–
Length of cervical canal (cm)	>2	2–1	1–0.5	<0.5
Position of cervix	Posterior	Central	Anterior	–
Station of presenting part	−3	−2	−1 or 0	Below spines

but the most common formulation in current use is PGE_2, inserted vaginally into the posterior fornix as a tablet or gel. Two doses are often required, given at least 6 hours apart. A controlled-release pessary is also available and this is left in place for up to 24 hours. Prostaglandins are recommended even when the cervix is favourable. Labour may ensue following the administration of prostaglandin, but ARM and oxytocin are often also necessary, particularly in primiparous women. Oxytocin is given intravenously, as a dilute solution. The response to oxytocin is highly variable and a strict protocol exists for its use. The starting infusion rate is low and defined increments follow every 30 minutes until 3–5 contractions are achieved every 10 minutes.

Mifepristone (an anti-progesterone) and misoprostol (another prostaglandin) can be used to induce labour, but complication rates seem higher and this drug combination is currently used in the UK only to induce labour following intrauterine fetal death.

'Membrane sweeping' describes the insertion of a gloved finger through the cervix and its rotation against the wall of the uterus. This safe technique strips off the chorionic membrane from the underlying decidua and releases natural prostaglandins. It can be uncomfortable for the woman, and is only possible if the cervix is beginning to dilate and efface. It can be performed more than once and evidence shows that it reduces the need for formal induction. It is usually only performed at term, and placenta praevia must be excluded before it is offered. It should be considered an adjunct to the normal processes of induction.

Complications of induction of labour

It is generally agreed that a woman is likely to experience more pain with an induced labour and the use of epidural analgesia is more common. The rates of instrumental delivery and Caesarean section are higher following induction, and not all of this increase can be explained by the underlying problems which necessitated the induction in the first place. Long labours augmented with oxytocin predispose to postpartum haemorrhage secondary to uterine atony. Fetal compromise is more common during induced labours and this, in part at least, is due to uterine hyperstimulation caused by the injudicious use of prostaglandins and oxytocin (Figure 14.38). A contraction frequency of >5 per 10 minutes should be treated by stopping the oxytocin and the administration of a tocolytic drug, most commonly the subcutaneous injection of the β_2-agonist terbutaline. Uterine hyperstimulation may precipitate a fetal bradycardia and the need for emergency Caesarean section if the fetal heart rate fails to resolve promptly. If ARM is performed while the fetal head is high then cord prolapse may occur, again precipitating the need for emergency delivery by Caesarean section. Women with a previous Caesarean section scar, or some other form of old uterine injury, are at greater risk of uterine rupture if they are induced. The risk of scar rupture increases from one in 200 in a spontaneous labour, to as high as one in 70 if induction of labour is performed using prostaglandins.

Induction of labour may fail and this is said to have occurred if an ARM is still impossible after the maximum number of doses of prostaglandin have been given, or if the cervix remains uneffaced and less than 3 cm dilated after an ARM has been performed and oxytocin has been running for 6–8 hours with regular contractions. When an induction fails, the options include attempting induction again at some point in the future, or performing a Caesarean section. Delaying delivery further is only acceptable if there is no major threat to fetal or maternal condition. This may be the case with a failed social induction, for example. Failed induction in the setting of pre-eclampsia or fetal growth restriction will usually necessitate a Caesarean delivery.

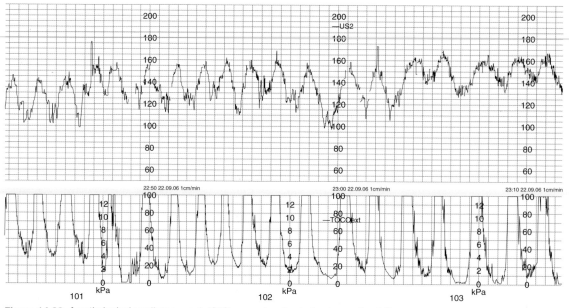

Figure 14.38 A pathological cardiotocograph (CTG) secondary to uterine hyperstimulation

Risks of induction of labour

- Greater pain in labour
- Uterine hyperstimulation
- Cord prolapse
- Greater risk of uterine rupture during VBAC

- Failure
- Increased need for Caesarean or instrumental delivery
- Fetal compromise

CASE HISTORY

Mrs B is a 33-year-old woman in her first pregnancy. She is 41 weeks gestation and a report of reduced fetal movements has prompted an ultrasound scan. Although the growth parameters of the fetus are on the 50th centile, there is oligohydramnios (reduced amniotic fluid). A CTG is normal.

An IOL has been discussed and a vaginal examination performed. The Bishop score is 2.

What risks do Mrs B and her baby face?

Oligohydramnios at term, in isolation, is a poor indicator of placental function. Reduced fetal movements is a worrying but insensitive marker of fetal compromise. However, this is a prolonged pregnancy and this is sufficient on its own to recommend IOL. The other features support this conclusion. Continuation of the pregnancy will increase the risks of intrauterine hypoxia, acidosis or even fetal death. Labour will carry a higher risk of compromising the fetus and there is a greater risk of meconium

passage and aspiration by the newborn. The reactive normal CTG gives no guarantee of future fetal well-being or its ability to tolerate contractions.

The unfavourable cervix increases the chances of long induction, which may ultimately be unsuccessful. Whether the labour is induced or spontaneous, this scenario carries a greater risk of assisted delivery, either instrumental or by Caesarean section. Women and their partners should be advised of these risks before embarking on the procedure, and the alternative policy of expectant management should be discussed objectively, even if the clinician does not favour it.

What care should Mrs B receive?

She should be given full psychological support from the midwifery and medical team and counselled against delaying the delivery of the fetus any further. Despite the concerns, there is a good chance of a normal birth and IOL should be recommended. Mrs B should receive vaginal prostaglandin, and is likely to need two doses, 6 hours apart. Electronic fetal heart rate monitoring should be instituted when significant contractions begin. ARM should be performed and an oxytocin infusion used if labour fails to establish or progress following the ARM. Pain relief should be offered as usual, although epidural anaesthesia might be encouraged in these circumstances, as the labour process may be long.

What ongoing care should she receive?

Attention should be paid to the need for continuity of care despite staff shift changes. A senior doctor should be involved and should review the situation at intervals to determine if it is safe to continue or whether emergency Caesarean section should be performed. If labour is prolonged and difficult, an H_2-blocker and an anti-emetic should be given orally to suppress gastric acid secretion and reduce the risks in the event of a general anaesthetic being necessary. Caesarean section should be performed if induction fails, the labour establishes but fails to progress, or if fetal monitoring suggests compromise.

Clinical risk management

Risk management is an approach to healthcare provision that aims to limit harm occurring to patients. Clinical risk management (CRM) can be applied to all areas of medicine, but the labour ward provides one of the best illustrations of its importance to modern health care.

Labour and delivery carry a serious risk of harm. Maternal trauma (both physical and psychological) and infant neurological injuries are examples of poor outcomes following birth that can potentially be avoided in many cases. Legal action is frequently taken after outcomes such as these, and this is expensive for the National Health Service in litigation payments, and distressing for the staff involved. The aim of CRM is to improve standards of care and subsequently reduce the harm occurring to women and their babies. This in turn should reduce the number of complaints made against hospital trusts and the financial costs of litigation.

Shoulder dystocia, for example, can result in Erb's palsy, intrapartum asphyxial damage and serious maternal perineal trauma. In the majority of cases, these poor outcomes following shoulder dystocia can be avoided by appropriate management. Regular staff education, and the performance of shoulder dystocia 'drills', should limit these outcomes. In these drills, the manoeuvres used to safely overcome shoulder dystocia are rehearsed to aid with recollection in the event of a real emergency. The use of guidelines and protocols drawn from evidence-based medicine is another tool of CRM. These help to reduce errors and to prevent bizarre or unusual decision-making.

Medical and midwifery staff are encouraged to report when things 'go wrong'. Once a 'near-miss' or a poor outcome has occurred, careful documentation is vital if claims of negligence are to be defended. Good communication between the staff and the patient involved may help to clear up misunderstandings and minimize the chances of a formal complaint or legal action. 'Root-cause analysis' is a technique that serves to examine in detail a poor outcome, or near-miss, so that every step of the patient-journey is scrutinized to see if the outcome could have been prevented. In this way, lessons are learned for the future and unit policies and guidelines can be adjusted accordingly. It is usually the case that a whole series of failings or errors need to occur together for a poor outcome to result. Institutional systems as a whole often contribute, and one single individual is rarely solely responsible for a poor outcome.

Audit of labour ward outcomes is an important tool in risk management. If guidelines are not being followed, and certain standards are not being met, this will be detected by audit and steps taken to address the problem. A repeat audit should show that improvements have occurred as a result of the actions taken.

Key points

Induction of labour and clinical risk management
- Every induction of labour should have a valid indication.
- The most common indication for induction of labour is prolonged pregnancy.
- A high Bishop score predicts an easier induction of labour.
- Clinical risk management aims to improve standards of intrapartum care and to reduce the number and severity of poor obstetric outcomes.

CHAPTER 15

OPERATIVE INTERVENTION IN OBSTETRICS

Philip N Baker

OVERVIEW

For any practitioner, the best outcome of pregnancy is a healthy mother and baby. Ideally, this outcome should follow a normal vaginal delivery with an intact perineum, however, 40–50 per cent of deliveries in the United Kingdom are associated with an episiotomy, or are effected by forceps, ventouse or Caesarean section. The indications and prerequisites for these procedures merit constant scrutiny, as do the optimal techniques to minimize complications.

Introduction

The anatomy of the birth canal and the fetal head must be understood as a prerequisite to becoming skilled in the safe use of the forceps or vacuum extractor, just as knowledge of the abdominal and pelvic anatomy must precede Caesarean section. The Royal College of Obstetricians and Gynaecologists recommends that obstetricians achieve experience in spontaneous vaginal delivery prior to commencing training in operative deliveries.

The goal of operative delivery is to expedite delivery with a minimum of maternal or neonatal morbidity. There has been an increasing awareness of the potential for morbidity for both the mother and the baby. The risk of traumatic delivery in relation to forceps, particularly rotational procedures, has been long established. In 1998, the US Food and Drug Administration issued a warning about the potential dangers of delivery with the ventouse or vacuum extractor; this followed several reports of infant fatality secondary to intracranial haemorrhage. In addition, there has been a growing recognition of the short- and long-term morbidity of pelvic floor injury following operative vaginal delivery. Caesarean section, particularly in the second stage of labour, also carries significant morbidity and implications for future births. It is not surprising, therefore, that there has been an increase in litigation relating to obstetric delivery. If we are to offer women the option of safe operative deliveries, we need to improve our approach to clinical care. The goal should be to minimize the risk of morbidity and, where morbidity occurs, to minimize the likelihood of litigation, without limiting maternal choice.

Episiotomy

Definition

An episiotomy is an incision through the perineum made to enlarge the diameter of the vulval outlet and assist childbirth.

Prevalence

Although episiotomies were first described almost 300 years ago, widespread use of the procedure increased during the twentieth century. By the early 1970s, rates were as high as 90 per cent and it was often advocated that there were two reasons for episiotomy; one was a primigravida and the other a previous episiotomy. In other words, every vaginal delivery should be accompanied by episiotomy. It was argued that this reduced the risk of tears and subsequent problems from prolonged bearing down, such as prolapse. The evidence for the latter was tenuous.

The uncritical liberal use of episiotomy was opposed by consumer groups including the National Childbirth Trust and these very high rates of episiotomy have been reversed. In the UK, rates approximate to the World Heath Organization (WHO) recommendation of 10 per cent of normal deliveries, however, there is considerable international variation (rates are 50 per cent in the United States and 99 per cent in Eastern Europe).

Technique

The question of informed consent needs to be addressed during antenatal care; when the fetal head is crowning, it is not possible to obtain true informed consent.

- An episiotomy is performed in the second stage, usually when the perineum is being stretched and it is deemed necessary.
- If there is not a good epidural, the perineum should be infiltrated with local anaesthetic.
- If an effective epidural anaesthetic is in place it should be topped up for delivery with the patient upright to get best coverage of the perineal area.
- The incision can be midline or at an angle from the posterior end of the vulva (a mediolateral episiotomy).
- A mediolateral episiotomy is usually recommended; a midline episiotomy is an incision in a comparatively avascular area and results in less bleeding, quicker healing and less pain, however, there is an increased risk of extension to involve the anal sphincter (third/ fourth-degree tear).
- A mediolateral episiotomy should start at the posterior part of the fourchette, move backwards and then turn medially well before the border of the anal sphincter, so that any extension will miss the sphincter (Figure 15.1).

Complications

Complications include haemorrhage, infection (prophylactic antibiotics may be indicated if contamination is suspected), extension to the anal sphincter (third/fourth-degree tears) and dyspareunia.

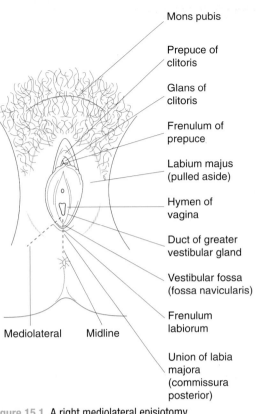

Figure 15.1 A right mediolateral episiotomy

Labels:
Mons pubis
Prepuce of clitoris
Glans of clitoris
Frenulum of prepuce
Labium majus (pulled aside)
Hymen of vagina
Duct of greater vestibular gland
Vestibular fossa (fossa navicularis)
Frenulum labiorum
Union of labia majora (commissura posterior)
Mediolateral   Midline

Perineal trauma

Definitions

1. First-degree trauma corresponds to lacerations of the skin/vaginal epithelium alone.
2. Second-degree tears involve perineal muscles and therefore include episiotomies.
3. Third-degree extensions involve any part of the anal sphincter complex (external and internal sphincters):
   i   Less than 50 per cent of the external anal sphincter is torn.
   ii More than 50 per cent of the external anal sphincter is torn.
   iii Tear involves the internal anal sphincter (usually there is complete disruption of the external sphincter).
4. Fourth-degree tears involve injury to the anal sphincter complex extending into the rectal mucosa.

An increased risk of perineal trauma is associated with:

- larger infants
- prolonged labour
- instrumental delivery.

Prevalence

Eighty-five per cent of women who have a vaginal delivery will have some degree of perineal trauma and 60–70 per cent will require suturing. Internal anal sphincter incompetence results in insensible faecal incontinence, whereas external anal sphincter incompetence causes faecal urgency. Third-degree tears are reported in approximately 2.8 per cent of primigravidae and 0.4 per cent of multigravidae.

Perineal repair

The following is recommended as a routine for perineal repair (Figure 15.2):

- Ensure adequate analgesia. This may be achieved by topping up an epidural or by infiltration with local anaesthetic.
- It is often useful to place a pad high in the vagina to prevent blood from the uterus from obscuring the view.
- Check the extent of cuts and lacerations. Sometimes, the anatomy is not clear and it becomes more apparent as the wound is repaired. If a tear is complex, a more experienced operator may be required.
- First repair the vaginal mucosa using rapidly absorbed suture material on a large, round body needle. Start above the apex of the cut or tear (as severed vessels retract slightly) and use a continuous stitch to close the vaginal mucosa.
- Interrupted sutures are then placed to close the muscle layer.
- Closure of the skin follows. Interrupted sutures can be used; however, a continuous subcuticular stitch produces more comfortable results.
- Perform a gentle vaginal examination to check for any missed tears or inappropriate apposition of anatomy. Remove the pad that was placed at the top of the vagina and check that no swabs have been left in the vagina.

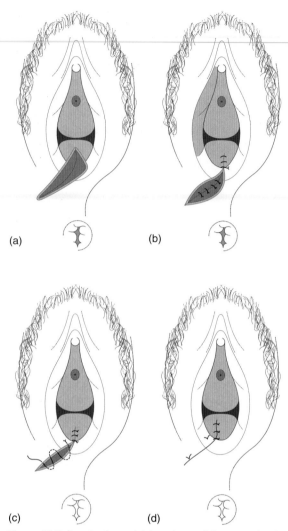

Figure 15.2 Repair of an episiotomy/second degree perineal tear. (a) The perineum prior to the repair; (b) continuous repair of the vaginal mucosa and interrupted repair of the muscle; (c) subcutaneous suture of the skin; (d) completed repair

- Finally, put a finger in the rectum to check that no sutures have passed through into the rectal mucosa and that the sphincter is intact. If sutures are felt in the rectum they must be removed and replaced.

Repair of third- and fourth-degree trauma should be performed or directly supervised by a trained practitioner. There must be adequate analgesia. In practice, this means either a regional or general anaesthetic, as local infiltration does not allow relaxation of the sphincter enough to allow a satisfactory repair. The lighting must be adequate and an assistant is usually needed.

Repair of the rectal mucosa should be performed first. The torn external sphincter is then repaired. It is important to ensure that the muscle is correctly approximated with long-acting sutures so that the muscle is given adequate time to heal. Some surgeons opt for an end-to-end repair, while others use an overlap technique; current evidence suggests that the outcome is similar with both methods. The remainder of the perineal repair is as for second-degree trauma.

Lactulose and a bulk agent, such as Fybogel, are recommended for 5–10 days. It is common sense to give a broad-spectrum antibiotic that will cover possible anaerobic contamination, such as metronidazole (this should be prescribed orally rather than per rectum). Adequate oral analgesia should also be prescribed.

All women who have sustained a third- or fourth-degree tear should be offered follow up by someone interested in this field. A team approach is best; physiotherapy should include augmented biofeedback as this has been shown to improve continence.

At 6–12 months, a full evaluation of the degree of symptoms should take place. This must include careful questioning with regard to faecal and urinary symptoms. Symptomatic women should be offered investigation including endoanal ultrasound and manometry (see Chapter 17, The puerperium).

Key points

- If an episiotomy is performed – a mediolateral incision reduces risk of extension to the anal sphincter.
- Following the repair of an episiotomy or perineal tear, a rectal examination should be performed, to ensure that the sphincter is intact and that sutures have not passed through into the rectal mucosa.
- Women who suffer third- or fourth-degree tears should undergo careful multidisciplinary follow up.

Operative vaginal delivery

Although the use of instruments to facilitate a birth was initially reserved for the extraction of dead infants via destructive techniques, from as early as 1500BC there exist reports of successful deliveries of live infants in obstructed labours. In the sixteenth and seventeenth centuries, the male midwife started to appear, and was frequently required to deal with obstructed labours.

The development of the modern obstetric forceps by the Chamberlens, a Huguenot family practising in England, dramatically changed the aim of intrapartum intervention in favour of delivery of a live infant. The Chamberlens kept their secret for more than a century, however, it is thought that Peter Chamberlen the Elder was the pioneer in the development of forceps. Hugh Chamberlen, son of Peter, unsuccessfully tried to persuade the great French obstetrician François Mauriceau to adopt obstetric forceps. Chamberlen's visit to Paris failed miserably when Mauriceau mischievously challenged him to deliver a baby in obstructed labour due to a rachitic pelvis; Chamberlen's futile efforts had disastrous effects for both mother and baby. That instrumental intervention in the process of labour has become more widely accepted is at least partially due to the work of William Smellie, a Scottish doctor practising in the poorer parts of London. Smellie was a great teacher of both midwives and physicians, and described the use of forceps in his *Treatise on the theory and practice of midwifery* published in 1752.

Definition

Delivery of a baby vaginally using an instrument for assistance.

Prevalence

In the UK, approximately 12 per cent of deliveries are assisted with forceps/ventouse. The incidence of instrumental intervention varies widely both within and between countries and may be performed as infrequently as 1.5 per cent, or as often as 26 per cent. These differences are often related to variations in labour ward management.

Many different strategies have been suggested and employed to help lower the rates of assisted delivery. A few of these are evidence based:

- provision of a caregiver in labour;
- active management of the second stage with syntocinon in nulliparous women with epidural analgesia;
- delayed pushing in nulliparous women with epidural analgesia.

Other techniques that are commonly used but have no evidence to support their usage are upright positions in labour and allowing epidural analgesia to wear off.

Indications for assisted vaginal delivery

Fetal

- The most common fetal indications are those concerning malpositions of the fetal head (occipito-transverse and occipito-posterior). Such positions occur more frequently with regional anaesthesia as a consequence of alterations in the tone of the pelvic floor that impede spontaneous rotation to the optimal occipito-anterior position. Epidural analgesia has been shown to be associated with longer first and second stages of labour, increased incidence of fetal malposition, increased use of oxytocin and increased incidence of instrumental vaginal deliveries. It is possible that the increasing incidence of instrumental deliveries may reflect the rising demand for regional anaesthesia.

- Fetal distress is a commonly cited indication for instrumental intervention, although it is infrequently the fetus that is actually distressed. 'Presumed fetal compromise' is a better term, especially when employed in conjunction with a precise description of the situation surrounding the intervention.

- The use of elective instrumental intervention for infants of reduced weight is more controversial. In infants of less than 1.5 kg, delivery with forceps offers no advantage over spontaneous delivery and may increase the incidence of intracranial haemorrhage. Ventouse carries the same risks, but in addition should be avoided in infants of less than 35 completed weeks of gestation.

Maternal

- The most common maternal indications for intervention are those of maternal distress, exhaustion or undue prolongation of the second stage of labour. Labour may be deemed to be prolonged if the second stage lasts >2 hours in a primigravida (3 hours if an epidural is *in situ*), or >1 hour in a multipara (2 hours if an epidural is *in situ*).

- Less common indications include medically significant conditions, such as aortic valve disease with significant outflow obstruction or myasthenia gravis.

The reasons cited for intervention are often imprecise as one or more factors may interact, e.g. delay in the second stage as a consequence of poor maternal effort and transitional malpositions.

Contraindications

The ventouse should not be used:

- in gestations of less than 35 completed weeks because of the risk of cephalohaematoma and intracranial haemorrhage.
- face or breech presentation.

There is minimal risk of fetal haemorrhage if the vacuum extractor is employed following fetal blood sampling or application of a spiral scalp electrode; no excess bleeding was reported in two randomized trials comparing deliveries performed with forceps or ventouse.

Forceps and vacuum extractor deliveries before full dilatation of the cervix are contraindicated, although possible exceptions occurs with the vacuum delivery of a second twin where the cervix has contracted or with a prolapsed cord at 9 cm if rapid delivery is anticipated.

Instrument choice

The Royal College of Obstetricians and Gynaecologists has issued clinical guidelines regarding the use of instruments to aid vaginal delivery, and has stated that obstetricians should be competent and confident in the use of both forceps and the ventouse; practitioners should use the most appropriate instrument for individual circumstances. The choice of instrument employed by the accoucheur should be based on a combination of indication, experience and training, and the last two of these issues are particularly pertinent, in the context of changes in 'junior doctors' hours' and working practices. It is certainly the case that only adequately trained or supervised practitioners should undertake any vacuum or forceps delivery.

The ventouse, when compared to the forceps is significantly more likely to:

- fail to achieve a vaginal delivery;
- be associated with a cephalohaematoma (subperiosteal bleed);
- be associated with retinal haemorrhage;

- be associated with maternal worries about the baby;

and is significantly less likely to be associated with:

- use of maternal regional/general anaesthesia;
- significant maternal perineal and vaginal trauma;
- severe perineal pain at 24 hours;

and is equally likely to be associated with:

- delivery by Caesarean section;
- low 5 minute Apgar scores.

The incidence of maternal injuries in deliveries performed with the ventouse is significantly reduced when compared with forceps; anal sphincter injury in particular is twice as common with forceps delivery. There is a paucity of long-term follow-up data, however, women enrolled in one of the largest randomized controlled trials showed no difference in the groups delivered by forceps or ventouse when assessed at approximately five years. Although the degree of rotation required is a significant indicator of a potentially difficult delivery, the data currently available from the published trials cannot be analysed separately to compare the ventouse and forceps (e.g. Kiellands) in their use for rotational deliveries.

Rotational instrumental vaginal delivery versus Caesarean section

Often, the decision is whether to perform a rotational vaginal delivery or Caesarean section. Caesarean section has been viewed as the less harmful of the two interventions, however, there are limited data comparing the morbidity of second-stage Caesarean section with instrumental vaginal delivery. Women who are delivered by Caesarean section in the second stage of labour are more likely to have a major haemorrhage of more than a litre and to need a hospital stay of more than 5 days. On the other hand, babies delivered by Caesarean section are less likely to have trauma than babies delivered by forceps but are more likely to require admission for intensive care. It is important to note that the experience of the operator is directly related to the chance of major haemorrhage whatever the mode of delivery. It should therefore be the aim at this stage in labour to deliver women vaginally, unless there are clear signs of cephalopelvic disproportion. It is undoubtedly the case that skilled obstetricians should supervise complex operative deliveries, whatever the time of day they occur. Although the psychological consequences of transferring a patient to an operating theatre in the second stage should not be underestimated, most mid-cavity procedures, which by their nature have a higher rate of complications than outlet or low deliveries, should be performed in theatre.

Prerequisites for any instrumental delivery

- Confirmed rupture of the membranes.
- The cervix must be fully dilated (except second twin and rare other situations).
- Vertex presentation with identification of the position.
- For occipitoanterior and transverse positions, no part of the fetal head should be palpable abdominally. For occipito-posterior positions, it is acceptable that one-fifth of the head may be palpable. The presenting part should be at +1 or more below the ischial spines.
- Adequate analgesia/anaesthesia.
- Empty bladder/no obstruction below the fetal head (contracted pelvis/pelvic kidney/ovarian cyst, etc.).
- A knowledgeable and experienced operator with adequate preparation to proceed with an alternative approach if necessary.
- An adequately informed and consented patient (consent must be sought though not necessarily written).

For forceps, all the prerequisites above apply, but in addition it is essential that the operator check the pair of forceps to ensure that a matching pair has been provided and that the blades lock with ease (both before and after application).

Basic rules

It has been suggested that failure rates of less than 1 per cent should be achieved with well-maintained apparatus and the use of the correct technique. However, this is probably an unrealistic target; most studies suggest failure rates of 10–15 per cent. Several factors contribute to delivery failure:

- inadequate initial case assessment – high head, misdiagnosis of the position and attitude of the head;

- failure due to traction in the wrong plane;
- poor maternal effort with inadequate use of Syntocinon to aid expulsive efforts in the second stage;
- failure to select the correct ventouse cup type and/or incorrect cup position.

Evaluation

A careful pelvic examination is essential to determine whether there are any 'architectural' contraindications to performing an instrumental vaginal delivery. If, for example, a contracted pelvis is the cause of failure to progress in the second stage, then due consideration must be paid to determining the type of instrument to be employed, or whether it may be more prudent to perform a Caesarean section. The shape of the subpubic arch, the curve of the sacral hollow, the presence of flat or prominent ischial spines, all contribute to the decision as to whether a vaginal delivery may be safely performed. Anthropoid (narrow), android (male/funnel-shaped) or platypelloid (squashed) pelvises all make instrumental deliveries more difficult and may preclude the use of rotational forceps.

With any difficult instrumental delivery, the risk of shoulder dystocia occurring after successful delivery of the fetal head should always be remembered, as should the subsequent and probable postpartum haemorrhage. As a consequence, the accoucheur must develop the skills necessary to anticipate such events and to manage the consequences in a logical and calm manner.

Analgesia

Analgesic requirements are greater for forceps than ventouse delivery. Where rotational forceps are needed, regional analgesia is preferred. For a rigid cup ventouse delivery, a pudendal block with perineal infiltration may be all that is needed and if a soft cup is used, analgesic requirements may be minimal. A requirement for haste should not preclude the use of analgesia. No operator would consider performing a Caesarean section without the appropriate anaesthesia and the same should be true for vaginal delivery.

Positioning

Instrumental deliveries are traditionally performed with the patient in the lithotomy position and using as aseptic a technique as is possible. The angle of traction needed requires that the foot of the bed be removed. In patients with limited abduction (such as those with symphysis pubis dysfunction), it may be necessary to limit abduction of the thighs to a minimum. It is the accoucheur's duty to ensure that the bladder is emptied.

Instrument types

Ventouse/vacuum extractors

The basic premise of such instruments is that a suction cup, of a silastic or rigid construction, is connected, via tubing, to a vacuum source (Figure 15.3). Either directly through the tubing or via a connecting 'chain', direct traction can then be applied to the presenting part to expedite delivery. Recent developments have removed the need for cumbersome external suction generators and have incorporated the vacuum mechanism into 'hand-held' pumps, e.g. OmniCup™. Such devices appear to be more acceptable to patients than standard equipment and have no obvious effects on instrumental delivery success or on the incidence of maternal or fetal complications, but large trials have yet to be performed.

Technique

Soft cups are significantly more likely to fail to achieve vaginal delivery than rigid cups, however, they are associated with less scalp injury. There appears to be no difference in terms of maternal injury. The soft cups are appropriate for straightforward deliveries with an occipitoanterior position; metal cups appear to be more suitable for 'occipitoposterior', transverse and difficult 'occipitoanterior' position deliveries where the infant is larger or there is a marked caput.

For successful use of the ventouse, determination of the flexion point is vital. This is located at the vertex, which, in an average term infant, is on the saggital suture 3 cm anterior to the posterior fontanelle and thus 6 cm posterior to the anterior fontanelle. The centre of the cup should be positioned directly over this, as failure to do so will lead to a progressive deflexion of the fetal head during traction, and an inability to deliver the baby.

The operating vacuum pressure for nearly all ventouse is between 0.6 and 0.8 kg/cm². It is prudent

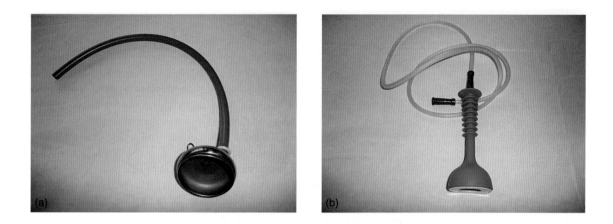

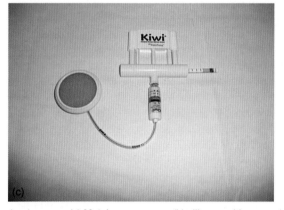

Figure 15.3 Ventouse/vacuum extractor cups: (a) Metal venouse cup; (b) silicone rubber cup; (c) OmniCup™

to increase the suction to 0.2 kg/cm² first and then to recheck that no maternal tissue is caught under the cup edge. When this is confirmed the suction can then be increased.

Traction must occur in the plane of least resistance along the axis of the pelvis – the traction plane (Figure 15.4). This will usually be at exactly 90° to the cup and the operator should keep a thumb and forefinger on the cup at the traction insertion to ensure that the traction direction is correct and to feel for slippage. Safe and gentle traction is then applied in concert with uterine contractions and voluntary expulsive efforts. With the ventouse, the operator should allow no more than two episodes of breaking the suction in any vacuum delivery, and the maximum time from application to delivery should ideally be less than 15 minutes. Rotation is achieved by the natural progression of the head through the pelvis.

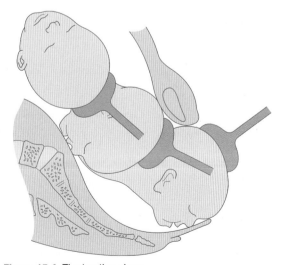

Figure 15.4 The traction plane

It is not acceptable to use a ventouse when:

- The position of the fetal head is unknown.
- There is a significant degree of caput that may either preclude correct placement of the cup or, more sinisterly, indicate a substantial degree of cephalopelvic disproportion.
- The operator is inexperienced in the use of the instrument.

Forceps

Types of forceps

The basic forceps design has not radically changed over many years and, all types in use today consist of two blades with shanks, joined together at a lock, with handles to provide a point for traction. The specific details of construction vary between the instruments. The blades may be fenestrated – open, pseudofenestrated (open with a protruding ridge), or solid. Likewise, the length of the shanks, the design of the lock (convergent, divergent or sliding) and the fashioning of the handles are instrument specific.

Non-rotational forceps are used when the head is occipitoanterior ±15°. Examples such as Neville Barnes or Simpson forceps (Figure 15.5) have a pelvic curve and an English or non-sliding lock. If the head is positioned >15° from the vertical, rotation must be accomplished before traction. Forceps designed for rotation, such as Kielland forceps, have minimal pelvic curve to allow rotation around a fixed axis; the sliding lock of the Kielland forceps (Figure 15.5) facilitates correction of asynclitism.

Technique

By convention, the left blade is inserted before the right with the accoucheur's hand protecting the vaginal wall from direct trauma. With proper placement of the forceps blades, they come to lie parallel to the axis of the fetal head and between the fetal head and the pelvic wall. The operator then articulates and locks the blades, checking their application before applying traction (Figure 15.6).

Traction should be applied intermittently in concert with uterine contractions and maternal expulsive efforts. The axis of traction changes during the delivery and is guided along the 'J'-shaped curve of the pelvis. As the head begins to crown, the blades are directed to the vertical, and the head is delivered.

(Specific techniques are required for rotational forceps deliveries and only those who have been properly trained in their use should employ them.)

It has been recommended that an episiotomy be cut whenever an instrumental vaginal delivery is performed. This is not based on any robust evidence. It is recognized in spontaneous vaginal delivery that episiotomy does not protect against third- and fourth-degree tears, but does reduce the incidence of anterior vaginal trauma. Perineal trauma will occur in most nulliparous women undergoing instrumental vaginal delivery and episiotomy should be considered in these women in order to limit multiple lacerations. In multiparae, particularly those requiring only a simple ventouse, an episiotomy may not be needed.

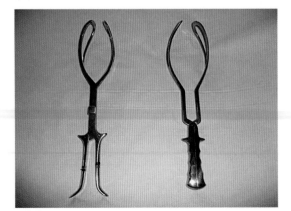

Figure 15.5 Kielland rotational forceps and Simpson non-rotational forceps

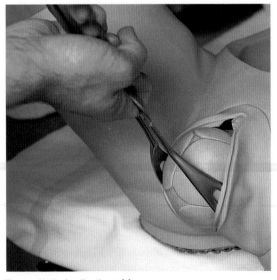

Figure 15.6 Application of forceps

Special considerations

Failure of the chosen instrument

Failures can occur when the choice of instrument is wrong (e.g. a silastic cup ventouse for a rotational delivery), when the positioning of the ventouse cup is wrong or when the position has been wrongly defined, leading to inappropriately large diameters presenting to the pelvis. Failure is also more common if the fetus is large or maternal effort is poor.

There have been no randomized studies assessing the best approach following a failure to deliver with the first choice of instrument. Observational studies show that the outcomes for babies are worse than if the instrument of first choice is successful, but this is hardly surprising. In addition, the rates of third- and fourth-degree tears are higher when a second instrument is used.

Unfortunately, there are no easy answers; the head may have descended to a point at which Caesarean section becomes hazardous. A policy of delivering all such women by Caesarean section will undoubtedly lead to increased maternal morbidity.

Where the first instrument fails, the following scenarios may pertain:

- The reason for failure was cup detachment and the head is occipitoanterior and on the perineum. A full reassessment should be made. If it is confirmed that this is still the case (i.e. occipitoanterior, head on the perineum), a simple lift out forceps is acceptable. If there are any concerns, senior help must be sought.

- The instrument failed because there was little or no descent with the first pull. Where there has been little or no descent, delivery must be by Caesarean section.

- The instrument failed because the position was wrongly defined. In this case, the next option will either be a rotational forceps or Caesarean section. Already the fetus will have been subjected to traction with probably minimal descent. Only after a full assessment by a senior person in theatre could further instrumentation be considered. In many cases, delivery by Caesarean section will be the safer option for the fetus.

Complications

Assisted deliveries with both vacuum and forceps can be associated with significant maternal and fetal complications.

Maternal deaths have been reported with vacuum deliveries, associated with cervical tears in women delivered before full dilatation. Traumatic vaginal delivery is considered the most important risk factor for faecal incontinence in women and may occur not only after recognized third-degree perineal tears, but also after apparently non-traumatic vaginal delivery.

Postpartum haemorrhage is more common in women needing instrumental vaginal delivery compared to women who deliver spontaneously, but less common than in women delivered by Caesarean section in the second stage. Measures to limit this include:

- prophylactic syntocinon infusion post delivery;
- prompt suturing;
- careful identification of high tears.

Underestimation of blood loss at instrumental vaginal delivery is common. Where possible, loss should be measured through the weighing of swabs and towels.

Fetal complications are no less important; the incidence of cephalhaematoma is increased with the use of the ventouse, and there are rare reports of severe intracranial injuries. Risks of perinatal trauma correlate with:

- the duration of the operative delivery;
- the station of the fetal head at the commencement of the delivery;
- the difficulty of the delivery;
- the condition of the baby at the time of commencement of the procedure.

It is important to remember that the risks of such damage significantly increase among babies who are exposed to multiple attempts at both vacuum and forceps delivery.

Clinical risk management in obstetrics

Instrumental vaginal delivery has never been free from criticism, and is certainly not without risks, although most instrumental deliveries have normal outcomes and give no reason for complaint. However, in today's litigious society, the risks of litigation against an accoucheur or the hospital in which they practise are increased by a bad outcome.

Common allegations against practitioners that are cited in lawsuits include (among others): inadequate indication, failure to exclude cephalopelvic disproportion, improper use of instruments with excessive use of force resulting in fetal or maternal injury, lack of informed consent (although this may not be fully possible in an emergency situation), and inadequate supervision. The fear of litigation must not dictate good medical practice, and assisted vaginal deliveries remain an appropriate intervention when practised with the appropriate safeguards.

Key points 🔑

- Careful assessment of each patient combining history and examination must be performed before any intervention is undertaken.
- The prerequisites for an instrumental delivery must all be met before either forceps or the ventouse are applied.
- Instruments should only be used by those trained to do so.
- Failure rates are higher with soft than rigid cups and with ventouse than forceps.
- Use of a second instrument increases the risks of fetal and maternal damage.
- Caesarean section in the second stage is associated with higher rates of haemorrhage than instrumental delivery.

Caesarean section

Definition

A Caesarean section, also known as C-section or Caesar, is a surgical procedure in which incisions are made through a mother's abdomen (laparotomy) and uterus (hysterotomy) to deliver one or more babies.

There are three theories about the origin of the name. The name is said to derive from a Roman legal code called *Lex Caesarea*, which allegedly contained a law prescribing that the baby be cut out of its mother's womb in the case that she dies before giving birth. The derivation of the name is also often attributed to an ancient story, told in the first century AD by Pliny the Elder, who claimed that an ancestor of Caesar was delivered in this manner. An alternative etymology suggests that the procedure's name derives from the Latin verb *caedere*, to cut, in which case the term 'Caesarean section' is redundant.

Caesar's mother, Aurelia, lived through childbirth and successfully gave birth to her son, ruling out the possibility that the Roman dictator and general was born by Caesarean section. However, the Catalan saint, Raymond Nonnatus (1204–40), received his surname (from the Latin *non natus*, not born) because he was born by Caesarean section; his mother died while giving birth to him. In 1316, the future Robert II of Scotland was delivered by Caesarean section and his mother, Marjorie Bruce, died (this may have been the inspiration for Macduff in Shakespeare's play Macbeth). The first recorded incidence of a woman surviving a Caesarean section was in 1500, in Siegershausen, Switzerland: Jakob Nufer, a pig gelder, is supposed to have performed the operation on his wife after a prolonged labour. For most of the time since the sixteenth century, the procedure had a high mortality. A Caesarean section was considered an extreme measure, performed only when the mother was already dead or considered to be beyond help. In Great Britain and Ireland, the mortality rate in 1865 was 85 per cent. Key steps in reducing mortality were:

- adherence to principles of asepsis;
- the introduction of uterine suturing by Max Sänger in 1882;
- extraperitoneal Caesarean section and then moving to low transverse incision;
- anaesthesia advances;
- blood transfusion;
- antibiotics.

On March 5, 2000, Inés Ramírez performed a Caesarean section on herself and survived, as did her son. She is believed to be the only woman to have performed a successful Caesarean section on herself.

Birth by Caesarean section has become a commonplace intervention on the modern labour ward. According to some, the Caesarean section rate has reached epidemic proportions and requires a dramatic rethink of obstetric management.

Prevalence

In the UK, more than 21 per cent of all babies are now delivered by Caesarean section. The principal aims must be to ensure that those women and babies who need delivery by Caesarean section are so delivered and that those who do not are saved from unnecessary intervention. In 1985, concern regarding the increasing frequency of Caesarean section led the World Health Organization to hold a consensus conference. This conference concluded that there were no health benefits above a Caesarean section rate of 10–15 per cent. The Scandinavian countries have managed to hold Caesarean section rates at this level with outcomes comparable or better than those countries with higher Caesarean section rates.

Factors that may contribute to an increase in the rates of Caesarean section

- **Inaccurate dating of the pregnancy.** Many practitioners combine the information obtained from a carefully taken history with that from a dating ultrasound scan, particularly when the date of the last menstrual period is uncertain. Such accurate dating reduces the anxiety experienced by many women when they pass their 'expected date of delivery' and also reduces the requests for 'early' induction of labour. In units that do not date pregnancy by ultrasound scanning before 20 weeks, an opportunity for accurate dating may be missed. This may be of particular importance in units that have a policy of offering routine induction of labour to women who are 41 weeks gestation or more.
- **Fetal monitoring.** Following its introduction in the 1970s, electronic fetal monitoring (EFM) was universally implemented without the appropriate trials. This has resulted in an increase in the incidence of Caesarean section without demonstrable improvement in perinatal outcome. Current recommendations are for intermittent auscultation to be performed in all 'low risk pregnancies', with continuous EFM in those pregnancies deemed to be 'high risk'.
- **Macrosomia.** Maternal concern about fetal size is a common problem that frequently engenders anxiety among obstetricians and midwives. Although there is evidence to suggest that birthweights are rising in developed countries, the amount (30 g over 12 years) is unlikely to be of any biological significance. Unfortunately, both clinical and ultrasonographic estimations of fetal size are prone to inaccuracy (especially in large term infants), and unnecessary inductions of labour and Caesarean deliveries are performed as a consequence.
- **Maternal request.** Traditionally, Caesarean sections have been reserved for situations guided by standard clinical indications. However, the request for delivery by an elective Caesarean section where there is not a compelling obstetric indication is becoming more common. There is huge heterogeneity in studies examining the effect of maternal request on Caesarean section rates; studies range from 2–28 per cent in the contribution of request as the primary reason, due in major part to the differing definitions of 'request'.
- The arguments surrounding this area are complex and combine ethical dilemmas, the fetal and maternal risks of vaginal and surgical deliveries and the financial consequences of permitting such preferences. During the antenatal period, the dialogue between patients and their doctors has increased over recent years. Policy documents such as *Changing childbirth* enshrined in practice the principle of total involvement of the pregnant woman in her own care. Implicit in this is the consideration of her wishes relating to delivery. Therefore, discussions must be accompanied by the careful imparting of information, counselling and advice, but should the patient's opinions differ from those of her healthcare providers, these cannot simply be ignored. The risks of Caesarean section and labour are different, and the risks of recurrent Caesarean deliveries are additive (increasing risk of placenta praevia, accreta, operative complications, etc.). However, many practitioners believe that if these risks are fully explained to the woman, she should be allowed to choose to accept one set of risks over the other.

Indications

There are many different reasons for performing a delivery by Caesarean section. The four major indications accounting for greater than 70 per cent of operations are:

1. previous Caesarean section
2. dystocia
3. malpresentation
4. suspected acute fetal compromise.

Other indications, such as multifetal pregnancy, abruptio placenta, placenta praevia, fetal disease and maternal disease are less common. No list can be truly comprehensive and whatever the indication, the overriding principle is that whenever the risk to the mother and/or the fetus from vaginal delivery exceeds that from operative intervention, a Caesarean section should be undertaken.

Absolute indications for recommending delivery by Caesarean section are few, almost all indications are relative and there will be circumstances where Caesarean section may be best for one woman but not another. Lack of consent in a woman with capacity to give consent will prohibit Caesarean section regardless of the clinical need.

Morbidity and mortality

Although Caesarean section is becoming increasingly safe and evidence is mounting regarding the risks of labour and vaginal delivery, pregnant women, their midwives and doctors need to understand and appreciate the maternal risks associated with the different modes of delivery. Confidential Enquiries into Maternal Deaths have enabled the risks associated with different methods of delivery to be analysed; case fatality rate for all Caesarean sections is five times that for vaginal delivery, although for elective Caesarean section the difference does not reach statistical significance. Some maternal deaths following Caesarean section are not attributable to the procedure itself, but rather to medical or obstetric disorders that lead to the decision to deliver using this approach. Many women who deliver vaginally encounter the same problems.

Repeat Caesarean section

In many units, Caesarean section rates for primigravidae of 24 per cent are seen. Consequently, the problem of management of a woman with a scarred uterus in subsequent pregnancies is a common antenatal problem. It is a vital part of antenatal care that women be given a clear understanding of the plan of management from early on in their pregnancy, with the caveat that this may need to be adapted if the pregnancy presents unexpected problems. The management in pregnancy following a Caesarean section should be to assess the available options and to select the appropriate choice for an individual woman. The dictum 'once a Caesarean section, always a Caesarean section' is not true; up to 70 per cent of women with a previous Caesarean section can achieve a vaginal delivery. Patient choice cannot and should not be ignored in decisions regarding management, and it is important to discuss the risks and benefits of elective Caesarean section as compared to trial of vaginal delivery.

From a maternal perspective, elective Caesarean section avoids labour with its risk of perineal trauma (urinary and faecal problems), the need to undergo emergency Caesarean section, and scar dehiscence/rupture with subsequent morbidity and mortality. However, elective Caesarean section carries maternal risks: increased bleeding, thromboembolism, febrile morbidity, prolonged recovery, long-term bladder dysfunction and increased risks of placenta praevia in subsequent pregnancies. From a fetal perspective,

an elective Caesarean section reduces the risk of scar rupture, but increases the risk of transient tachypnoea/respiratory distress syndrome. There is remarkably little evidence to inform practice with regard to management of previous Caesarean section: there are no randomized trials and much of the data relate to observational studies.

Consideration of the risk of scar rupture is probably the most important consideration when determining whether delivery should be by elective Caesarean section or by trial of vaginal delivery. Most published studies do not differentiate between scar dehiscence and rupture, however, analysis of observational and comparative studies indicates that the excess risk of uterine rupture following trial of labour compared with women undergoing repeat elective Caesarean section is considerably lower than 1 per cent; indeed, some studies do not demonstrate any increased risk.

Providing the first operation was carried out for non-recurrent cause, and providing the obstetric situation close to term in the succeeding pregnancy is favourable, then it is appropriate to offer a trial of labour to any woman with a previous uncomplicated lower uterine segment Caesarean section and no other adverse obstetric feature. The factors to be weighed when determining the recommended mode of delivery depend on the balance between the desires of the mother, the risks of a repeat operation, the risks to her child of labour, and the risk of labour on the strength of the old scar.

Procedure

Informed consent

Full informed consent must always be obtained prior to operation. The level of information discussed must be commensurate with the urgency of the procedure, and a common sense approach is needed. However, although it is often difficult to impart complete and thorough information when Caesarean sections are performed as emergency procedures, mothers must understand what is being planned and why. Where possible, all women must be educated in pregnancy about Caesarean section and the occasions under which it may be urgently needed. It is important to remember that no other adult may give consent for another (although it is good practice to keep relatives fully informed). Where there is incapacity to consent (as may occur with conditions such as eclampsia), the doctor is expected to act in the patient's best interests.

The national consent forms require both the risks and benefits to be discussed with patients and recorded on the consent form. Common medical practice is to highlight risks but not benefits. It is important to remember that the operation is being offered because of perceived benefits, both maternal and fetal in many cases.

Surgical basics

The bladder should be emptied before the procedure. A left lateral tilt minimizes compression of the maternal inferior vena cava and reduces the incidence of hypotension (with its consequent reductions in placental perfusion).

The Pfannenstiel incision

The skin and subcutaneous tissues are incised using a transverse curvilinear incision two fingerbreadths above the symphysis pubis extending from and to points lateral to the lateral margins of the abdominal rectus muscles. Subcutaneous tissues are separated by blunt dissection and the rectus sheath is incised transversely along the middle 2 cm. This incision is then extended with scissors before the fascial sheath is separated from the underlying muscle by further blunt dissection. Separation is performed cephalad to permit adequate exposure of the peritoneum in a longitudinal plane. The recti are separated, the peritoneum incised and the abdominal cavity entered. The transverse Pfannensteil incision has the advantages of improved cosmetic results, decreased analgesic requirements and superior wound strength.

The infra-umbilical incision

A vertical skin incision is indicated in cases of extreme maternal obesity, suspicion of other intra-abdominal pathology necessitating surgical intervention, or where access to the uterine fundus may be required (classical Caesarean section). The lower midline incision is made from the lower border of the umbilicus to the symphysis pubis, and may be extended caudally toward the xiphisternum. Sharp dissection to the anterior rectus sheath is performed and is then freed of subcutaneous fat. The rectus sheath is then incised taking care to avoid damage to any underlying bowel, and extended inferiorly to the vesical peritoneal reflection and superiorly to the upper limit of the abdominal incision. The vertical incision provides greater ease of access to the pelvic and intra-abdominal organs and may be enlarged more easily; however, the incidence of wound dehiscence is increased.

Uterine incision

A lower uterine segment incision is used in over 95 per cent of Caesarean deliveries due to ease of repair, reduced blood loss and low incidence of dehiscence or rupture in subsequent pregnancies (Figure 15.7). The loose reflection of vesico-uterine serosa overlying the uterus is divided laterally, the underlying lower uterine segment is reflected with blunt dissection, the developed bladder flap is retracted and the lower uterine segment is opened in a transverse plane for a distance of 1–2 cm; the incision is extended laterally to allow delivery of the fetus without extension into the broad ligament or uterine vessels. There are relatively few absolute indications for classical section (which incorporates the upper uterine segment, Figure 15.7). These include a lower uterine segment containing fibroids or a lower segment covered with dense adhesions, both of which may make entry difficult. Other indications include placenta praevia, transverse lie with the back down, fetal abnormality (e.g. conjoined twins), or Caesarean section in the presence of a carcinoma of the cervix (so as to avoid damage to the cervix and its vascular and lymphatic supply).

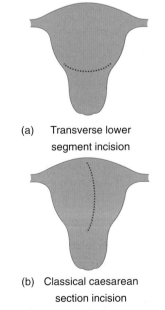

(a) Transverse lower segment incision

(b) Classical caesarean section incision

Figure 15.7 Uterine incisions for Caesarean section. (a) Transverse lower segment incision. (b) classical Caesarean section incision

Once the uterus is incised, the membranes are ruptured if still intact, and the accoucheur's hand is positioned below the presenting part. If cephalic, the head is flexed and delivered by elevation though the uterine incision either manually, or with forceps. Fundal pressure is applied to aid delivery; this should not commence until the presenting part is located within the incision – for fear of converting the lie from longitudinal to transverse. Once the fetus is delivered, an oxytocic (5 IU Syntocinon i.v.) is administered to aid uterine contraction and placental separation. The placenta is delivered by combined cord traction; manual removal significantly increases the intraoperative blood loss and postoperative infectious morbidity.

Closure of the uterus should be performed in either single or double layers with continuous or interrupted sutures. The initial suture should be placed just lateral to the incision angle, and the closure continued to a point just lateral to the angle on the opposite side. A running stitch is often employed and this may be locked to improve haemostasis. If a second layer is used, an inverting suture or horizontal suture should overlap the myometrium. Once repaired, the incision is assessed for haemostasis and 'figure-of-eight' sutures can be employed to control bleeding. Peritoneal closure is unnecessary. Abdominal closure is performed in the anatomical planes with high strength, low reactivity materials, such as polyglycolic acid or polyglactin.

Complications

Caesarean section is a major abdominal surgical procedure and carries significant risks.

Intraoperative complications

Bowel damage

Bowel damage may occur during a repeat procedure or if adhesions are present from previous surgery.

Caesarean hysterectomy

The most common indication for Caesarean hysterectomy is uncontrollable maternal haemorrhage; life-threatening haemorrhage requiring immediate treatment after 1 in 1000 deliveries. The most important risk factor for emergency postpartum hysterectomy is a previous Caesarean section – especially when the placenta overlies the old scar, increasing the risks of placenta accreta (see Chapter 16, Obstetric emergencies).

Other indications for hysterectomy are atony, uterine rupture, extension of a transverse uterine incision and fibroids preventing uterine closure and haemostasis. This operation, while a major undertaking, should not be left too late, as the risk of operative complications, maternal morbidity and mortality increase with increasing haemorrhage.

Haemorrhage

Haemorrhage may be a consequence of damage to the uterine vessels, or may be incidental as a consequence of uterine atony or placenta praevia. In patients with an anticipated high risk of haemorrhage, e.g. known cases of placenta praevia, blood should be routinely crossmatched. There are many manoeuvres to manage haemorrhage; these range from bimanual compression, oxytocin infusion, administration of prostaglandins, conservative surgical procedures, such as uterine compression sutures to the more radical, but life saving, hysterectomy.

Placenta praevia

The proportion of patients with a placenta praevia increases almost linearly after each previous Caesarean section, and as the risks of such a complication increases with increasing parity, future reproductive intentions are very relevant to any individual decision for operative delivery.

Urinary tract damage

The risk of bladder injury is increased after prolonged labours where the bladder is displaced caudally, after previous Caesarean section where scarring obliterates the vesicouterine space, or where a vertical extension to the uterine incision has occurred. If damage is suspected, then transurethral instillation of methylene blue-coloured saline will help to delineate the defect. When such an injury is observed, repair with 2-0 Vicryl as a single continuous or interrupted layer is appropriate. The urinary catheter should remain *in situ* for 7–10 days. Damage to the ureters is uncommon as reflection of the bladder displaces them rostrally.

Post-operative complications

Infection and endometritis

Women undergoing Caesarean section have a 5–20-fold greater risk of an infectious complication when compared with a vaginal delivery. Complications include fever, wound infection, endometritis, bacteraemia and urinary tract infection. Other common causes of postoperative fever include haematoma, atelectasis and deep vein thrombosis. Labour, its duration and the presence of ruptured membranes appear to be the most important risk factors, with obesity playing a particularly important role in the occurrence of wound infections. The most important source of microorganisms responsible for post-Caesarean section infection is the genital tract, particularly if the membranes are ruptured preoperatively. Even in the presence of intact membranes, microbial invasion of the intrauterine cavity is common, especially with preterm labour. Infections are commonly polymicrobial and pathogens isolated from infected wounds and the endometrium include *Escherichia coli*, other aerobic Gram-negative rods, and Group B streptococcus. General principles for the prevention of any surgical infection include careful surgical technique, skin antisepsis; prophylactic antibiotics should be administered to reduce the incidence of postoperative endometritis.

Pulmonary emboli and deep vein thrombosis

Deaths from pulmonary embolism remain the leading direct cause of maternal death, and Caesarean section is a major risk factor. The signs and symptoms of pulmonary emboli and deep vein thrombosis are as detailed in Chapter 8, Antenatal obstetric complications. The incidence of such complications can undoubtedly be reduced by the peri-operative administration of prophylactic heparin and the prompt initiation of treatment when required (see Chapter 8, Antenatal obstetric complications).

Psychological

All difficult deliveries carry increased maternal psychological and physical morbidity. The compromised postpartum psychological functioning in women delivered by Caesarean section may be secondary to delayed contact with the baby; a factor that in most cases should be amenable to remedy.

Key points

- The increasing rate of delivery by Caesarean section continues to be an issue of great concern to many midwives, obstetricians, politicians and society as a whole.

- Maternal satisfaction is an important part of childbirth and must be taken into consideration when implementing any changes in childbirth policy. There is a need for national debate on whether maternal choice is a valid indication for Caesarean section.

- It is appropriate to offer a trial of labour to any woman with a previous uncomplicated lower uterine segment Caesarean section and no other adverse obstetric feature.

- Although Caesarean section continues to be associated with considerable morbidity and mortality, thromboembolism prophylaxis and prophylactic antibiotics have reduced the risks of thrombotic and infective complications.

CASE HISTORY

Mrs B, a 26-year-old primigravid woman, went into spontaneous labour at 40 weeks gestation. There was no relevant past medical history and findings on examination were unremarkable; the symphseal fundal height was deemed to be equivalent to the gestational age. Delay in the first stage of labour led to artificial rupture of the membranes (clear liquor drained) and then to the instigation of an oxytocin infusion. Two successive vaginal examinations, 4 hours apart, identified a cervical dilatation of 9 cm. The cardiotocograph (CTG) tracing was adjudged to show a normal fetal heart rate pattern. An epidural was *in situ* and was effective. The management plan was for a further examination after an interval of 2 hours; if the cervix was not fully dilated, delivery was to be by Caesarean section.

When the examination was repeated, the cervix was fully dilated, with the fetal head at the level of the ischial spines and in the right occipitio-transverse position. There was marked caput and moulding. Clear liquor drained and there was a normal, reactive fetal heart rate pattern.

Were the prerequisites for an operative vaginal delivery met?

The findings on abdominal examination are crucial to any consideration of this question. On examination, >1/5th of the fetal head was palpable. The prerequisites for a forceps/ventouse delivery were thus not met. The appropriate management plan was for transfer to theatre for probable Caesarean section delivery.

Following an epidural 'top up' and transfer to theatre, the abdominal and vaginal examinations were repeated. On abdominal examination, the fetal head was no longer palpable and on vaginal examination the fetal head was below the level of the ischial spines and in the occipito-anterior position.

continued ➤

How should the delivery be effected?

On the assumption that the delivery was to be performed by an appropriately trained and experienced obstetrician, and that informed consent was elicited, the prerequisites for an operative delivery were now met. Such a delivery, following delay in the first stage of labour, and in the presence of marked caput and moulding should optimally be performed in theatre.

Use of either forceps or the ventouse would be reasonable. Although the ventouse is associated with less perineal trauma, the obstetrician opted to use forceps as the presence of caput and moulding indicated that the ventouse was more likely to fail.

What type of forceps should be used?

The fetal head had rotated to the occipito-anterior position prior to the application of forceps. Non-rotational forceps (for example, Neville Barnes or Simpsons forceps), with a pelvic curve, were applied.

The forceps were positioned and 'locked'. Traction was applied with a contraction, and with maternal pushing. There was no descent of the fetal head. Following traction with another contraction, there was no descent of the fetal head.

What is the appropriate management plan?

There has been a failed trial of an operative vaginal delivery, with no descent of the fetal head. Delivery must be by Caesarean section.

A lower segment Caesarean section was performed, through a Pfannenstiel incision. Although there was difficulty delivering a deeply impacted fetal head, there was no significant extension of the uterine incision. The infant birth weight was 4.35 kg. Closure of the uterus and abdomen was unremarkable.

What complications should be anticipated after delivery?

There was a significant risk of postpartum haemorrhage due to uterine atony. In addition to prophylactic antibiotic and anticoagulant therapy (to reduce the likelihood of infective and thrombotic complications), the bolus dose of oxytocin at delivery was followed by an intravenous infusion of oxytocin over 4 hours.

No postoperative complications ensued and Mrs B was discharged home, with her baby, 4 days after the Caesarean section. She was given a hospital follow-up appointment to discuss the events of the labour and delivery.

CHAPTER 16

OBSTETRIC EMERGENCIES

Clare Tower

OVERVIEW

Obstetric emergencies occur not infrequently and can have catastrophic consequences for the mother, baby and their family. In the United Kingdom, CMACE (Centre for Maternal and Child Enquiries) produces regular confidential reports on all maternal deaths and perinatal deaths. Unfortunately, each report includes a substantial number of cases in which there has been substandard care. The maternal mortality report which reviewed all deaths between 2003 and 2005 found evidence of substandard care in 64 per cent of maternal deaths occurring directly as a result of obstetric complications. In order to improve the care of women and their babies, there has been an increasing use of a structured approach to obstetric emergencies. In other words, by using the same principles in each emergency situation, it is hoped that outcomes improve and staff can cope better with a stressful and traumatic situation.

In the UK, the maternal mortality rate is currently 14 per 100 000 maternities, a rate which has stayed constant over recent years. It is expected that this rate may increase in the future due to rising obesity, maternal age and more women, particularly from overseas, with complex medical problems. The most common reasons for maternal death in the UK are thrombosis, pre-eclampsia and eclampsia, amniotic fluid embolus and haemorrhage, as shown in Table 16.1.

Definition

An emergency is defined as a serious situation or occurrence that happens unexpectedly and demands immediate action. Although the definition implies that it is unforeseen, preparation and prevention should always be used to reduce the risks of emergencies occurring. For example, an eclamptic fit is an obstetric emergency that may be prevented by the administration of magnesium sulphate to women with severe pre-eclampsia. In obstetrics, emergencies can be classified as maternal (occurring antenatally and post-natally) and fetal. The causes are summarized in Table 16.2.

Table 16.1 Causes of maternal death 2003–2005

	No.	Rate per 100 000 maternities
Direct deaths		
Thrombosis (cerebral and pulmonary)	41	1.94
Pre-eclampsia/ eclampsia	18	0.85
Haemorrhage	14	0.66
Amniotic fluid embolus	17	0.80
Early pregnancy deaths	14	0.66
Genital tract sepsis	18	0.85
Other direct deaths	4	0.19
Anaesthetic deaths	6	0.28

continued

Table 16.1 Continued

	No.	Rate per 100 000 maternities
Cardiac	48	2.27
Psychiatric	18	0.85
Malignancies	10	0.47
Others	87	4.12
Coincidental	55	2.60

Direct deaths are defined as those resulting from obstetric complications, Indirect deaths as those resulting from pre-existing disease that has been worsened by pregnancy.

Source. Lewis G (ed.). The Confidential Enquiry into Maternal and Child Health (CEMACH). Saving Mothers Lives: reviewing maternal deaths to make motherhood safer, 2003–2006. The Seventh Report on Confidential Enquiries into Maternal Deaths in the United Kingdom. London: CEMACH, 2007.

The structured approach to obstetric emergencies

Developing a structured approach to emergencies that can be practised within a 'drill-type' scenario provides staff with an ordered sequence of actions that can help in a stressful and sometimes chaotic situation. While many of the fetal obstetric emergencies require the use of specific drill, the maternal emergencies can make use of the common ABC approach used for all adult emergencies. When called to any emergency situation, the first action should be to call for help. After this, a systematic evaluation and resuscitation should be conducted in the following order:

1. **A**irway
2. **B**reathing and ventilation
3. **C**irculation with volume replacement and control of bleeding
4. **D**isability
5. **E**nvironment and exposure.

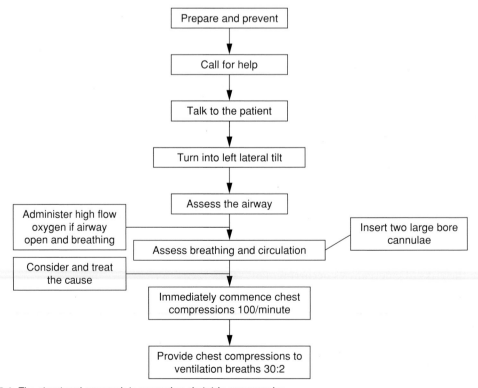

Figure 16.1 The structured approach to managing obstetric emergencies

Conducting a structured assessment

The stuctured assessment should be conducted according to Figure 16.1.

Approach

On approaching the patient, first speak to them to find out whether they are able to respond. In addition to being an important form of communication, this also reveals important information. If the patient responds appropriately, they must have an open airway and be able to move sufficient air to speak. Furthermore, it also gives useful information about neurological status. In contrast, if the patient is unable to respond, it should trigger the immediate call for help and assessment of airway, breathing and circulation. In pregnant patients (20 weeks or more) and in the immediate postpartum period, the enlarged uterus compresses the inferior vena cava, thus reducing venous return to the heart when the patient is lying flat on their back. It is therefore extremely important to tilt the patient to the left to aid resuscitation (left lateral tilt, Figure 16.2). This will lift the heavy uterus away from the abdominal vessels, improving the venous return to the heart and aiding the resuscitation attempt.

Table 16.2 Causes of obstetric emergencies

Maternal		Fetal	
Haemorrhage	Antepartum	Placenta previa	Bradycardia
		Abruption	Abruption
	Postpartum	Uterine atony	Cord prolapse
		Trauma	Shoulder dystocia
		Retained placenta	Vasa previa
		Disseminated Intravascular coagulaopathy (DIC)	
Hypertensive disorders	Pre-eclampsia		
	Eclampsia		
Uterine causes	Inversion		
	Rupture		
Sudden maternal collapse	Amniotic fluid embolus		
	Pulmonary embolus		
	Shock- including sepsis, haemorrhage, anaphylaxis, etc.		
	Cardiac causes, e.g. myocardial infarct		
	Intracranial events – bleeds, thrombosis		
	Biochemical causes – e.g. hypoglycaemia		
	Anaesthetic events		

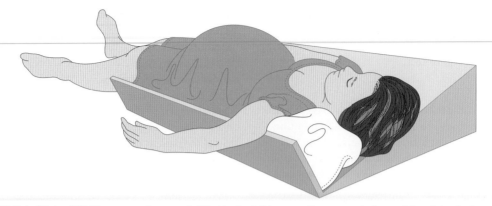

Figure 16.2 Left lateral tilt. The pregnant woman is tilted to the left to move the pregnant uterus of the abdominal vessels, thus improving cardiac output. There are various methods of achieving this; many hospitals have special wedge-shaped cushions ('the Cardiff wedge'), but pillows, blankets or even an individual kneeling can also be used.

Assessing the airway (A)

First, check in the mouth for any obstructing material, such as blood or vomit, and remove using suction. Such obstruction is uncommon in obstetric patients. Next, open the airway by using either the head tilt and chin lift, or a jaw thrust. The head tilt and chin lift is carried out by placing a hand on the forehead and gently tilting back, and two fingers of the other hand under the chin and gently lifting. The alternative manoeuvre, the jaw thrust, involves placing the fingers of each hand behind the two angles of the mandible and pushing upwards.

Assessing breathing (B) and circulation (C)

Having opened the airway, the breathing should be assessed for 10 seconds by looking for chest movement and listening and feeling for signs of air movement. Although experienced clinicians may also feel the carotid pulse at this stage, the current resuscitation guidelines advise that lack of breathing also indicates a lack of circulation. If the airway is open and the patient breathing, high flow oxygen should be administered via a face mask.

If there is no circulation, or there is some uncertainty, cardiopulmonary resuscitation (CPR) should be commenced immediately. This begins immediately with 30 chest compressions followed by two ventilation breaths. Administering chest compressions should be conducted with the patient in the left lateral position. Both hands should be placed on top of one another with straight arms, in the middle of the lower half of the sternum in the midline and the sternum be depressed by 4–5 cm at a rate of 100 per minute. Providing chest compressions is tiring, and in the hospital situation, help is readily available. Therefore, it is recommended that the person doing chest compression should change every 2 minutes.

Ventilation breaths, usually provided via a bag and mask in hospital with high flow oxygen, should last 1 second and the chest should be seen to rise with each breath. This can be continued until the arrival of skilled help, when more definitive airway management in the form of intubation can be performed. After intubation, ventilation should be at a rate of ten breaths per minute and does not need to be synchronized with chest compressions.

If a circulation is present but no breathing (respiratory arrest), then ventilation breaths with high flow oxygen should be given at a rate of ten breaths per minute, with a regular check on the circulation via the carotid pulse every ten breaths. If the patient begins to breathe spontaneously, they should be placed in the recovery position and closely monitored.

Two large bore cannulae (16- or 14-gauge, usually grey or orange) should be inserted into both antecubital fosse to allow blood to be taken for full blood count, cross-matching, and biochemistry, fluid resuscitation and drug administration.

As soon as possible, the defibrillator pads should be applied to assess the cardiac rhythm, treat accordingly and specific treatment initiated. The reversible causes of cardiac arrest can be remembered as the 'four Hs and the four Ts' and are given below (those in italics signify those most likely in pregnancy):

Four Hs	Four Ts
Hypovolaemia due to haemorrhage or sepsis	*Thromboembolism*
Hypoxia	*Toxicity due to drugs, e.g. anaesthetic*
Hyperkalemia and other metabolic disorders	Tension pneumothorax
Hypothermia	Cardiac tamponade

A detailed description of advanced resuscitation is beyond the scope of this book, but can be found in the suggested further reading.

Difficulties in resuscitation due to pregnancy

In addition to compression of the large abdominal blood vessels described above, some other physiological changes of pregnancy can also make resuscitation of the collapsed pregnant woman more difficult. The pregnant uterus presses on the diaphragm, therefore reducing the lung functional residual capacity and making the lungs more difficult to ventilate. Larger breasts compound this problem. Furthermore, pregnancy causes the oesophageal sphincter to become more relaxed, therefore increasing the likelihood of aspiration of the stomach contents into the lungs. It is important that the airway is secured early to prevent this.

The fetus

The presence of a fetus within the uterus makes resuscitation of the mother more difficult due to aortocaval compression, obstruction to ventilation and increased oxygen requirements. In the emergency situation, it is always the welfare of the mother that takes precedence. If resuscitation has not been successful by 4 minutes, an immediate Caesarean section should be conducted, with the aim of having the baby delivered by 5 minutes. The aim of this is primarily to increase the likelihood of successfully resuscitating the mother, and, for the sake of speed, does not require the patient to be in an operating theatre.

Cardiorespiratory arrest in obstetrics is rare. However, many obstetric emergencies occur that have not yet progressed to this dire stage. The principles of management (summarized in Figure 16.1) remain the same, and if successful will prevent the most serious sequelae.

Management of specific obstetric emergencies

Haemorrhage

Obstetric haemorrhage can occur antenatally or post-natally, and both can present as obstetric emergencies.

Antepartum haemorrhage

Antepartum haemorrhage (APH) is any bleeding occurring in the antenatal period after 24 weeks gestation. It complicates 2–5 per cent of pregnancies. Most cases involve relatively small quantities of blood loss, but they often signify that the pregnancy is at increased risk of subsequent complications, including postpartum haemorrhage. At term, APH can be difficult to distinguish from a 'show' which is the release of the cervical mucus in the early stages of labour. The causes of APH are placental abruption (one third), placenta praevia (one third) and other causes (one third). Thus, placental bleeding is responsible for approximately two thirds of APHs. When assessing patients presenting with an APH, a digital examination should not be conducted until an ultrasound scan has identified the location of the placenta (see below under Diagnosis).

Placenta praevia

Aetiology and epidemiology

Placenta praevia is defined as a placenta that has implanted into the lower segment of the uterus. It is now classified as either major, in which the placenta is covering the internal cervical os, or minor, when the placenta is sited within the lower segment of the uterus, but does not cover the cervical os (Figure 16.3). This has replaced the older I–IV classification system. The incidence in the UK is approximately 5 per 1000 and is increasing due to the rising Caesarean section rate and increasing maternal age. It is more

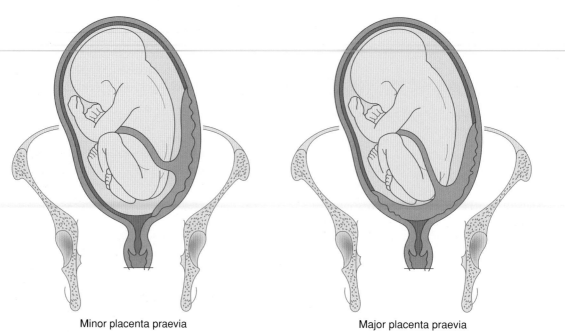

Minor placenta praevia   Major placenta praevia

Figure 16.3 Placenta praevia

common in older (often multiparous) women and in women with previous uterine surgery. In women who have had a previous caesearean section, there is a risk that the placenta implants into, and thus invades, into the previous scar. This is called a 'morbidly adherent placenta' and there are three types:

1. **Placenta accreta**. Placenta is abnormally adherent to the uterine wall.

2. **Placenta increta**. Placenta is abnormally invading into the uterine wall.

3. **Placenta percreta**. Placenta is invading through the uterine wall.

The risk of a morbidly adherent placenta increases with increasing numbers of previous Caesarean sections.

Diagnosis

The mother will present with painless bleeding, often recurrent in the third trimester, and ultrasound scans will demonstrate the abnormal location of the placenta. The bleeding occurs due to separation of the placenta as the lower segment develops in the third trimester. Contractions can also precipitate bleeding by a similar mechanism. On abdominal palpation, the uterus will be soft and non-tender and the presenting part will be free as it cannot enter the pelvis due to obstruction by the placenta. A digital examination is contraindicated as this can precipitate bleeding. Approximately 10 per cent of cases of placenta praevia can also be complicated by placental abruption (see below under Placental abruption).

Management

The patient should be initially resuscitated using the structured approach of ABC. If the bleeding is relatively minor and the fetus uncompromised, the patient should be admitted for observation and not allowed home until at least 24 hours has passed without further bleeding. Women with major placenta praevia who have had recurrent bleeding should be admitted as inpatients from 34 weeks, and those who have not bled need a careful risk assessment before being managed at home. Major bleeding will require fluid resuscitation and delivery of the fetus by Caesarean section by a senior obstetrician. The risk to the fetus is mainly prematurity due to early Caesarean section. There is considerable risk of serious maternal haemorrhage, either as APH or during Caesarean section when the placental bed may not contract, or due to morbid adherence. This may lead to massive postpartum haemorrhage (PPH). The indications for delivery are reaching 37–38 weeks gestation, a massive (>1500 mL) bleed, or continuing significant bleeding of lesser severity. Cases of minor placenta praevia can be considered for a vaginal delivery if the placenta is a minimum of 2 cm away from the cervical os.

Placental abruption

Aetiology and epidemiology

A placental abruption is separation of a normally sited placenta from the uterine wall. In most cases, the separation reaches the edge of the placenta, tracks down to the cervix and is revealed as vaginal bleeding. The remaining cases are concealed, and present as uterine pain and potentially maternal shock or fetal distress without obvious bleeding. The fetus is at risk because of hypoxia following placental separation and premature delivery. The mother is at risk of hypovolaemic shock, clotting disorders and consequent more widespread organ damage. The aetiology and pathophysiological consequences of placental abruption are discussed in further detail in Chapter 10, Pre-eclampsia and other disorders of placentation.

Diagnosis

Placental abruption typically presents as vaginal bleeding associated with pain. The pain can be constant, or as frequent short-lasting contractions caused by the irritable effect of blood within the uterus. The patient may report reduced fetal movements and the cardiotocograph may demonstrate a non-reassuring fetal heart rate pattern. Constant pain associated with a uterus that is very hard on palpation is known as a Couvelaire uterus and is due to a large volume of blood within the myometrium.

Management

The patient should be initially resuscitated using the structured approach of ABC. Management depends on recognition of the problem, realization that true blood loss may be far greater than the blood loss seen, and rapid institution of major haemorrhage management (see below under Postpartum haemorrhage). In very severe cases, the fetus will be dead and vaginal delivery can be accelerated by artificial rupture of the membranes once the mother is reasonably stable. If the fetus is alive, delivery without compromising the mother's resuscitation is urgent and this will usually be by Caesarean section.

Other causes of antepartum haemorrhage

Other causes of APH include cervical bleeding (ectropion, post-coital), genital tract infection, genital tract tumours, a show and vasa praevia. With the exception of vasa previa, these generally cause insignificant amounts of blood loss. Vasa praevia is rupture of fetal vessels running within the membranes, often near to the cervical os and damaged when the membranes rupture. It is a rare condition, but it is catastrophic for the fetus as it is fetal blood that is lost. Risk factors include placenta praevia, a velamentous placental insertion and multiple pregnancy. Although relatively small amounts of bleeding are seen, this can represent a large proportion of the total fetal blood volume. Hence, the fetus can rapidly exsanguinate and there is a high risk of fetal death. The cardiotocograph will rapidly become abnormal with a fetal tachycardia, followed by deep decelerations. Although tests for fetal haemoglobin are possible (rarely used in UK practice), the best solution is a high index of suspicion and rapid Caesarean section.

Postpartum haemorrhage

Postpartum haemorrhage (PPH) is probably one of the most common obstetric emergencies. In the UK Confidential Enquiry 2003–5, haemorrhage was the third most common cause of death. It is defined as:

- **Primary PPH.** Loss of ≥500 mL blood from the genital tract within 24 hours of delivery;
- **Secondary PPH.** Loss of ≥500 mL blood from the genital tract between 24 hours and 12 weeks post delivery.

It is considered to be minor if the blood loss is between 500 and 1000 mL and major if it is greater than 1000 mL. In practice, blood losses between 500 and 1000 mL are relatively common, and can usually be tolerated well by the woman. Thus, it has been suggested that losses over 1000 mL should trigger emergency PPH protocols. However, it should be remembered that estimation of blood loss is notoriously inaccurate, and if a woman demonstrates evidence of cardiovascular compromise, such as tachycardia, or if there is continued bleeding, then protocols should be instituted even if estimated losses are less than 1000 mL. In common with other

Table 16.3 Risk factors for postpartum haemorrhage

Maternal		Fetal
Pre-existing	Raised maternal age	Large baby
	Primiparity	Multiple pregnancy
	Grand multiparity	Polyhydramnios
	Uterine fibroids	Shoulder dystocia
	Previous caesarean	
	Bleeding disorders	
	Obesity	
	Antepartum haemorrhage	
	Previous PPH	
Intrapartum	Prolonged labour	
	Caesarean section	
	Instrumental delivery	
	Pyrexia in labour	
	Episiotomy	

obstetric emergencies, PPH can often be predicted and preventative measures undertaken if significant risk factors are present (Table 16.3).

Aetiology and epidemiology

The causes of PPH can be remembered as the four 'Ts':

Tone	Uterine atony
Tissue	Retained placenta and/or membranes
Trauma	Injury to vagina, perineum and uterine tears at Caesarean section
Thrombin	Clotting disorders

Uterine atony, or failure of the uterus to contract after the delivery of the placenta ('tone'), is the most common cause of PPH and can cause torrential loss of blood immediately following delivery. It can be predicted, and therefore steps taken to prevent it, by the use of oxytocic infusions and active management of the third stage of labour. A retained placenta ('tissue') can also prevent a uterus from contracting efficiently until the tissue is removed. Occasionally, parts of the placenta or membranes can be retained, and this can be identified by careful examination of the placenta following delivery. Almost all types of delivery can cause some degree of genital tract trauma in the form of perineal and vaginal tears, although this is most common following a forceps delivery. Rarely, the cervix can be torn if delivery has occurred before the cervix is fully dilated. More rarely, abnormal blood clotting ('thrombin') can contribute to an excessive blood loss. This can occur in women with an underlying disorder such as Von Willebrand's disease, or platelet disorders. It more commonly arises in women who have developed a consumptive coagulopathy as a result of another obstetric complication, such as a massive placental abruption, an unidentified dead fetus, amniotic fluid embolus or massive haemorrhage.

Diagnosis

Early recognition of blood loss and rapid action is vital in the management of PPH. Appreciation of risk factors, accurate estimation of blood loss and recognition of the maternal signs of cardiovascular compromise are vital. These include a tachycardia, low blood pressure, symptoms of nausea, vomiting and feeling faint, pallor and slow capillary refill (greater than 2 seconds). It is important to recognize that young, fit women have the capacity to tolerate large amounts of blood loss without demonstrating many clinical symptoms. The earliest symptom will be a tachycardia and often blood pressure does not fall until massive haemorrhage has occurred (often 1200–1500 mL of blood).

Management

In practice, diagnosis and management of PPH occur simultaneously. The structured ABC approach outlined above should be instituted. This management is summarized in Table 16.4. Rapid fluid resuscitation should occur at the same time as assessing and treating the cause. Since uterine atony is the most common cause, the uterus should be massaged to

Table 16.4 Management of severe postpartum haemorrhage

Summon help from:	senior obstetrician anaesthetist senior midwife porter
Oxygen by mask initially	
2 × 14-gauge intravenous lines	
Full blood count and clotting studies	
Test for renal function and liver function tests	
Cross-match at least 6 units of blood	
Fluid resuscitation intravenously	
Notify blood bank and consult haematologist	
Foley catheter into the bladder and fluid balance chart	
Transfuse blood as soon as possible – uncross-matched same group as mother or, in extreme cases, O negative	
Central venous pressure and arterial lines	
May need fresh frozen plasma, platelets and cryoprecipitate (consult haematologist)	
Eliminate the cause – deliver the baby and placenta, manage postpartum haemorrhage	

encourage contraction and oxytocics given. In the first instance, this would be a further bolus of the drug used to manage the third stage (oxytocin or Syntometrine) and an infusion of oxytocin (40 IU in 500 mL saline over 4 hours). Bimanual compression and more potent drugs can also be used. These include ergometrine, prostaglandin F2α or misoprostol. The bladder should be catheterized as an empty bladder aids uterine contraction. A vaginal examination should be conducted to expel clots which will prevent contraction of the uterus and assess for genital tract trauma. Any identified tears will need prompt compression to limit blood loss followed by repair. The placenta should be delivered if retained and inspected. If bleeding continues, the patient should be transferred to theatre to allow a further thorough examination under anaesthetic. This will also allow the use of further measures, including uterine tamponade using uterine balloons, radiological occlusion of the uterine vessels, laparotomy for bilateral iliac artery ligation, uterine compression sutures, and, as a last resort, hysterectomy. Massive PPH will require

correction of clotting factors using fresh frozen plasma, platelets and cryoprecipitate.

Secondary PPH is a rare cause of massive bleeding. It is usually the result of retained products of conception and/or uterine infection. Although bleeding can be life threatening, it is usually slight or moderate.

> **Key points**
>
> **Massive haemorrhage**
> - Summon senior multidisciplinary help
> - Resuscitate
> - Replace and maintain fluid volume
> - Investigate status and cause of bleeding
> - Arrest blood loss

Hypertensive disorders

Pre-eclampsia is a disease of pregnancy characterized by a blood pressure of 140/90 mmHg or more on two separate occasions after the 20th week of pregnancy in a previously normotensive woman. This is accompanied by significant proteinuria (300 mg in 24 hours). Eclampsia is the same condition that has proceeded to the presence of convulsions. Imminent eclampsia (the development of seizures), or fulminating pre-eclampsia, is the transitional condition characterized by increasing symptoms and signs. Pre-eclampsia is discussed in detail in Chapter 10, Pre-eclampsia and other disorders of placentation. The management of severe or fulminating pre-eclampsia and eclampsia is included in this chapter.

Aetiology and epidemiology

Eclampsia is relatively rare in the UK, occurring in approximately 1:2000 pregnancies. It may occur antepartum (40 per cent), intrapartum (20 per cent) or postpartum (40 per cent). Severe pre-eclampsia is more common than eclampsia, occurring in 5:1000 pregnancies. Other risk factors are discussed in Chapter 13, Perinatal infections.

Diagnosis

Severe pre-eclampsia is identified by a blood pressure of 160/110 mmHg or more and the presence of proteinuria on 'dipstick' testing. A 24-hour urine collection for quantification of proteinuria may be started, but in practice there may not be time to wait for its completion before effecting delivery. The symptoms and signs of severe pre-eclampsia are:

Symptoms

- Frontal headache
- Visual disturbance (blurred vision and flashing lights)
- Epigastric pain
- General malaise and nausea
- Restlessness

Signs

- Agitation
- Hyper-reflexia and clonus
- Facial (especially periorbital) oedema
- Right upper quadrant tenderness
- Poor urine output
- Papilloedema

In addition, the fetus may appear small, with oligohydramnios and reduced fetal movements. The cardiotocograph may demonstrate signs of hypoxia with a fetal tachycardia, reduced variability and decelerations. Eclampsia is obvious as a grand mal convulsion. However, other causes of fits such as epilepsy have to be considered. Preceding pre-eclampsia suggests eclampsia, but in approximately one-third of cases the eclamptic fit precedes other signs. After the convulsion, the blood pressure is frequently normal for a while, but proteinuria will usually still be present. Any convulsion in pregnancy should be considered to be eclamptic until proved otherwise.

Management

In the same way as other emergencies, the structured ABC approach outlined above should be used. Call for help from senior obstetric and anaesthetic colleagues. Depending upon the results of clotting studies and the severity of the disease, a consultant haematologist may need to be informed.

In a woman with severe pre-eclampsia, the airway and breathing are likely to be secure. However, if a seizure has occurred, these will need assessment and treatment. Seizures occurring due to eclampsia are usually short-lasting and self-limiting. However, the patient should be moved to the side (recovery position) and oxygen applied. Large bore intravenous cannulae should be sited and blood taken for full blood count, clotting studies, renal and liver function tests and cross-matching. The mother's condition needs to be stabilized urgently, before considering delivery in antenatal cases. Stabilizing the mother's condition will involve blood pressure control, prevention and treatment of fits and management of fluid balance.

Intravenous magnesium sulphate is used to treat and prevent fits. The MAGPIE trial showed that administration of magnesium sulphate halved the risk of seizures. An initial loading dose of 4 g is given, followed by an infusion of 1 g/hour. Magnesium sulphate can also lower blood pressure and cause some maternal side effects, such as flushing. It is important to recognize that overdose of magnesium sulphate can cause respiratory and cardiac depression. This can be reversed using calcium gluconate.

The blood pressure should be reduced to safe levels. In common with previous reports, the UK Confidential Enquiry 2003–5 found that deaths in association with pre-eclampsia and eclampsia occur as result of intracranial haemorrhage, largely due to poor blood pressure control. In particular, systolic hypertension greater than 160 mmHg must be treated. Antihypertensives can be either labetalol (can be given orally while intravenous access is obtained), oral nifedipine or intravenous hydrallazine. If given intravenously, a bolus is initially used followed by an infusion that can be titrated to obtain a safe blood pressure. Maternal observations should be conducted frequently until the mother has stabilized (every 5–15 minutes depending on condition) and continuous fetal monitoring used. A gradual reduction of the blood pressure is optimal to avoid precipitating fetal distress (in the form of a bradycardia) secondary to sudden drops in maternal blood pressure that reduce uterine blood flow.

Management of fluid balance can be problematic. In pre-eclampsia, there is intense peripheral vasoconstriction accompanied by a decrease in the plasma volume, together with redistribution of the extracellular fluid. The urine output falls, and over-enthusiastic efforts to provide a fluid challenge may cause pulmonary and cerebral oedema. A strict input/output balance (this needs catheterization) must be maintained, using either blood products or crystalloids, as appropriate. In the absence of bleeding, no more than 80 mL/hour of fluids (oral and intravenous) should be given. Renal failure is uncommon and if it occurs is usually reversible.

Timing of delivery depends upon the gestation, the presence of other complicating factors, the severity of the disease and the stability of the patient's condition. In general, if the patient has disease severe enough to warrant antihypertensive and anticonvulsant therapy, delivery should follow stabilization of the maternal condition.

When it is clear that early delivery is likely, if the gestation is less than 34 weeks, steroids should be given to improve lung maturity and decrease neonatal complications. Steroid administration must not delay delivery that is necessary for the control of severe maternal problems, although recent evidence indicates that steroids also benefit the mother with pre-eclampsia.

Delivery is often by Caesarean section, although if labour is well established, vaginal delivery is possible. If at all possible, clotting disorders must be corrected before delivery (by whatever means) is attempted. Postpartum, both fulminating pre-eclampsia and eclampsia may occur. Management is as for the antenatal case except that delivery has already taken place.

HELLP syndrome

HELLP syndrome – a combination of haemolysis, elevated liver enzymes and low platelets – is seen in 5–10 per cent of cases of severe pre-eclampsia. It is more common in multiparous women. It may be associated with disseminated intravascular coagulation, placental abruption and fetal death.

Key points

Hypertensive disorders

- Fulminating pre-eclampsia and eclampsia are dangerous.
- Recognize women at risk.
- Manage minor hypertensive problems to prevent progression.
- In the serious case:
  - call for help
  - prevent or control convulsions with magnesium sulphate
  - control the blood pressure
  - tightly control fluid balance
  - minimize or avoid organ damage
  - control coagulopathy
  - deliver a healthy baby safely.

Uterine causes of obstetric emergency

Uterine rupture

Aetiology and epidemiology

Uterine rupture, or a tear in the uterus, usually happens due to a previous uterine injury. It is rare, occurring with an incidence of 0.03–0.3 per cent. It occurs mainly in association with a previous Caesarean section. This is because scar tissue does not have the same inherent strength as myometrium. However, scarring can also exist as a result of previous uterine surgery, such as a surgical evacuation of retained products of conception resulting in a perforation. The vast majority of cases occur during labour, usually during late first stage or the active second stage. The risk factors for uterine rupture are given in Table 16.5.

Diagnosis

The patient may complain of abdominal pain ('scar tenderness', often not masked epidural analgesia) and vaginal bleeding. Haematuria may be present if the uterus has ruptured into the bladder. Typically, contractions stop and decelerations are present on the cardiotocograph. If the rupture occurs in the late second stage of labour, it may not be recognized immediately. In this scenario, the fetus has usually delivered by ventouse or forceps for an abnormal cardiotocograph (CTG). In the immediate post-natal period, the mother bleeds internally and shows signs of circulatory collapse while complaining of abdominal discomfort.

Management

Immediate resuscitation of ABC is required as previously outlined. Immediate laparotomy to deliver

Table 16.5 Risk factors for uterine rupture

Previous Caesarean section
Previous uterine surgery
Induction and augmentation of labour
High parity
Macrosomic fetus
Placenta percreta
Fetal version, e.g. breech extraction
Congenital uterine anomaly, e.g. unicornuate uterus

the baby and repair the uterine is required. Frequently, the only safe treatment is hysterectomy.

Uterine inversion

Aetiology and epidemiology

Uterine inversion is a rare complication occurring during the third stage of labour. It has a reported incidence of between 1:2000 and 1:6000. The uterine fundus descends either the uterine cavity, through the cervix, and very rarely beyond the introitus (Figure 16.4). It is caused by traction on the umbilical cord before the placenta has separated and can occur after vaginal deliveries or Caesarean section. Associated factors are a fundal placenta, a short cord and a morbidly adherent placenta.

Diagnosis

The prolapsed uterus stretching the cervix causes vagal stimulation, thus the woman will demonstrate signs of cardiovascular collapse and shock. Although haemorrhage is commonly present, the symptoms will be out of proportion to the estimated blood loss. The inverted uterus may be obvious at the introitus, but other signs include the lack of a palpable uterus in the abdomen or the feeling of a 'dimple' in the uterine fundus on abdominal examination.

Management

Resuscitate the patient using the structured ABC approach. It is very important not to remove the placenta if it is still attached as this will increase the bleeding. Immediately replace the uterus through the cervix by manual compression. If that fails, hydrostatic pressure can be applied by pouring warmed saline into the vagina, usually via a silc cup ventouse. Tocolysis may be helpful to relax the cervical ring. Surgery, to reposition the uterus from above, should be used as a last resort. After replacement, uterine contraction is maintained with an oxytocic.

Sudden maternal collapse

Sudden collapse, as in non-pregnant adults, occurs due to a multitude of reasons. Some will be benign, such as a vasovagal attack (simple faint) or an epileptic fit in a known epileptic, but other causes are life threatening and are outlined in Table 16.2.

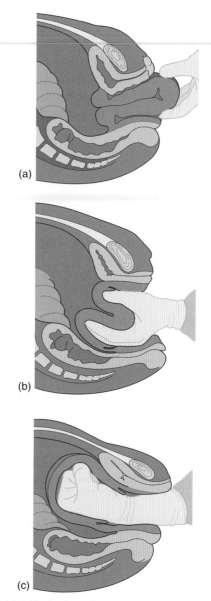

(a)

(b)

(c)

Figure 16.4 Uterine inversion

The management approach should be the same, structured ABC approach. The causes of particular relevance to pregnant women are discussed in more detail below.

Pulmonary embolism

Aetiology and epidemiology

Thrombosis is consistently the most common cause of maternal death in the UK, and the UK Confidential

Enquiry 2003–5 reported 33 deaths caused by pulmonary embolism (PE). The most recent data (Table 16.1) suggest an incidence of between 10.6 and 16.1 per 100 000 maternities in the UK. It is important to recognize that although PE is more common in the puerperium, it can occur at any time in the antenatal and post-natal period. The diagnosis and management of thromboembolic events is discussed in detail in Chapter 8, Antenatal obstetric complications, thus this chapter will focus on the emergency situation.

Diagnosis and management

PE can be a cause of sudden cardiorespiratory collapse. In this situation, diagnosis and management should occur simultaneously. Urgent resuscitation using the structured ABC approach is needed. If PE is suspected, anticoagulation should be instituted.

Amniotic fluid embolism

Aetiology and epidemiology

Amniotic fluid embolism is a rare cause of maternal collapse specific to pregnancy, believed to be caused by amniotic fluid entering the maternal circulation. This causes acute cardiorespiratory compromise and severe disseminated intravascular coagulation. In some cases, there may be an abnormal maternal reaction to amniotic fluid as the primary event. It is difficult to diagnose in life, and is typically diagnosed at post-mortem, with the presence of fetal cells (squames or hair) in the maternal pulmonary capillaries. It caused 18 deaths in the 2003–5 maternal mortality report.

Diagnosis and management

In the case of sudden collapse, management should be the structured ABC approach. Symptoms occurring just before the collapse may be helpful in diagnosis. The 2003–5 maternal mortality report suggested that women may report the following symptoms:

- breathlessness
- chest pain
- feeling cold
- lightheadedness
- restlessness, distress and panic
- pins and needles in the fingers
- nausea and vomiting.

The prognosis is poor, with around 30 per cent of patients dying in the first hour and only 10 per cent surviving overall. Management is supportive, requiring intensive care and there are no specific therapies available.

Fetal emergencies

The fetus may be severely affected by any of the preceding maternal emergencies that occur before delivery. However, there are some emergencies that directly affect the fetus without major immediate physical compromise of the mother. Major abnormalities of the fetal heart rate, in particular prolonged fetal bradycardia, call for immediate delivery, usually by Caesarean section. This is discussed further in Chapter 14, Labour. This chapter will discuss two specific causes of fetal emergency: cord prolapse and shoulder dystocia.

Umbilical cord accidents (cord prolapse)

Aetiology and epidemiology

A cord presentation is defined as the presence of umbilical cord below the fetal presenting part when the membranes are intact. Cord prolapse is the presence of the cord below the presenting part when the membranes are ruptured (Figure 16.5). It has an incidence of 1:500 deliveries and occurs when the fetal presenting part does not fit well into the maternal pelvis, giving 'space' for the cord to prolapse when the membranes rupture. It is associated with risk factors outlined in Table 16.6.

Diagnosis

Most commonly, it is diagnosed by seeing the cord at the introitus, or feeling it during a vaginal examination. However, an abnormal fetal heart rate pattern may suggest it, as compression of the umbilical vein between the presenting part and the pelvis, reduces or stops the flow of oxygenated blood to the fetus, causing deep variable decelerations, then bradycardia if the situation is not relieved.

Management

Immediate management aims to minimize the pressure of the fetal presenting part on the cord,

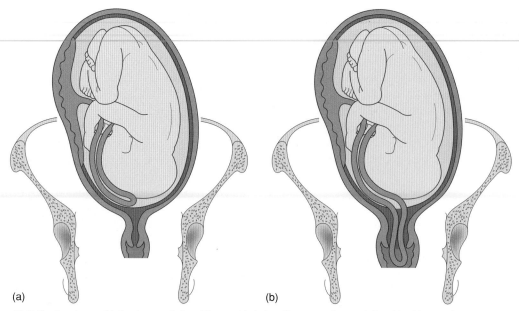

(a)   (b)

Figure 16.5 Cord prolapse. (a) Cord presentation. The cord is below the presenting part (head in this case but commonly a malpresentation) with the membranes intact. (b) Cord prolapse. The membranes have ruptured and the cord is below the presenting part. In this case, it has prolapsed into the vagina

Table 16.6 Risk factors for cord prolapse

Maternal causes	Fetal causes
Pelvic tumours (e.g. fibroids in the lower segment)	Prematurity
Narrow pelvis	Malpresentation, e.g. breech, transverse lie Multiple pregnancy Polyhydramnios Placenta praevia Large baby

while plans are made to deliver the baby. This is achieved by moving the woman on to all fours with the head down, applying pressure vaginally to push the presenting part out of the pelvis, or by filling the bladder with 500 mL of saline. There should be minimal handling of the cord, as this causes spasm which will worsen blood flow. However, if the cord is beyond the introitus it should be replaced into the vagina to keep it warmer. Emergency Caesarean section is required unless the cervix is fully dilated and an assisted vaginal delivery can be safely and easily performed. Fetal outcome depends upon the gestation, other complicating factors such as intrauterine growth restriction, and for how long the cord has been compressed. With a term baby and a prompt diagnosis in hospital, the prognosis is usually excellent. If the cord prolapse occurs outside hospital, the fetus is likely to be dead by the time of admission. Total cord compression for longer than 10 minutes will cause cerebral damage and, if continued for around 20 minutes, death. These times will be shorter in a fetus that is already compromised for reasons such as prematurity or fetal growth restriction.

Shoulder dystocia

Aetiology and epidemiology

Shoulder dystocia is defined by the Royal College of Obstetricians and Gynaecologists (RCOG) as the need for 'additional obstetric manoevres to release the shoulders after gentle downward traction has failed'.

Table 16.7 Risk factors for shoulder dystocia

Maternal	Fetal	Intrapartum
Diabetes	Macrosomia	Long first stage of labour
Short stature	Postmaturity	Long second stage of labour
Previous shoulder dystocia		Instrumental delivery
Obesity		Induction of labour
		Use of oxytocin

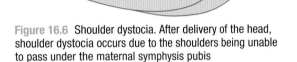

Figure 16.6 Shoulder dystocia. After delivery of the head, shoulder dystocia occurs due to the shoulders being unable to pass under the maternal symphysis pubis

The incidence is approximately 0.6 per cent in the UK and it results in excessive morbidity for both mother and fetus. There is a risk of fetal hypoxia, death and fetal trauma, in the form of fractures (usually long bones of the arm or clavicle), or brachial plexus injury. For the mother, there is an increased risk of bleeding and perineal trauma, including third and fourth degree tears. It is very difficult to predict shoulder dystocia, although the well-recognized risk factors are given in Table 16.7. Unfortunately, none of these risk factors are clinically useful predictors. Approximately half of shoulder dystocias occur in infants of 'normal' weight (i.e. less than 4 kg).

During vaginal delivery, the fetal head and shoulders rotate to make use of the widest pelvic diameters. After delivery of the head, restitution occurs and the shoulders rotate into the anteroposterior (AP) diameter. This makes use of the widest AP diameter of the pelvic outlet. However, if the shoulders have not entered the pelvic inlet, the anterior shoulder may become caught above the symphysis pubis. Occasionally, both shoulders (or rarely, the posterior shoulder) may remain above the pelvic brim (see Figure 16.6).

Diagnosis

Diagnosis is usually obvious when the shoulders fail to deliver during the next contraction after delivery of the head. It is sometimes preceded by the 'turtle sign', which is the head appearing to be pulled back on to the perineum at delivery.

Management

Shoulder dystocia is very alarming and its management should be practised in 'drill-type' training. The high-risk of litigation necessitates that meticulous notes are kept, and no more than gentle traction is ever applied to the fetal head. Thus, on recognition, the emergency buzzer should be activated and help summoned. This should include senior obstetricians, midwifery staff, a paediatrician and an individual to document the times at which the specific manoeuvres are used. The vessels in the fetal neck are occluded after delivery of the head, and cerebral damage will occur if delivery is delayed significantly. The fetus may already be compromised because of the prolongation of labour. After 5 minutes, there is the risk of cerebral damage. However, inappropriate traction, particularly downward traction on the head causing lateral flexion of the head on the neck, will cause stretching of the brachial plexus and nerve damage. Erb's palsy is a likely consequence.

Shoulder dystocia is managed by a sequence of manoeuvres designed to facilitate delivery while minimizing the risk of fetal damage. The basic principle of all the manoeuvres is to reduce the anterior–posterior diameter of the shoulders and gain the maximum space in the maternal pelvis:

- Call for help.

- Ensure personnel are available to 'scribe'. Document the time the head delivered, which shoulder is anterior (this is the arm most vulnerable to injury) and the times at which each manoeuvre is employed.

- Drop the level of the delivery bed as low as it will go, and flatten the back of the bed so the woman is completely flat. Remove the foot of the bed to allow access.

- Assess for and perform an episiotomy, if needed.

- Using one assistant on each of the mother's legs, flex and abduct the legs at the hip (thighs to abdomen, known as MacRoberts manoeuvre). This flattens the lumbosacral spine and will facilitate delivery is around 90 per cent of cases.

- If this fails, suprapubic pressure should be applied by another assistant. This should be applied over the posterior aspect of the anterior fetal shoulder and will act to push the shoulders together. It can be used in a constant and then rocking motion.

- If both these fail, then internal manoeuvres are necessary. The order of these will depend on the skill and experience of the person conducting the delivery and the individual case. These manoeuvres have been named after famous obstetricians, but it is the process rather than the name that is important:

  - An attempt can be made to rotate the baby, so that the shoulders enter the diagonal to allow delivery. The first procedure is usually to insert a hand behind the anterior shoulder, and push it towards the chest (Rubin II). This will adduct the shoulders then push them into the diagonal. This can be combined with pressure on the anterior aspect of the posterior shoulder to aid rotation (Woods' screw). If this fails, an attempt can be made to rotate the baby in the opposite direction (reverse Woods'

screw). Delivery of the posterior arm can be attempted passing a hand into the vagina, in front of the posterior shoulder and deliver the posterior arm by swinging it in front of the fetal chest.

If these all fail, the patient can be moved on to all fours as this increases the anterior–posterior diameter of the inlet. In this position, the posterior arm can be delivered.

After this, manoeuvres of last resort include a symphysiotomy, in which the maternal symphysis is divided, Zavanelli's, in which the head is reduced back into the vagina and a Caesarean section performed and intentional fracture of the fetal clavicle.

After delivery of the baby, the risks of maternal morbidity should be remembered: prevent the PPH and check for vaginal trauma.

Women will require debriefing after the delivery, and most obstetricians would suggest a Caesarean section in the next pregnancy.

Summary

Obstetric emergencies occur not uncommonly. The approach to them should be structured and regularly practised in training drills. In many cases, risk factors exist to enable prediction of emergencies and preventative steps to be taken. Documentation is crucial and lessons can be learnt from many emergency situations. For these reasons, most hospitals utilize an incident reporting system to allow reviews of these cases. Debriefing of the patient and their family after the event is vital.

Key points

- Use a structured approach to all emergencies.
- Call for help.
- Use the A (airway), B (breathing), C (circulation) approach to all maternal emergencies.
- Use drill-type training sessions.
- Documentation is vital.
- Debrief the patient and the family afterwards.

Additional reading

Grady K, Howell C, Cox C (eds). *Managing obstetric emergencies and trauma.* The MOET Course Manual, 2nd edn. London: RCOG Press, 2007.

Lewis G (ed.). The Confidential Enquiry into Maternal and Child Health (CEMACH). Saving Mothers Lives: reviewing maternal deaths to make motherhood safer, 2003–2006. The Seventh Report on Confidential Enquiries into Maternal Deaths in the United Kingdom. London: CEMACH, 2007.

Magpie Trial Collaborative Group. Do women with pre-eclampsia, and their babies, benefit from magnesium sulphate? The Magpie Trial: A randomised placebo-controlled trial. *Lancet* 2002; **359**: 1877–90.

Royal College of Obstetricians and Gynaecologists. Placenta praevia and placenta praevia accreta: Diagnosis and management. Green-top Guidelines No. 27. London: RCOG, 2005.

Royal College of Obstetricians and Gynaecologists. Shoulder dystocia. Green-top Guidelines No. 42. London: RCOG, 2005.

Royal College of Obstetricians and Gynaecologists. Postpartum haemorrhage. Prevention and management. Green-top Guidelines No. 52. London: RCOG, 2009.

CHAPTER 17

THE PUERPERIUM

Louise C Kenny

OVERVIEW

The puerperium refers to the 6-week period following completion of the third stage of labour, when considerable adjustments occur before return to the pre-pregnant state. During this period of physiological change, the mother is also vulnerable to psychological disturbances, which may be aggravated by adverse social circumstances. Adequate understanding and support from her partner and family are crucial. Difficulty in coping with the newborn infant occurs more frequently with the first baby, and vigilant surveillance is therefore necessary by the community midwife, general practitioner and health visitor. The degree of care provided by the health service varies from country to country. In the United Kingdom, a mother who has delivered in hospital may be discharged within 6 hours of an uncomplicated birth, although she may request to stay longer. Irrespective of duration or the place of birth, or the length of hospital stay, however, a midwife must visit her at least once daily for a minimum of 10 days after delivery. Thereafter, the health visitor takes on responsibility for continuing care, particularly of the infant, but the midwife may continue making home visits, if necessary, for up to 4 weeks after delivery. In the Netherlands, a doctor or midwife provides care for the first 5 days, but maternity aides are available to help mothers care for their older children and cope with household duties. In North America, there is more dependence on private health care, and very little organized care after discharge from hospital. There is therefore a lack of consensus as to what constitutes ideal postpartum care, and protocols differ from one centre to the next.

Physiological changes

Uterine involution

Involution is the process by which the postpartum uterus, weighing about 1 kg, returns to its pre-pregnancy state of less than 100 g. Immediately after delivery, the uterine fundus lies about 4 cm below the umbilicus or, more accurately, 12 cm above the symphysis pubis. However, within 2 weeks, the uterus can no longer be palpable above the symphysis. Involution occurs by a process of autolysis, whereby muscle cells diminish in size as a result of enzymatic digestion of cytoplasm. This has virtually no effect on the number of muscle cells, and the excess protein produced from autolysis is absorbed into the bloodstream and excreted in the urine. Involution appears to be accelerated by the release of oxytocin in women who are breastfeeding, as the uterus is smaller than in those who are bottle-feeding. The height of the uterine fundus is measured daily to ascertain the trend in involution.

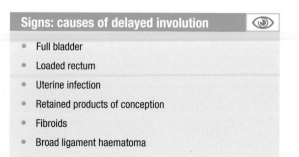

Signs: causes of delayed involution

- Full bladder
- Loaded rectum
- Uterine infection
- Retained products of conception
- Fibroids
- Broad ligament haematoma

A delay in involution in the absence of any other signs or symptoms, e.g. bleeding, is of no clinical significance.

Genital tract changes

Following delivery of the placenta, the lower segment of the uterus and the cervix appear flabby and there may be small cervical lacerations. In the first few days, the cervix can readily admit two fingers, but by the end of the first week it should become increasingly difficult to pass more than one finger, and certainly by the end of the second week the internal os should be closed. However, the external os can remain open permanently, giving a characteristic appearance to the parous cervix.

Lochia

Lochia is the blood-stained uterine discharge that is comprised of blood and necrotic decidua. Only the superficial layer of decidua becomes necrotic and is sloughed off. The basal layer adjacent to the myometrium is involved in the regeneration of new endometrium and this regeneration is complete by the third week. During the first few days after delivery, the lochia is red; this gradually changes to pink as the endometrium is formed, and then ultimately becomes serous by the second week. Persistent red lochia suggests delayed involution that is usually associated with infection or a retained piece of placental tissue. Offensive lochia, which may be accompanied by pyrexia and a tender uterus, suggests infection and should be treated with a broad-spectrum antibiotic. Retained placental tissue is associated with increased red blood cell loss and clots, and this may be suspected if the placenta and membranes were incomplete at delivery (see Chapter 14, Labour and Chapter 16, Obstetric emergencies). Management includes the use of antibiotics and evacuation of retained products under regional or general anaesthesia.

Puerperal disorders

Daily maternal observations include temperature, pulse, blood pressure, urinary function, bowel function, breast examination and feeding, assessment of uterine involution, appearance of lochia, perineal inspection, examination of legs and pelvic floor exercises. These observations should be made more frequently in high-risk women or if an abnormality has been detected, for example the presence of maternal pyrexia. In the UK, it is traditional to check haemoglobin levels on day 3 unless otherwise indicated, and most women who are particularly symptomatic should be transfused if their haemoglobin level at this time is <8 g/dL.

Perineal complications

Perineal discomfort is the single major problem for mothers, and about 80 per cent complain of pain in the first 3 days after delivery, with a quarter continuing to suffer discomfort at day 10. Discomfort is greatest in women who sustain spontaneous tears or have an episiotomy, but especially following instrumental delivery. A number of non-pharmacological and pharmacological therapies have been used empirically with varying degrees of success. However, local cooling (with crushed ice, witch hazel or tap water) and topical anaesthetics, such as 5 per cent lignocaine gel, provide short-term symptomatic relief. Effective analgesia following perineal trauma can be achieved with regular paracetamol. If necessary, diclofenac given rectally or orally may also be added. Codeine derivatives are not preferable, as they have a tendency to cause constipation.

Infections of the perineum are generally uncommon considering the risk of bacterial contamination during delivery; therefore, when signs of infection (redness, pain, swelling and heat) occur, especially when associated with a raised temperature, these must be taken seriously. Swabs for microbiological culture must be taken from the infected perineum, and broad-spectrum antibiotics (see below) should be commenced. If there is a collection of pus, drainage should be encouraged by removal of any skin sutures; otherwise infection would spread, with increasing morbidity and a poor anatomical result.

Spontaneous opening of repaired perineal tears and episiotomies is usually the result of secondary infection. Surgical repair should never be attempted in the presence of infection. The wound should be irrigated twice daily and healing should be allowed to occur by secondary intention. If there is a large, gaping wound, secondary repair should only be performed when the infection has cleared, there is no cellulitis or exudate present and healthy granulation tissue can be seen.

Bladder function

Voiding difficulty and over-distension of the bladder are not uncommon after childbirth, especially if regional anaesthesia (epidural/spinal) has been used. It is now known that after epidural anaesthesia the bladder may take up to 8 hours to regain normal sensation. During this time, about 1 L of urine may be produced and therefore if urinary retention occurs, considerable damage may be inflicted on the detrusor muscle. Over-stretching of the detrusor muscle can dampen bladder sensation and make the bladder hypocontractile, particularly with fibrous replacement of smooth muscle. In this situation, overflow incontinence of small amounts of urine may erroneously be assumed to be normal voiding. Fluid overloading prior to epidural analgesia, the antidiuretic effect of high concentrations of oxytocin during labour, increased postpartum diuresis (particularly in the presence of oedema) and increased fluid intake by breastfeeding mothers all contribute to the increased urine production in the puerperium. Therefore, an intake/output chart alone may not detect incomplete emptying of the bladder.

Women who have undergone a traumatic delivery, such as a difficult instrumental delivery, or who have suffered multiple/extended lacerations or a vulvovaginal haematoma, may find it difficult to void because of pain or periurethral oedema. Other causes of pain, such as prolapsed haemorrhoids, anal fissures, abdominal wound haematoma or even stool impaction of the rectum, may interfere with voiding. The midwife needs to be particularly vigilant after an epidural or spinal anaesthetic to avoid bladder distension. The distended bladder should either be palpable as a suprapubic cystic mass or it may displace the uterus laterally or upwards, thereby increasing the height of the uterine fundus.

In order to minimize the risk of over-distension of the bladder in women undergoing a Caesarean section under regional anaesthesia, a urinary catheter may be left in the bladder for the first 12–24 hours. The benefit of leaving a catheter *in situ* for about 12 hours after epidural insertion should be evaluated against a vigorously enforced postpartum voiding protocol and the small risk of urinary tract infection. However, any woman who has not passed urine within 4 hours of delivery should be encouraged to do so before resorting to catheterization. In general, a clean-catch specimen of urine should be sent for microscopy, culture and sensitivity, and if the residual urine in the bladder is <300 mL, a catheter should be left in to allow free drainage for 48 hours.

Although vaginal delivery is strongly implicated in the development of urinary stress incontinence, it rarely poses a problem in the early puerperium. Therefore, any incontinence should be investigated to exclude a vesicovaginal, urethrovaginal or, rarely, ureterovaginal fistula. Obstetric fistulae are rare in the UK, but are a source of considerable morbidity in developing countries. Pressure necrosis of the bladder or urethra may occur following prolonged obstructed labour, and incontinence usually occurs in the second week when the slough separates. Small fistulae may close spontaneously after a few weeks of free bladder drainage; large fistulae will require surgical repair by a specialist.

Bowel function

Constipation is a common problem in the puerperium. This may be due to an interruption in the normal diet and possible dehydration during labour. Advice on adequate fluid intake and increase in fibre intake may be all that is necessary. However, constipation may also be the result of fear of evacuation due to pain from a sutured perineum, prolapsed haemorrhoids or anal fissures. Avoidance of constipation and straining is of utmost importance in women who have sustained a third-degree or fourth-degree tear. A large, hard bolus of stool in this situation would disrupt the repaired anal sphincter and cause anal incontinence. It is important to ensure that these women are prescribed lactulose and ispaghula husk (Fybogel, Regulan) or methylcellulose immediately after the repair, for a period of 2 weeks.

The high prevalence of anal incontinence and faecal urgency following childbirth has only recently been recognized. One prospective study using anal endosonography has identified evidence of occult anal sphincter trauma in one-third of primiparous women, although only 13 per cent admitted to defaecatory symptoms by 6 weeks postpartum. Larger, retrospective, short-term studies of parous women indicate a prevalence of between 6 and 10 per cent. Long-term anal incontinence following primary repair of a third-degree or fourth-degree tear occurs in 5 per cent of women, and anovaginal/rectovaginal fistulae occur in 2–4 per cent of these women (Figure 17.1). It is therefore important to consider a fistula as a cause of anal incontinence in the postpartum period,

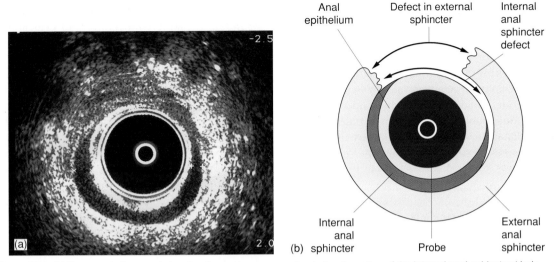

Figure 17.1 (a) Transanal ultrasound showing the anal mucosa and anterior disruption of the internal anal sphincter (dark band) following a third-degree tear at delivery. (b) Diagrammatic representation of part (a)

particularly if the woman complains of passing wind or stool per vagina. Approximately 50 per cent of small anovaginal fistulae will close spontaneously over a period of 6 months, but larger fistulae will require formal repair.

Secondary postpartum haemorrhage

Secondary postpartum haemorrhage (PPH) is defined as fresh bleeding from the genital tract between 24 hours and 6 weeks after delivery (see Chapter 16, Obstetric emergencies, for primary PPH). The most common time for secondary PPH is between days 7 and 14, and the cause is most commonly attributed to retained placental tissue. Associated features include crampy abdominal pain, a uterus larger than appropriate, passage of bits of placental tissue or tissue within the cervix and symptoms and signs of infection. The management of heavy bleeding includes an intravenous infusion, cross-match of blood, Syntocinon, an examination under anaesthesia and evacuation of the uterus. Antibiotics should be given if placental tissue is found, even without evidence of overt infection. If blood loss is not excessive, the use of pelvic ultrasound to exclude retained products is contentious; distinction between retained products and blood clot can be extremely difficult. Other causes of secondary PPH include endometritis, hormonal contraception, bleeding disorders, e.g. von Willebrand's disease, and rarely choriocarcinoma.

Obstetric palsy

Obstetric palsy, or traumatic neuritis, is a condition in which one or both lower limbs may develop signs of a motor and/or sensory neuropathy following delivery. Presenting features include sciatic pain, foot-drop, parasthesia, hypoaesthesia and muscle wasting. The mechanism of injury is unknown and it was previously attributed to compression or stretching of the lumbosacral trunk as it crosses the sacroiliac joint during descent of the fetal head. It is now believed that herniation of lumbosacral discs (usually L4 or L5) can occur, particularly in the exaggerated lithotomy position and during instrumental delivery. An orthopaedic opinion should be sought and management includes bed rest with a firm board beneath the mattress, analgesia and physiotherapy. Peroneal nerve palsy can occur when the nerve is compressed between the head of the fibula and the lithotomy pole, resulting in unilateral foot-drop. The development of urinary and faecal incontinence is most likely due to structural damage to the anal sphincter muscle and supporting fascia.

Symphysis pubis diastasis

Separation of the symphysis pubis can occur spontaneously in at least 1 in 800 vaginal deliveries. Deliberate surgical separation of the pubis in labour (symphysiotomy) is rarely performed in extreme cases of shoulder dystocia. Spontaneous separation is usually noticed after delivery and has been associated with forceps delivery, rapid second stage of labour or severe abduction of the thighs during delivery. Common signs and symptoms include symphyseal pain aggravated by weight-bearing and walking, a waddling gait, pubic tenderness and a palpable interpubic gap. Treatment includes bed rest, anti-inflammatory agents, physiotherapy and a pelvic corset to provide support and stability.

Thromboembolism

The risk of thromboembolic disease rises five-fold during pregnancy and the puerperium. The majority of deaths occur in the puerperium and are more common after Caesarean section. If deep vein thrombosis or pulmonary embolism is suspected, full anticoagulant therapy should be commenced and a lower limb compression ultrasound and/or lung scan should be carried out within 24–48 hours (see Chapter 8, Antenatal obstetric complications and Chapter 16, Obstetric emergencies).

Puerperal pyrexia

Significant puerperal pyrexia is defined as a temperature of 38°C or higher on any two of the first 10 days postpartum, exclusive of the first 24 hours (measured orally by a standard technique). A mildly elevated temperature is not uncommon in the first 24 hours, but any pyrexia associated with tachycardia merits investigation. In about 80 per cent of women who develop a temperature in the first 24 hours following a vaginal delivery, no obvious evidence of infection can be identified. The reverse holds true for women delivering by Caesarean section, when a wound infection should be considered. Common sites associated with puerperal pyrexia include chest, throat, breasts, urinary tract, pelvic organs, Caesarean or perineal wounds and legs (Table 17.1).

Chest complications

Chest complications are most likely to appear in the first 24 hours after delivery, particularly after general anaesthesia. Atalectasis may be associated with fever and can be prevented by early and regular chest physiotherapy. Aspiration pneumonia (Mendleson's syndrome) must be suspected if there is wheezing, dyspnoea, a spiking temperature and evidence of hypoxia.

Genital tract infection

Genital tract infection following delivery is referred to as puerperal sepsis and is synonymous with older descriptions of puerperal fever, milk fever and childbed fever. It was not realized until the mid-nineteenth century that the high maternal mortality and morbidity were due to poor hygiene of the birth attendants; the establishment of lying-in hospitals and overcrowding perpetuated the condition to epidemic proportions. Until 1937, puerperal sepsis was the major cause of maternal mortality. The discovery of sulphonamides in 1935 and the simultaneous reduction in the virulence of the haemolytic streptococcus resulted in a dramatic fall in maternal mortality. The Confidential Enquiry into Maternal and Child Health (UK) reported that, in 2003–5, genital tract sepsis accounted for 14 per cent of direct causes of maternal death. Although some of these cases followed miscarriage or occurred antenatally after preterm prelabour rupture of membranes (PPROM), the majority of deaths occurred post-natally, indicating that puerperal fever was a significant factor in maternal death.

Aetiology of genital tract infections

A mixed flora normally colonizes the vagina with low virulence. Puerperal infection is usually polymicrobial and involves contaminants from the bowel that colonize the perineum and lower genital tract. The organisms most commonly associated with puerperal genital infection are listed in the box below. Following delivery, natural barriers to infection are temporarily removed and therefore organisms with a pathogenic potential can ascend from the lower genital tract into the uterine cavity. Placental separation exposes a large raw area equivalent to an open wound, and retained products of conception and blood clots within the uterus can provide an excellent culture medium for infection. Furthermore, vaginal delivery is almost invariably associated with lacerations of the genital tract (uterus, cervix and vagina). Although these lacerations may not need surgical repair, they can become a focus for infection similar to iatrogenic wounds, such as Caesarean section and episiotomy.

Table 17.1 Diagnosis and management of puerperal pyrexia

Symptoms	Diagnosis	Special investigations	Management
Cough	Chest infection	Sputum M, C and S	Physiotherapy
Purulent sputum	Pneumonia	Chest x-ray	Antibiotics
Dyspnoea			
Sore throat	Tonsillitis	Throat swab	Antibiotics
Cervical lymphadenopathy			
Headaches	Meningitis	Lumbar puncture	Antibiotics
Neck stiffness (epidural/spinal anaesthetic)			
Dysuria	Pyelonephritis	Urine M, C and S	Antibiotics
Loin pain and tenderness			
Secondary PPH	Metritis	Pelvic ultrasound	Antibiotics
Tender bulky uterus	Retained placental		Uterine tissue
Pelvic/calf pain/ tenderness	Deep vein thrombosis	Doppler/venogram of legs	Heparin
Chest pain	Pulmonary embolism	Chest x-ray and blood gases	Lung perfusion scan angiogram
Painful engorged breasts	Mastitis Abscess	Milk M, C and S	Express milk Antibiotics Incision and drainage

M, C and S, microscopy, culture and sensitivity; PPH, postpartum haemorrhage.

Organisms commonly associated with puerperal genital infection

Aerobes
- Gram-positive
  - Beta-haemolytic streptococcus, groups A, B, D
  - *Staphylococcus epidermidis* and *aureus*
  - Enterococci – *Streptococcus faecalis*
- Gram-negative
  - *Escherichia coli*
  - *Haemophilus influenzae*
  - *Klebsiella pneumoniae*
  - *Pseudomonas aeruginosa*
  - *Proteus mirabilis*

- Gram-variable
  - *Gardenella vaginalis*

Anaerobes
- *Peptococcus* sp.
- *Peptostreptococcus* sp.
- *Bacteroides* – *B. fragilis, B. bivius, B. disiens*
- *Fusobacterium* sp.

Miscellaneous
- *Chlamydia trachomatis*
- *Mycoplasma hominis*
- *Ureaplasma urealyticum*

Signs of puerperal pelvic infection 👁

- Pyrexia and tachycardia
- Uterus – boggy, tender and larger
- Infected wounds – Caesarean/perineal
- Peritonism
- Paralytic ileus
- Indurated adnexae (parametritis)
- Bogginess in pelvis (abscess)

Symptoms of puerperal pelvic infection 📋

- Malaise, headache, fever, rigors
- Abdominal discomfort, vomiting and diarrhoea
- Offensive lochia
- Secondary PPH

Table 17.2 Investigations for puerperal genital infections

Investigations	Abnormalities
Full blood count	Anaemia, leukocytosis, thrombocytopenia
Urea and electrolytes	Fluid and electrolyte imbalance
High vaginal swabs	Infection screen and blood culture
Pelvic ultrasound	Retained products, pelvic abscess
Clotting screen (haemorrhage or shock)	Disseminated intravascular coagulation
Arterial blood gas	Acidosis and hypoxia (shock)

Chlamydia trachomatis puerperal parametritis may develop in one-third of women who had a pre-existing infection, but presentation is usually delayed. Investigations for puerperal genital infections are shown in Table 17.2.

There are a number of factors that determine the clinical course and severity of the infection, namely the general health and resistance of the woman, the virulence of the offending organism, the presence of haematoma or retained products of conception and the timing of antibiotic therapy and associated risk factors. The common methods of spread of puerperal infection are as follows:

- An ascending infection from the lower genital tract or primary infection of the placental site may spread via the Fallopian tubes to the ovaries, giving rise to a salpingo-oophoritis and pelvic peritonitis. This could progress to a generalized peritonitis and the development of pelvic abscesses.
- Infection may also spread by contiguity directly into the myometrium and the parametrium, giving rise to a metritis or parametritis, also referred to as pelvic cellulitis. Pelvic peritonitis and abscesses may also occur.
- Infection may also spread to distant sites via lymphatics and blood vessels. Infection from the uterus can be carried by uterine vessels into the inferior vena cava via the iliac vessels or, directly, via the ovarian vessels. This could give rise to a septic thrombophlebitis, pulmonary infections or a generalized septicaemia and endotoxic shock.

Common risk factors for puerperal infection

- Antenatal intrauterine infection
- Caesarean section
- Cervical cerclage for cervical incompetence
- Prolonged rupture of membranes
- Prolonged labour
- Multiple vaginal examinations
- Instrumental delivery
- Manual removal of the placenta
- Retained products of conception
- Non-obstetric, e.g. obesity, diabetes, human immunodeficiency virus (HIV)

In contrast to pelvic inflammatory disease unrelated to pregnancy, tubal involvement in puerperal sepsis is in the form of perisalpingitis, which, rarely, causes tubal occlusion and consequent infertility. Tubo-ovarian abscesses are also a rare complication of puerperal sepsis.

Mild to moderate infections can be treated with a broad-spectrum antibiotic, e.g. co-amoxiclav or a cephalosporin, such as cefalexin, plus metronidazole. Depending on the severity, the first few doses should be given intravenously.

With severe infections, there is a release of inflammatory and vasoactive mediators in response to the endotoxins produced during bacteriolysis. The resultant local vasodilatation causes circulatory embarrassment and hence poor tissue perfusion. This phenomenon is known as septicaemic/septic/endotoxic shock, and delay in appropriate management could be fatal.

Necrotizing fasciitis is a rare but frequently fatal infection of skin, fascia and muscle. It can originate in perineal tears, episiotomies and Caesarean section wounds. Perineal infections can extend rapidly to involve the buttocks, thighs and lower abdominal wall. A variety of bacteria can be involved, but anaerobes predominate and *Clostridium perfringens* is usually identified. In addition to general signs of infection, there is extensive necrosis, crepitus and inflammation. As well as the measures usually taken to manage septic shock, wide debridement of necrotic tissue under general anaesthesia is absolutely essential to avoid mortality. Split-thickness skin grafts may be necessary at a later date.

Prevention of puerperal sepsis

Increased awareness of the principles of general hygiene, a good surgical approach and the use of aseptic techniques have contributed to the decline in severe puerperal sepsis. However, the risk of sepsis is higher following Caesarean section, particularly when performed after the onset of labour. There is now overwhelming evidence that prophylactic antibiotics during emergency Caesarean section reduce the risk of post-operative infection, namely wound infection, metritis, pelvic abscess, pelvic thrombophlebitis and septic shock. A single intraoperative dose of antibiotics (amoxiclav or cephalosporin plus metronidazole) should be given after clamping of the umbilical cord to avoid unnecessary exposure of the baby to antibiotics. The benefit of prophylaxis for elective Caesarean section is of greater significance in units where the background infectious morbidity is high.

The breasts

Anatomy

The breasts are largely made up of glandular, adipose and connective tissue (Figure 17.2). They lie superficial

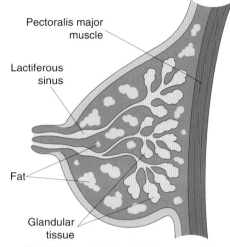

Figure 17.2 The breast during lactation

to the pectoralis major, external oblique and serratus anterior muscles, extending between the second and sixth rib from the sternum to the axilla. A pigmented area called the areola, which contains sebaceous glands, surrounds the nipple. During pregnancy, the areola becomes darker and the sebaceous glands become prominent (Montgomery's tubercles). The breast is comprised of 15–25 functional units arranged radially from the nipple and each unit is made up of a lactiferous duct, a mammary gland lobule and alveoli. The lactiferous ducts dilate to form a lactiferous sinus before converging to open in the nipple. Contractile myoepithelial cells surround the ducts as well as the alveoli.

Physiology

The human species is unique in that most of the breast development occurs at puberty and is therefore primed to produce milk within 2 weeks of hormonal stimulation. It is hypothesized that, unlike animals, female breasts have an erotic role to attract the male to procreate. The control of mammary growth and development is not fully understood and many hormones may contribute to this process. In general, oestrogens stimulate proliferation of the lactiferous ducts (possibly with adrenal steroids and growth hormones), while progesterone is responsible for the development of the mammary lobules. During early pregnancy, lactiferous ducts and alveoli proliferate, while in later pregnancy the alveoli hypertrophy in preparation for secretory activity. The lactogenic hormones prolactin and human placental lactogen probably modulate these changes during pregnancy.

Colostrum

Colostrum is a yellowish fluid secreted by the breast that can be expressed as early as the 16th week of pregnancy, but is replaced by milk during the second postpartum day. Colostrum has a high concentration of proteins but contains less sugar and fat than breast milk, although it contains large fat globules. The proteins are mainly in the form of globulins, particularly immunoglobulin (Ig) A, which plays an important role in protection against infection. Colostrum is also believed to have a laxative effect, which may help empty the baby's bowel of meconium.

Breast milk

The major constituents of breast milk are lactose, protein, fat and water (Table 17.3). However, the composition of breast milk is not constant; early lactation differs from late lactation, one feed differs from the next, and the composition can even change during a feed. Artificial infant formulas cannot therefore be identical to breast milk. Compared to cow's milk, breast milk provides slightly more energy, has less protein but more fat and lactose. The major protein fractions are lactalbumin, lactoglobulin and caseinogen. Lactalbumin is the major protein in breast milk, whereas caseinogen forms 90 per cent of the protein in cow's milk. The mineral content (particularly sodium) is much higher in cow's milk, which can therefore be dangerous if given to a baby who is dehydrated from gastroenteritis. In addition to IgA, breast milk contains small amounts of IgM and IgG and other factors such as lactoferrin, macrophages, complement and lysozymes. Although breast milk contains a lower concentration of iron, its absorption is better than from cow's milk or iron-supplemented infant formula (>75 per cent, 30 per cent and 10 per cent, respectively). The improved bioavailability may be related to lactoferrin, an iron-binding glycoprotein, which also inhibits bacterial growth. With the exception of vitamin K, all other vitamins are found in breast milk and therefore vitamin K is given to the baby to minimize the risk of haemorrhagic disease (see Chapter 19, Neonatology).

Table 17.3 Comparison between human and cow's milk

	Human breast milk	Cow's milk
Energy (kcal/mL)	75	66
Lactose (g/100 mL)	6.8	4.9
Protein (g/100 mL)	1.1	3.5
Fat (g/100 mL)	4.5	3.7
Sodium (mmol/L)	7	22
Water (mL/100 mL)	87.1	87.3

Prolactin

Prolactin is a long-chain polypeptide produced from the anterior pituitary; levels rise up to 20-fold during pregnancy and lactation. Peak levels of prolactin are reached within 45 minutes of suckling, but return to normal immediately after weaning and in non-breastfeeding mothers. The exact mechanism of action is not fully understood, but prolactin appears to have a direct action on the secretory cells to synthesize milk proteins. Prolactin is essential for lactation and it is hypothesized that nipple stimulation prevents the release of prolactin-inhibiting factor from the hypothalamus, thereby initiating the production of prolactin by the anterior pituitary. This theory is supported by the fact that lactation can be arrested with bromocriptine, a dopamine agonist that inhibits prolactin. A similar phenomenon occurs following pituitary necrosis (Sheehan's syndrome) when prolactin production ceases.

Oxytocin

Once milk has been produced under the influence of prolactin, it has to be delivered to the infant. The milk-ejection or let-down reflex is initiated by suckling, which stimulates the pulsatile release of oxytocin from the posterior pituitary. Oxytocin contracts the myoepithelial cells surrounding the alveoli, as well as the myoepithelial cells lying longitudinally along the lactiferous ducts, thereby aiding the expulsion of milk. Oxytocin release can also be stimulated by visual, olfactory or auditory stimuli, e.g. hearing the baby cry, but can be inhibited by stress. Oxytocin can also stimulate uterine contractions, giving rise to the 'after-pains' of childbirth.

Breastfeeding

Women who opt to breastfeed tend to decide before or very early in their pregnancy. This decision is usually based on previous experience, influence of family or friends, culture and custom. A new mother who is unprepared for breastfeeding may find it a frustrating task and turn to bottle-feeding. There is now evidence to suggest that antenatal classes and literature on breastfeeding given antenatally may be beneficial.

The most common reasons mothers give for abandoning breastfeeding are inadequate milk production and sore and cracked nipples. Both these problems can be overcome by correct positioning of the baby on the breast (Figure 17.3). The mouth should be placed over the nipple and areola so that suction created within the baby's mouth draws the breast tissue into a teat which extends as far back as the junction of the soft and hard palate. The tongue applies peristaltic force to the underside of the teat against the support of the hard palate. In this way,

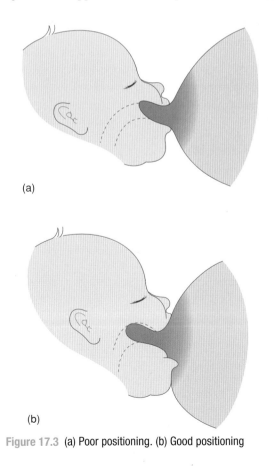

(a)

(b)

Figure 17.3 (a) Poor positioning. (b) Good positioning

there should be no to-and-fro movement of the teat in and out of the baby's mouth, thus minimizing friction. The mother should also be taught how to implement the rooting reflex. When the skin around the baby's mouth is touched, the mouth begins to gape. At this point, the mother should reposition the baby so that the lower rim of the baby's mouth fits well below the nipple, allowing a liberal mouthful of breast tissue. When the baby is properly attached, breastfeeding should be pain free. The use of creams and ointments for cracked nipples has not been shown to be beneficial and the use of a nipple shield merely reduces milk production.

Although no study has identified the threshold of the critical time limit for successful breastfeeding, early suckling appears to be beneficial. However, this should not be rushed, and perhaps should be done initially under supervision when the mother is comfortable and in privacy.

There is no scientific evidence to justify a rigid breastfeeding schedule. Babies should be fed on demand and left on the breast until feeding finishes spontaneously. An imposed time limit on feeding can have a deleterious effect on calorie intake.

Supplementary feeds of formula, glucose or water are often given to breastfed infants in the belief that the baby is still hungry or thirsty. However, this is a misconception, as this practice merely increases the risk of total abandonment of breastfeeding.

Test-weighing infants before and after a feed to establish the ideal quantity of milk intake is an archaic practice that should be abandoned, as inappropriate action could prove hazardous.

Advantages of breastfeeding

- Readily available at the right temperature and ideal nutritional value.
- Cheaper than formula feed.
- Associated with a reduction in:
  - childhood infective illnesses, especially gastroenteritis,
  - fertility with amenorrhoea,
  - atopic illnesses, e.g. eczema and asthma,
  - necrotizing enterocolitis in preterm babies,
  - juvenile diabetes,
  - childhood cancer, especially lymphoma,
  - pre-menopausal breast cancer.

Non-breastfeeding mothers

There are various reasons why a woman may choose not to breastfeed, ranging from personal choice to stillbirth. Previously, women infected with HIV were discouraged from breastfeeding. The most recent recommendations from the World Health Organization reflect an understanding that the risk of vertical transmission of HIV via breastfeeding is less than the risk of death by malnutrition or sepsis for the majority of infants who have to rely on formula feeds in developing countries.

Non-breastfeeding mothers may suffer considerable engorgement and breast pain. Dopamine receptor stimulants, such as bromocriptine and cabergoline, inhibit prolactin and thus suppress lactation. However, both have been associated with an increased risk of hypertension and stroke. Furthermore, fluid restriction and a tight brassiere have been shown to be equally effective as bromocriptine usage by the second week and therefore this is the method of choice for the suppression of lactation.

Breast disorders

Blood-stained nipple discharge

Blood-stained nipple discharge of pregnancy is typically bilateral and believed to be due to epithelial proliferation. It usually occurs in the second or third trimester of pregnancy and rarely persists beyond three months postpartum. As the condition is self-limiting, no investigation or treatment is necessary, and the woman should be reassured.

Painful nipples

The nipple can become very painful if the covering epithelium is denuded or if a fissure develops giving rise to 'cracked nipples'. The cause is usually attributed to poor positioning of the baby on the breast, although thrush (candidiasis) may also cause soreness. Cracked nipples are also associated with an increased risk of a breast abscess developing. Treatment involves resting the affected nipple and manually expressing milk. Breastfeeding should then be reintroduced gradually.

Galactocele

A galactocele is a retention cyst of the mammary ducts following blockage by inspissated secretions. It is identified as a fluctuant swelling with minimal pain and inflammation. It usually resolves spontaneously but may also be aspirated; with increasing discomfort, surgical excision may become necessary.

Breast engorgement

Engorgement of the breasts usually begins by the second or third postpartum day and if breastfeeding has not been effectively established, the over-distended and engorged breasts can be very uncomfortable. Breast engorgement may give rise to puerperal fever of up to 39°C in 13 per cent of mothers. Although the fever rarely lasts more than 16 hours, other infective causes must be excluded. A number of remedies for the treatment of breast engorgement, such as manual expression, firm support, applying an ice bag and an electric breast pump, have all been recommended in the past, but allowing the baby easy access to the breast is the most effective method of treatment and prevention.

Mastitis

Inflammation of the breast is not always due to an infective process. Mastitis can occur when a blocked duct obstructs the flow of milk and distends the alveoli. If this pressure persists, the milk extravasates into the perilobular tissue, initiating an inflammatory process. The affected segment of the breast is painful and appears red and oedematous (Figure 17.4). Flu-like symptoms develop associated with a tachycardia and pyrexia. In the first few postpartum days, about 15 per cent of women will develop a temperature of up to 39°C, lasting less than 24 hours, due to breast engorgement. By contrast, in infective mastitis, the pyrexia develops later and persists for longer. In general, suppurative mastitis usually presents in the third to fourth postpartum week and is usually unilateral. Symptoms include rigors, fever, pain and reddened, swollen breasts. The most common infecting organism is *Staphylococcus aureus*, which is found in 40 per cent of women with mastitis. Other bacteria include coagulase-negative staphylococci and *Streptococcus viridans*. The most common sources of infection are, first, from the baby's nose or throat and,

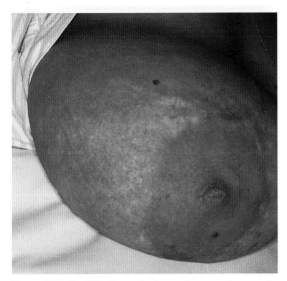

Figure 17.4 Mastitis demonstrating redness, oedema and engorged veins

second, from an infected umbilical cord. Management includes isolation of the mother and baby, ceasing breastfeeding from the affected breast, expression of milk either manually or by electric pump, and microbiological culture and sensitivity of a sample of milk. Flucloxacillin can be commenced while awaiting sensitivity results.

About 10 per cent of women with mastitis develop a breast abscess. Treatment is by a radial surgical incision and drainage under general anaesthesia.

Contraception

The exact mechanism of lactational amenorrhoea is poorly understood, but the most plausible hypothesis is that during lactation there is inhibition of the normal pulsatile release of luteinizing hormone from the anterior pituitary. Breastfeeding therefore provides a contraceptive effect, but it is not totally reliable, as up to 10 per cent of women conceive during this period. However, it has recently been shown that a mother who is still in the phase of postpartum amenorrhoea while fully breastfeeding her baby has a less than 2 per cent chance of conceiving in the first six months. Although this is comparable to some other forms of contraception (see Chapter 7, *Gynaecology by Ten Teachers*, 18th edn), most women in developed countries use some sort of additional contraception, such as barrier methods. If an intrauterine

contraceptive device is preferred, it is best to wait at least 4–8 weeks to allow for involution. Care needs to be exercised in breastfeeding mothers, as there have been reports of increased rates of uterine perforation. The combined oral contraceptive pill enhances the risk of thrombosis in the early puerperium and can have an adverse effect on the quality and constituents of breast milk. The progesterone-only pill (the minipill) is therefore preferable and should be commenced about day 21 following delivery, prior to which there may be puerperal breakthrough bleeding. Injectable contraception, such as depot medroxyprogesterone acetate (Depo-Provera) given three-monthly or norethisterone enantate (Noristerat) given two-monthly, is also very effective. However, injectable contraception given within 48 hours of delivery for convenience can cause breakthrough bleeding and therefore should preferably be given 5–6 weeks postpartum.

Sterilization can be offered to mothers who are certain that they have completed their family. Tubal ligation can be performed during Caesarean section or by the open method (mini-laparotomy) in the first few postpartum days. However, it is better delayed until after 6 weeks postpartum, when it can be done by laparoscopy. This allows the mother to spend more time in comfort with her newborn baby and, furthermore, laparoscopic clip sterilization is less traumatic and associated with a lower failure rate.

Women who are not breastfeeding should commence the pill within 4 weeks of delivery, as ovulation can occur by 6 weeks postpartum.

Pelvic floor exercises

It is a widespread belief that pelvic floor exercises tone up the muscles of the pelvic floor and should therefore be advocated in the postpartum period. However, large randomized trials to evaluate their benefit in preventing genital prolapse, urinary incontinence or anal incontinence are lacking. There is also no evidence that antenatal exercises prevent incontinence or prolapse. However, as general exercise is known to strengthen striated muscle, and pelvic floor exercises are unlikely to be harmful, women are still taught post-natal exercises. This should also serve to cultivate a feeling of pelvic floor awareness, so that women with pelvic floor dysfunction seek medical help sooner.

Perinatal death

- **Stillbirth**: a baby born with no signs of life
- **Perinatal death**: stillbirth >24 weeks gestation or death within 7 days of birth
- **Live birth**: any baby that shows signs of life irrespective of gestation.

Bereavement counselling following perinatal death requires special expertise and is best left to a senior clinician and a trained bereavement counsellor. Inappropriate management of this traumatic period can have a devastating effect on the woman's emotional and marital life. Effective communication and support are crucial and women should be encouraged to make contact with organizations, such as SANDS (Stillbirth and Neonatal Death Society).

The grieving process can be facilitated by practices such as seeing and holding the dead baby, naming the baby, and taking hand/foot prints and photographs. Coming to terms with the perinatal death of a twin is even more difficult because the mother has to mourn one baby and celebrate the arrival of the other.

A post-mortem is the most important diagnostic test, even though there may be no positive findings. Couples who decline a post-mortem may do so because of religious reasons or because they fear mutilation. In this situation, a partial post-mortem should be discussed whereby an autopsy of a single organ or a tissue biopsy can be performed. A full-body x-ray or, preferably, magnetic resonance imaging (MRI) may be useful in some cases (Table 17.4).

If the baby was stillborn, a stillbirth certificate should be completed by the attending doctor; otherwise, the paediatrician should complete the certificate. The certificate should be given to the parents to register the death with the Registrar of Births and Deaths. Funeral arrangements can be made privately or by the hospital.

Every mother who has lost a baby should have the 6-week post-natal visit at hospital.

The post-natal examination

This is carried out at about 6 weeks postpartum by the general practitioner or by the obstetrician if delivery had been complicated. The examination includes an assessment of the woman's mental and physical health, as well as the progress of the baby. In particular, direct questions must be asked about urinary, bowel and sexual function. Incontinence and dyspareunia are embarrassing issues that women do not volunteer to discuss readily. Weight, urine analysis and blood pressure are checked and a complete general, abdominal and pelvic examination is performed. If a cervical smear is due, it can be taken, although it is preferable to take one after three months postpartum. Contraception and pelvic floor exercises are also discussed.

Table 17.4 Investigations into perinatal death

Investigations	Reason
Full blood count	Anaemia, leukocytosis
Clotting screen	Disseminated intravascular coagulation
Kleihauer test	Fetomaternal transfusion
Virology, infection screen	Cytomegalovirus, parvovirus
Autoantibody screen (anti-cardiolipin and lupus anticoagulant)	Antiphospholipid syndrome, systemic lupus erythematosus
Blood and placenta culture	Infections such as *Listeria monocytogenes*
Antibodies in rhesus-negative women	Haemolytic disease
Toxoplasma antibodies	Toxoplasmosis
Skin biopsy/cardiac blood/placental biopsy	Chromosome analysis
Full-body x-ray or MRI	To identify congenital defects

MRI, magnetic resonance imaging.

CASE HISTORY

An 18-year-old woman with a BMI of 35 who had a forceps delivery after a prolonged second stage of labour 8 days previously presented with heavy, fresh vaginal bleeding and clots. She felt unwell and complained of abdominal cramps.

On examination, she had a temperature of 38.2°C and there was mild suprapubic tenderness. Vaginal examination revealed blood clots, but no products of conception. The cervix admitted only the tip of a finger and the uterus was tender and measured 14 weeks in size. A review of the delivery notes revealed that the placenta was delivered complete, but the membranes were noted to be ragged.

What is the most likely diagnosis?

Secondary PPH due to endometritis or infected retained products of conception.

What are the most relevant risk factors?

- Obesity.
- Prolonged labour.
- Instrumental delivery.

How should the patient be managed?

- Blood cultures.
- Intravenous broad-spectrum antibiotics, e.g. cephalosporin and metronidazole.
- Although a pelvic ultrasound may confirm the diagnosis, it has the potential to mislead and is not a prerequisite when the diagnosis is obvious.
- Surgical evacuation of retained products in the uterus.

Key points

- The puerperium refers to the 6-week period following childbirth.
- Care during this transition period is crucial before the woman returns to her pre-pregnant state.
- Perineal discomfort is a major complaint following vaginal delivery and therefore adequate analgesia should be prescribed.
- Common disorders include puerperal sepsis, thromboembolism, bowel and bladder dysfunction.

CHAPTER 18

PSYCHIATRIC DISORDERS AND THE PUERPERIUM

Alec McEwan

OVERVIEW

Overall, the incidence of mild mental health problems is not significantly different during pregnancy, although the risk of developing an antepartum serious new-onset psychiatric disorder is reduced. However, the risk of bipolar or severe depressive illness is greatly increased postpartum. Women with previous serious mental health problems are at high risk of a recurrence during both the antepartum and postpartum periods. It is vital for all healthcare professionals providing maternity and psychiatric care to understand how pregnancy may interact with mental health and to understand key themes in the detection of those at risk, and their subsequent management during and after the pregnancy. A multidisciplinary approach, supervised by specialist perinatal mental health teams, is vital to optimize care, limit morbidity and help prevent the tragic cases detailed in the maternal mortality reports. The problems of substance and alcohol misuse during pregnancy overlap significantly with mental health issues, and coordination is required between specialist services and providers of maternity care.

The significance of mental ill health to pregnancy, childbirth and motherhood

Childbirth contributes a substantial risk to the mental health of women. Although the antenatal period is not generally considered a high-risk time for the onset of new severe psychiatric disease, milder disorders do affect a significant minority of pregnant women (see Table 18.1) and up to a third of women presenting with severe depression in the antepartum period have no previous history. However, in the year following childbirth, women who were previously well have a greatly elevated risk of being admitted to a psychiatric hospital, being referred to a psychiatrist, suffering from a psychotic illness or developing severe depression. This risk is higher than their lifetime risk, and is much greater than for other women, or men. More than 80 per cent of women with postpartum psychiatric disease will be suffering from their first-ever psychiatric illness.

Pregnant women with pre-existing mental illness, or those who book with a previous history, are at significant risk of an antenatal or post-natal recurrence or exacerbation. Pregnancy, childbirth and the stresses of life as a new parent may destabilize conditions that had previously been under control. Certain pharmacological treatments may be contraindicated in pregnancy and suitable alternatives have to be found. Optimizing the new relationship between mother and baby may require help from specialist services.

The impact of psychiatric disease in pregnancy has been emphasized repeatedly by the Confidential Enquiries into Maternal and Child Health (CEMACH). The most recent report, 'Saving mothers' lives', covers the triennium 2003–5. It reports on 37 suicides occurring during pregnancy, or within one year of delivery. Most suicides occurred in association with post-natal mental illness. A further 22 women died from overdose of drugs of abuse, of which at least six

Table 18.1 Incidence of postpartum mental disorders

Depression	15–30%
Major depressive illness	10%
Moderate/severe depressive illness	3–5%
Referral to a psychiatrist	2%
Admission to a psychiatric unit	0.4%
Admission with puerperal psychosis	0.2%

may have been intentional, rather than accidental. Of special note, suicide during pregnancy is unusually violent (shootings, hangings), in contrast with suicide attempts in younger women, which commonly take the form of overdose and are less frequently successful. This emphasizes the severity of mental health problems occurring after delivery, when most maternal suicides take place. The number of suicides has fallen since the last triennium and it is hoped that recommendations made in these reports are having a positive impact.

Psychiatric disease is also commonly found in cases of violent maternal death. Life-threatening medical disorders may arise as a direct result of substance misuse, or may be misdiagnosed as perinatal mental health problems leading to delay in appropriate treatment, and, in some cases, death.

Pregnancy therefore impacts significantly on the incidence and presentation of psychiatric disorders, but it also poses unique treatment challenges. The safety of the fetus must also be considered, and the focus of therapy may ideally be away from drug treatments and toward psychological alternatives. However, failure to treat mental health issues rapidly may put both mother and baby at greater risk and drug treatment is often required. Strategies which are safe for the fetus are best recommended by specialist perinatal psychiatrists with particular skills in this field.

Normal emotional and psychological changes during pregnancy

Diagnosing mental illness in pregnancy is complicated by the wide variety of 'normal' emotional and behavioural changes which may occur. Common patterns include the following:

- Antenatal
  - mixed feelings about being pregnant
  - fears of being unable to cope
  - increased emotional lability
  - minor depressive symptoms (most marked in the first trimester)
  - anxiety and fears regarding delivery
  - obsessional thoughts regarding the safety of the baby (more common in the third trimester, particularly in women who have specific pregnancy complications).
- Post-natal
  - The 'pinks': for the first 24–48 hours following delivery, it is very common for women to experience an elevation of mood, a feeling of excitement, some overactivity and difficulty sleeping.
  - The 'blues': as many as 80 per cent of women may experience the 'post-natal blues' in the first 2 weeks after delivery. Fatigue, short temperedness, difficulty sleeping, depressed mood and tearfulness are common but usually mild, and resolve spontaneously in the majority of cases.

The following psychological disruptions should not be considered normal during pregnancy and require further assessment:

- panic attacks;
- episodes of low mood of prolonged duration (>2 weeks);
- low self-esteem;
- guilt or hopelessness;
- thoughts of self-harm or suicide;
- any mood changes that disrupt normal social functioning;
- 'biological' symptoms (e.g. poor appetite, early wakening);
- change in 'affect'.

Screening for mental health problems during and after pregnancy

Not all mental illness associated with pregnancy is predictable, however, identifiable risk factors do exist, as do screening methods designed to detect early psychiatric disease. Prophylactic treatments and management strategies can be instituted to prevent the onset of symptoms, or detect problems at an earlier and more easily treatable stage. It is the responsibility of all healthcare professionals looking after pregnant women to identify these risk factors, institute plans of surveillance and care, and refer to specialist services where necessary.

The National Institute for Health and Clinical Excellence (NICE) Clinical Guideline No. 45 'Antenatal and postnatal mental health' sets out screening questions that all pregnant women should be asked (Table 18.2). If the answers to these questions raise concerns, then the woman should be referred back to her GP, to her own psychiatrist, if she has one, or to a specialist perinatal mental health team depending on the severity of the symptoms or previous history.

Management of pregnancy in women with pre-existing psychiatric disease

Women with pre-existing mental health issues usually come to the attention of the maternity services at booking and appropriate screening questions should form part of all routine booking histories, as detailed in Table 18.2. Ideally, women with pre-existing psychiatric problems should receive pre-pregnancy counselling from a specialist in perinatal mental health. Issues to discuss include the impact of the pregnancy on the condition and the risk of relapse or deterioration. The long-term capacity for successful parenthood must be considered for women with schizophrenia, and other severe illnesses. Attention must be paid to the safety of medications during pregnancy, and the risk of relapse if they are withdrawn before conception. To minimize the risk of harm to the fetus from exposure to psychotropic drugs,

Table 18.2 Screening questions for mental health during and after pregnancy

At 'booking' (with midwife, GP or hospital obstetrician):

Is there a past history of severe mental illness (including schizophrenia, bipolar disorder, postpartum psychosis and severe depression)?

Have you ever received treatment from a psychiatrist or specialist mental health team?

Have you ever been admitted as an inpatient for psychiatric care?

Do you have a family history of mental health problems, particularly perinatal or bipolar illness?

At booking, and in the post-natal period (at least twice):

During the past month, have you often felt down, depressed or hopeless?

During the past month, have you often been bothered by having little interest or pleasure in doing things?

Are these feelings something you need or want help with?

the threshold for psychological treatments should be lower and access to these treatments should be straightforward. The mental health services should be involved at an early point in the pregnancies of women who have either ongoing disease or a past history of significant mental illness. Women requiring inpatient care during or after pregnancy should ideally be admitted to specialized regional 'mother-and-baby' units.

CASE I

A 28-year-old woman with obsessive-compulsive disorder had successfully been treated by her psychiatrist with a combination of psychotherapy and the SSRI, paroxetine. She had recently married and approached her doctor for pre-pregnancy advice. Paroxetine was gradually withdrawn in view of its teratogenic properties. She remained well and conceived seven months later. During the pregnancy, she became increasingly preoccupied with her body image and these concerns intensified as the pregnancy became more noticeable. She was spending excessive amounts of time in front of mirrors and could not be reassured by her midwife that her appearance was normal. Her psychiatrist suggested cognitive–behavioural therapy and a brief course seemed to help keep her symptoms under control.

She managed well through labour, however, she deteriorated in the post-natal period, becoming severely obsessive about cleanliness and the risks of infection to her new baby. Repeated handwashing and checking of electricity switches and gas cooker knobs began to interfere with normal post-natal routines. She was successfully breastfeeding and, when medications finally became necessary, fluoxetine was chosen over the more typical choices of citalopram or clomipramine because the quantities reaching breast milk are less. She continued this treatment for a further 12 months and was gradually withdrawn from the medication thereafter.

Depression

At least one in ten women will suffer some form of depression throughout their lifetime. There is no evidence that pregnancy reduces the risk of a relapse or improves the mood of women with active depression. Depression has a negative impact on pregnancy outcomes by adversely affecting diet, attendance for antenatal care, levels of smoking, alcohol consumption, self-harm and domestic violence. Existing family relationships suffer, and bonding with a new baby may be incomplete. There are biological reasons why depression might directly impact on placental function and predispose to fetal growth restriction and preterm labour.

Psychological treatments, including self-help approaches, cognitive–behavioural therapy, counselling and interpersonal psychotherapy may replace or supplement drug treatment. Withdrawing medication risks causing a relapse, but this may be possible under supervision. Alternatively, drug therapies can be minimized, rationalized, or safer alternatives used. There is ample experience with the use of tricyclic antidepressant drugs (TCAs) during pregnancy and women can be reassured that they carry no teratogenic risk and that they are safe to take while breastfeeding. The situation with selective serotonin reuptake inhibitors (SSRIs) is less clear. Studies have shown a possible increase in the number of congenital abnormalities with certain preparations, and a link with increased risk of preterm labour and low birthweight. However, their use in younger women is increasing. Minimization of the dose of all antidepressant drugs in the late third trimester will limit the levels in the newborn infant and help to prevent anticholinergic, serotonergic and extrapyramidal side effects in the neonate. Electroconvulsive therapy is not absolutely contraindicated in pregnancy, and may be needed in catatonic states.

Women with a history of severe depression not related to pregnancy carry between a 1:3 and 1:5 risk of a major postpartum depressive illness. If the previous depression occurred in the postpartum period, the recurrence risk is as high as 50 per cent. At the very least, skilled monitoring should be planned for the post-natal period. Prophylactic medications should also be considered.

Schizophrenia

Although older antipsychotic medications may have impaired fertility, this is not the case with newer drugs. Women with schizophrenia may be at greater risk of unplanned pregnancies as a result of their illness. Fluphenazine, trifluoperazine, haloperidol, chlorpromazine and flupenthixol do not have convincing teratogenic effects and the risks to the woman of stopping these drugs suddenly, with the real risk of disease relapse, are considered greater than any theoretical risks of fetal exposure. Under the guidance of a mental health specialist, it may be possible to reduce the dose in the third trimester to minimize levels in the newborn and prevent symptoms of withdrawal or toxicity.

Pre-pregnancy counselling is particularly important. Schizophrenia may seriously limit parenting skills and there is a significant risk that an affected mother will not ultimately remain the primary carer of her own child. Extra social support and surveillance will usually be necessary, but this is often tolerated poorly by affected individuals. Schizophrenia demonstrates multifactorial inheritance and the offspring of affected parents are at increased risk of developing the condition themselves.

Post-natally, the woman and her baby may benefit from an inpatient stay in a specialized mother and baby unit under the review and encouragement of a perinatal mental health team. Breastfeeding is to be encouraged to promote bonding with the newborn, and neuroleptic drugs in moderate doses are not a contraindication to this.

Bipolar affective disorder

This condition, also known as 'manic depression', is usually controlled with a combination of mood-stabilizing drugs (lithium, carbamazepine and sodium valproate), antidepressants and neuroleptics. Lithium carries a risk of causing cardiac defects if used in the first trimester and may cause fetal hypothyroidism, polyhydramnios and diabetes insipidus if used in the third trimester. Carbamazepine and valproate are also recognized teratogens. Stopping these medications abruptly before or just after conception carries a risk of causing a relapse. If the illness is stable, the mood stabilizers may be reduced and replaced by antidepressants with or without antipsychotics. Ideally, this is done following pre-pregnancy counselling. Ultimately, the fetal risks of continuing certain preparations may have to be accepted if the maternal risks of stopping treatment are thought to be too great.

Postpartum relapse occurs in approximately 50 per cent of women with bipolar illness and it is important that preventive therapy is commenced immediately after delivery. Lithium is contraindicated in breastfeeding, and the woman may be advised to bottle-feed so that it can be used in the postpartum period. Alternatively, a neuroleptic or antidepressant can be used for prophylaxis.

Anxiety disorders

Pregnancy, the anticipation of labour and the arrival of a new baby may all exacerbate an existing anxiety disorder. Cognitive–behavioural therapy may limit the need for drug treatment. Benzodiazepine use during the first trimester may be associated with an increased risk of cleft lip and/or palate, although the evidence is somewhat contradictory. Neonatal withdrawal effects are evident in the babies born to women who have used regular higher doses during pregnancy, and their use should be limited where possible. Breastfeeding may help to reduce the severity of the neonatal withdrawal (neonatal abstinence syndrome), as small amounts do reach breast milk.

CASE 2

A recent Eastern European immigrant to the United Kingdom, with minimal English, was seen by her GP at 12 weeks gestation. The only history of note was that her father had suffered a long-standing psychiatric illness which the woman believed to be 'schizophrenia'. He had died when she was young in a road traffic accident. Her pregnancy proceeded without complication, and she went home on the second post-natal day following a normal delivery at term.

Within a couple of weeks, her partner reported to the community midwife that he had concerns about her mood. She seemed agitated, fearful, and unduly concerned about the well-being of the baby and refused any help offered by him. The GP saw her, without an interpreter, and diagnosed 'post-natal depression'. He commenced tricyclic antidepressants, however, a week later she became frankly delusional and believed that her partner was trying to kill the baby. She was hardly sleeping and eating very little. Admission to a mother-and-baby unit was organized where puerperal psychosis was diagnosed. She was treated initially with antipsychotics (trifluoperazine) and with appropriate help from the specialist nursing and midwifery staff was able to re-establish breastfeeding and was not separated from the baby. Later information from her family in Poland suggested that her father had suffered with a bipolar illness. This information should have prompted review by a specialist in perinatal mental health, had it been known at booking. A post-natal plan, including regular review by a community psychiatric nurse, might have led to earlier intervention and may have prevented her deterioration to such a severe state.

Psychotropic medications during pregnancy and breastfeeding

Teratogenicity

The mood stabilizers carry particular concern. Lithium increases the risks of fetal cardiac defects, while valproate is strongly implicated in the causation of neural tube defects. Both valproate and carbamazepine can cause the 'fetal anticonvulsant syndrome'.

The antidepressant paroxetine (an SSRI) is linked with an increase in fetal cardiac defects, and use of benzodiazepines may increase facial clefting.

Amitriptyline, imipramine (both tricyclic antidepressants) and fluoxetine (an SSRI) do not seem to be overtly teratogenic.

Other antenatal side effects

Monoamine oxidase inhibitors (rarely used now) are contraindicated in pregnancy because of their vasoconstrictive properties, which may impair placental function. Chronic use of antipsychotic drugs may cause glucose intolerance and diabetes during pregnancy.

Neonatal effects

Lithium may cause fetal and neonatal hypothyroidism and SSRIs have been linked with persistent pulmonary hypertension. Benzodiazepine use later in pregnancy may cause depressed respiratory effort at birth, hypotonicity and poor feeding (the 'floppy baby syndrome'). Anticholinergic, extrapyramidal and serotonergic side effects may be evident in the newborns of women taking these drugs in higher doses during the third trimester. A neonatal abstinence syndrome is also seen with maternal use of TCAs and SSRIs. The neonate may be irritable, jittery, slow to feed, restless and show poor sleep with occasional convulsions.

Breastfeeding

TCAs and older 'typical' antipsychotics are present in only small amounts in breast milk and do not contraindicate breastfeeding. SSRIs are found in higher quantities and those with shorter half-lives, e.g. sertraline, may be preferable. Women needing lithium should not breastfeed, for fear of neonatal toxicity, but carbamazepine and valproate are safe.

CASE 3

A 36-year-old woman, with a previous history of moderately severe depressive illness treated with fluoxetine, booked at 8 weeks gestation with her midwife. Her only other pregnancy had been complicated by pre-eclampsia and preterm birth of the baby at 30 weeks by Caesarean section. He had done well, but she had subsequently suffered with a post-natal depressive disorder. She had fully recovered and declined referral in this next pregnancy to her psychiatrist, or the perinatal mental health team.

She later approached her GP at 24 weeks gestation with symptoms suggestive of a mild depressive disorder and a series of counselling appointments, with brief psychotherapy, was accepted. Despite these measures, she continued to be very tearful and anxious about the outcome of this pregnancy. Amitriptyline was commenced and continued into the post-natal period. With her consent, the perinatal health team became involved and a community psychiatric nurse visited on a regular basis after the birth of the baby. She was encouraged to attend a local post-natal group, and baby massage sessions, where she found further support and new friendships. By six months, she was coping well with two small children and was able to stop the antidepressants.

New-onset psychiatric disease in pregnancy

Women with no personal history of psychiatric disease are nevertheless at risk of mental illness during pregnancy. The 'common' symptoms of pregnancy (e.g. hyperemesis, poor sleep, backache), and ambivalence toward the pregnancy, may combine with social factors and relationship difficulties to cause depressive illness where there has been none previously. Indeed, one-third of women with major depression during pregnancy have no preceding history. 'Biological' factors are of far greater significance in the aetiology of severe depression in the postpartum period. This is the highest risk time for new-onset disease and the umbrella term of 'post-natal depression' should be abandoned and replaced by more specific and descriptive terms which can differentiate between affective disorders of differing aetiologies and severities.

Antenatal

The normal emotional changes occurring during pregnancy (see under Normal emotional and psychological changes during pregnancy, p. 273) may become exaggerated and potentially harmful. Anxiety associated with panic attacks and specific phobias relating to labour (tokophobia) or needles may require treatment with cognitive or behavioural therapy, benzodiazepines or SSRIs. Depression may have its onset during the pregnancy and is a strong risk factor for postpartum depression. Both pharmacological and non-drug treatment may be necessary.

Post-natal

The greater part of new-onset psychiatric illness presents in the puerperium. Affective (mood) disorders account for the majority and these vary in severity from the mildest (minor depression) to moderate and severe depressive illness and, in the extreme, puerperal psychosis (a variant of manic depression or bipolar disorder). As discussed in the overview, the post-natal period represents perhaps the highest risk period in a woman's life for the development of a psychiatric disorder. Although a previous history of moderate to severe depression or bipolar disorder is a significant risk factor, for many women this represents their first episode of mental illness.

Puerperal psychosis

This very severe disorder affects between 1:500 and 1:1000 women after delivery. It rarely presents before the 3rd postpartum day (most commonly the 5th), but usually does so before 4 weeks. The onset is characteristically abrupt, with a rapidly changing clinical picture.

Risk factors for postpartum psychosis

- Previous history of puerperal psychosis
- Previous history of severe non-postpartum depressive illness
- Family history (first/second-degree relative) of bipolar disorder/affective psychosis

---

Symptoms of puerperal psychosis

- Restless agitation
- Insomnia
- Perplexity/confusion
- Fear/suspicion
- Delusions/hallucinations
- Failure to eat and drink
- Thoughts of self-harm
- Depressive symptoms (guilt, self-worthlessness, hopelessness)
- Loss of insight

Management

The patient should be referred urgently to a psychiatrist and will usually require admission to a psychiatric unit. If possible, this should be a mother and baby unit under the supervision of a specialist perinatal mental healthcare team. These units prevent separation of the baby from its mother and this may help with bonding and the future relationship.

Treatments include:

- acute pharmacotherapy with neuroleptics, such as chlorpromazine or haloperidol;
- treatment of mania with lithium carbonate;
- electroconvulsive therapy (ECT) – particularly for severe depressive psychoses;
- antidepressants (which will take 10–14 days to be effective) as a second-line treatment.

Recovery usually occurs over 4–6 weeks, although treatment with antidepressants will be needed for at least six months. These women remain at high risk of pregnancy-related and non-pregnancy-related recurrences. The risk of recurrence in a future pregnancy is approximately 1 in 2, particularly if the next pregnancy occurs within two years of the one complicated by puerperal psychosis. Women with a previous history of puerperal psychosis should be considered for prophylactic lithium, started on the first postpartum day.

Postpartum (non-psychotic) depressive illness

Depression can be classified as 'minor' or 'major'. Major depression can be divided into 'mild', 'moderate' and 'severe' categories. It is important to distinguish postpartum depression of any degree from the postpartum 'blues'.

Between 10 and 15 per cent of women will suffer with some form of depression in the first year after the delivery of their baby. At least 7 per cent will satisfy the criteria for mild major depressive illness (see Symptom box) and many more could be described as having minor depression; 3–5 per cent will suffer a severe major post-natal depressive episode. Without treatment, most women will recover spontaneously within 3–6 months; however, 1 in 10 will remain depressed at one year.

Clinical features

In contrast to puerperal psychosis, non-psychotic postpartum depression usually presents later in the post-natal period, most commonly around 6 weeks, with a more gradual onset. The 6-week post-natal check is an ideal opportunity to detect early postpartum non-psychotic depression, but the signs are often missed. The Edinburgh Postnatal Depression Scale is an example of a screening technique, but there are others. NICE recommends that all women are asked about their mood at least twice in the postpartum period by midwives, obstetricians, health visitors or GPs, ideally at 6 weeks and 3–4 months after the birth. Particular attention should be paid to the assessment of women with risk factors for post-natal depressive illness. Indeed, women deemed at highest risk should be under close surveillance by a specialist community psychiatric nurse, with early admission to the local mother and baby unit if there are signs of concern.

Severe post-natal affective disorders usually present earlier than milder forms, and in this group, biological risk factors may be more important than psychosocial factors.

Treatment options include:

- remedy of social factors;
- non-directive counselling;
- interpersonal psychotherapy;
- cognitive–behavioural therapy;
- drug therapy.

The earlier the onset of the depression and the more severe it becomes, the more likely it is that formal psychiatric intervention will be needed. However, randomized trials have demonstrated the benefits of non-directive counselling from specially trained midwives and health visitors in the management of milder disorders. Even simple encouragement to join a local post-natal group may prevent social isolation and limit depression.

If pharmacotherapy is deemed necessary, tricyclic antidepressants or SSRIs are appropriate. There is good evidence to support the safety of the former in breastfeeding, less so for the latter. However, SSRIs in usual doses are probably safe.

There has been a vogue in the past for treating post-natal depression with progestogens in the erroneous belief that the fall in progesterone levels postpartum is the cause of post-natal depression. There is no good evidence to support this, and it may even be harmful if the use of other effective treatments is delayed because of it. This practice should therefore be avoided. High-dose oestrogen regimens have been tried in research trials, but these are not used routinely.

Women with a past history of severe post-natal depressive illness may be candidates for some form of prophylactic treatment, and the help of a specialist in perinatal mental health care should be sought before delivery.

Symptoms of severe post-natal depressive disorder

- Early-morning wakening
- Poor appetite
- Diurnal mood variation (worse in the mornings)
- Low energy and libido
- Loss of enjoyment
- Lack of interest
- Impaired concentration
- Tearfulness
- Feelings of guilt and failure
- Anxiety
- Thoughts of self-harm/suicide
- Thoughts of harm to the baby

Adverse sequelae of post-natal depressive illness

Immediate
- Physical morbidity
- Suicide/infanticide
- Prolonged psychiatric morbidity
- Damaged social attachments to infant
- Disrupted emotional development of infant

Later
- Social/cognitive effects on the child
- Psychiatric morbidity in the child
- Marital breakdown
- Future mental health problems

Risk factors for post-natal depressive illness

- Past history of psychiatric illness
- Depression during pregnancy
- Obstetric factors (e.g. Caesarean section/fetal or neonatal loss)
- Social isolation and deprivation
- Poor relationships
- Recent adverse life events (bereavement/illness)
- Severe post-natal 'blues'

Understanding the pathophysiology of postpartum affective disorders

The importance of psychosocial factors in the aetiology of non-psychotic mild and moderate postpartum depressive illness is in contrast to the biological factors (e.g. family history) predisposing to puerperal psychosis and severe postpartum depressive illness.

The constancy of incidence across cultures and the temporal relationship with childbirth would tend to suggest a neuroendocrine basis for the more severe conditions. Changes in cortisol, oxytocin, endorphins, thyroxine, progesterone and oestrogen have all been implicated in the causation. Comparable dramatic changes in steroidal hormones outside the postpartum period have a well-known association with affective psychoses and mood disorders. A plausible recent theory is that the sudden fall in oestrogen postpartum triggers a hypersensitivity of certain dopamine receptors in a predisposed group of women and may be responsible for the severe mood disturbance which follows. The occurrence and the severity of the 'post-natal blues' are thought to be related to both the absolute level of progesterone and the relative drop from a prepartum level. However, there is no clear association between the 'postpartum blues' and affective psychoses, and no evidence as yet to implicate progesterone in the aetiology of puerperal psychosis or severe post-natal depression.

Depression is a characteristic feature of hypothyroidism, which may occur as a consequence of postpartum thyroiditis. The other features of hypothyroidism may be missed, and checking thyroid function is important in women with milder depressive symptoms in the first year following childbirth as correction with thyroid supplements may elevate the mood.

Key points

- All women should be asked at booking about personal or family history of psychiatric illness.
- Close collaboration is recommended between obstetrician and psychiatrist for women with mental illness, a previous history of severe mental ill health, or a strong family history of bipolar affective disorder.
- Women with previous serious mental illness should be appropriately counselled regarding the recurrence risks associated with pregnancy.
- All women should be screened for depression, at least twice, in the postpartum period.
- Specialist perinatal psychiatric services should be available to all women.
- The prescribing of psychoactive drugs in pregnancy and breastfeeding should be done with care under the guidance of a psychiatrist with particular interest in pregnancy-related mental illness.
- Breastfeeding rarely needs to be avoided in women using psychotropic medications.
- There is an adequate range of drugs available to safely treat the pregnant or lactating woman who is mentally ill.

CHAPTER 19

NEONATOLOGY

Janet M Rennie

OVERVIEW

More than half a million babies are born every year in the United Kingdom, 4 million in the United States, 25 million in India and over 130 million worldwide. In the industrialized countries of the world, less than 1 per cent of these babies will die, and at least half the deaths are among premature babies with a birth weight of 1.5 kg. The picture is very different in the least developed countries, where the death rate is between 2 and 8 per cent. The countries of sub-Saharan Africa suffer the highest perinatal mortality rates in the world, around 80 per 1000 live births. Throughout the world, babies are still dying from prematurity, infections, congenital malformations, and hypoxia or trauma acquired intrapartum.

The challenge of neonatology

Neonatology is a relatively new subspecialty which has achieved some spectacular successes, most notably that of halving the mortality for very premature babies. Complex surgery can be performed safely, artificial nutrition maintained for weeks, and even the tiniest babies can be intubated and ventilated. Challenges remain; while therapeutic hypothermia holds promise for the treatment of some babies with perinatal hypoxic ischaemia, not all can benefit. Infectious diseases are still a problem. Advances in fetal medicine facilitate the antenatal diagnosis of a whole range of disorders, including cystic adenomatoid malformation of the lung, arachnoid cysts and other malformations of the brain, and dilatation of the renal pelvis. For many of these conditions, there is very little information about the natural history of the disorder if left untreated, and this makes counselling and management difficult. Early discharge and choice about the place of delivery have fragmented the provision of 'well baby' care. This means that all those who come into contact with newborns need to be informed about issues such as prophylaxis against vitamin K deficiency bleeding, the promotion of breastfeeding, the management of jaundice, the prevention of hypoglycaemia and the implementation of child health screening policies. The occasional baby with a rare medical condition needs identification and a fast track to highly specialized and appropriate services.

Organization and provision of neonatal care

About 10 per cent of all babies are admitted to UK neonatal units, with figures for different hospitals ranging from 4 to 35 per cent. Most of these admissions are for 'special care', for example jaundice requiring phototherapy or blood glucose monitoring. About 2 per cent of babies need full intensive care, mainly because they are born very prematurely and need artificial ventilation for respiratory distress syndrome (RDS). Table 19.1 gives examples taken from the current UK definitions of special care, high dependency care and intensive care. The UK Department of Health reviewed the neonatal service in 2003, and recommended the development of managed care networks. The Department of Health has also expressed government policy in the Maternity

Table 19.1 Categories of babies requiring neonatal care

Level 1 intensive care (maximal intensive care)

Care given in an intensive care nursery that provides continuous supervision by a suitably trained nurse, ideally 1:1, with immediate medical aid available.

Examples of babies who need intensive care are those:

1. receiving any respiratory support via a tracheal tube,
2. who are <29 weeks gestation and, <48 hours old.

Level 2 intensive care (high-dependency intensive care)

Care given in an intensive care nursery that provides care by specially trained nursing staff, who may care for two babies at a time.

Examples of babies who need level 2 intensive care are those:

1. requiring parenteral nutrition,
2. having convulsions,
3. having frequent apnoeic attacks,
4. requiring oxygen treatment and weighing <1500 g.

Special care

Care given in a special care nursery that provides care and treatment exceeding normal routine care. Nurses may care for four babies at a time. Some aspects of special care may be undertaken by a mother supervised by qualified nursing staff

Examples of babies who need special care are those:

1. being tube fed,
2. undergoing phototherapy,
3. receiving special monitoring (for example, frequent glucose or bilirubin estimations).

Normal care

Provided for babies who themselves have no medical reason to be in hospital.

Examples include:

1. maternal psychiatric illness requiring close observation of mother and baby,
2. social problems, such as homelessness.

Source: British Association of Perinatal Medicine.

Services National Service Framework (2004). The current model of neonatal services consists of three levels of care. A level 1 service provides neonatal intensive high dependency care only in an emergency; a level 2 service provides high dependency care and some intensive care, but not for the most extremely preterm babies, and a level 3 service provides all levels of care and is staffed by individuals with no other commitments. Gradually, cooperative perinatal networks are becoming established in the UK, with the goal of equality of access and shared clinical guidelines. Transport services have evolved and most regions now have dedicated specialist teams, a vast improvement on the situation a decade ago. A national neonatal audit programme has been established and the first report was published in 2008.

Delivery room care

The transition from intrauterine to extrauterine life

The vast majority of babies achieve a remarkably smooth transition from intrauterine to extrauterine life, making their first respiratory efforts within 10 seconds of birth. Fetal lungs are filled with 'lung liquid', a fluid that is important for normal lung development and growth. During labour, the production of lung liquid ceases and reabsorption begins. Lung liquid is squeezed out of the thorax during vaginal delivery. Finally, the baby takes his first gasp, establishing an air–liquid interface which moves rapidly down through the lungs. The last vestiges of lung liquid are then absorbed by the lymphatics and the pulmonary capillaries. At the same time as the lungs are filled with air, the blood supply to them increases dramatically. Pulmonary blood flow is low in fetal life because a high resistance is actively maintained in the pulmonary capillaries. Immediately after birth, the pulmonary vascular resistance starts to fall. The fall is driven by the release of vasoactive substances, including prostaglandins and nitric oxide, and by the presence of oxygenated blood in the pulmonary capillaries themselves.

Infants who fail to breathe after birth may do so as a result of a deprivation of oxygen and blood supply to the brain before birth (hypoxia–ischaemia or asphyxia), or because they have a central nervous system or muscle disease, or because they are systemically ill with infection. The possible placental and other mechanisms of hypoxia–ischaemia are discussed in Chapter 10, Pre-eclampsia and other disorders of placentation. Our understanding of the newborn's response to asphyxia is based on the classic primate experiments of Dawes. The changes in respiration and heart rate following asphyxia are illustrated in Figure 19.1. At birth, the asphyxiated infant may have taken his last gasp (terminal apnoea) or be in the phase of primary apnoea. A baby in terminal apnoea is unlikely to recover without intubation and positive-pressure ventilation, whereas a baby in primary apnoea can auto-resuscitate by gasping, and responds quickly to simple resuscitation.

All professionals who attend deliveries must be able to recognize when a baby is not establishing normal respiration and circulation, and be trained to initiate resuscitation. Certain situations are clearly

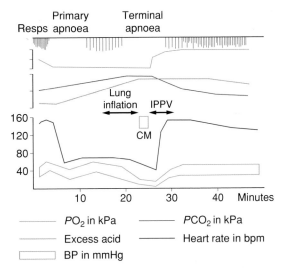

Figure 19.1 The response to asphyxia. (IPPV, intermittent positive-pressure ventilation; CM, cardiac massage.) (Reproduced with permission from the Northern Region handbook.)

high risk, and a person with intubation skills should be present at the delivery. Examples of such situations are given in Table 19.2, but about 20–30 per cent of babies who require resuscitation do not fall into high-risk categories. Our inability to predict which babies will fail to make a successful transition to extrauterine life is the reason why all those who attend deliveries have a responsibility to maintain their neonatal resuscitation skills. In the UK, the Resuscitation Council has developed a Newborn Life Support

Table 19.2 Deliveries at which a trained neonatal resuscitator should be present

Preterm deliveries

Vaginal breech deliveries

Thick meconium staining of the amniotic fluid

Significant fetal distress

Significant antepartum haemorrhage

Serious fetal abnormality (e.g. hydrops, diaphragmatic hernia)

Rotational forceps or vacuum deliveries

Caesarean section – unless elective and under regional anaesthesia

Multiple deliveries

Course, and there are similar such courses in the United States and Europe.

The Apgar score

The Apgar score is a tool which assists in the recognition of an infant who is failing to make a successful transition to extrauterine life. This is exactly what the score was designed to do, and in this respect it performs admirably. The reason for a low Apgar score may not be asphyxia, but the baby certainly has a problem, and the sooner it is recognized and treated the better. The original Apgar score (Table 19.3) includes an item (grimace) that reports the infant's response to a suction catheter. Frequent deep suction of the oropharynx can cause bradycardia, and although regular recording of the Apgar score is to be encouraged, this item carries less weight than the heart rate, colour or breathing pattern. The Apgar score is usually recorded at 1 and 5 minutes. If the Apgar score is still low at 5 minutes, further observations should be made at intervals. The Apgar score cannot replace a detailed narrative describing the baby's condition, the resuscitative efforts and the response to resuscitation. Recording the Apgar score is helpful because it has become an internationally recognized shorthand way of summarizing the condition of babies at birth and their response to resuscitation.

Resuscitation

Babies fall into one of three categories within a minute of birth:

1. A healthy baby; born blue but who cries within seconds, with good tone and activity with a heart rate of more than 100 beats per minute (bpm) and who rapidly turns pink. Leave this baby alone, preferably with his mother. If the baby has been given to you at the resuscitaire, dry him, wrap him in a warm towel and give him back to his mother. Do not suck him out; this risks producing a vagal bradycardia and cools him.

2. Not breathing regularly, but with a heart rate of more than 100 bpm and remaining centrally cyanosed. Dry the baby and place him under a radiant heat source wrapped in a warm, dry towel. Drying often provides enough stimulation to induce breathing, but gentle rubbing can also be used. If there is no response, begin active resuscitation using five 'inflation breaths' via a bag and mask (see below under Lung inflation through a facemask, p. 285), continue with regular breaths, and call for help.

3. Not breathing or has a heart rate of less than 100 bpm or is pale. These babies are usually completely floppy. This baby is in need of prompt resuscitation and will not recover without it. Dry him quickly, place him on the resuscitation surface in a warm, dry towel and call for help. Initiate basic resuscitation with mask ventilation. If the heart rate remains less than 60 bpm, commence chest compressions. If there is not a rapid response, proceed to intubation as soon as a person with the necessary skill arrives. Stay to help; a full-blown resuscitation is a job for at least two people.

Remember that, while time is of the essence in neonatal resuscitation, this is no excuse for rough

Table 19.3 The Apgar score

	Score	0	1	2
A	**A**ppearance: central trunk colour	White or blue all over	Pink with blue extremities	Pink all over
P	**P**ulse rate[a]	Absent	<100 bpm	>100 bpm
G	**G**rimace (response to stimulation)	Nil	Grimace	Cry or cough
A	**A**ctivity (muscle tone)	Limp	Some flexion	Well flexed, active movement
R	**R**espiratory effort	Absent	Gasping or irregular	Regular or strong cry

[a]Best to record the actual rate.

handling or sloppy thermal care. Remember, too, that the parents will be extremely anxious; watch what you say to other team members in their hearing and always spare some time to talk to them as soon as possible. Throwing the laryngoscope down, tipping the flat batteries on the floor and stamping on them may seem appropriate at the time, but will create an image that will never fade from the parents' minds. Even if you intubate the baby within seconds with the reserve laryngoscope, if he does badly, the episode will be replayed time and time again, and if you are unlucky, you may be faced with an unpleasant hour or two facing a cross-examination on your actions.

Further information and a useful algorithm are available from the UK Resuscitation Council (www. resus.org.uk).

Lung inflation through a facemask

Position the baby face upwards on a resuscitation surface; a head-down slope is not necessary. The head should be supported in a neutral position to keep the tongue from obstructing the back of the pharynx: use a small folded towel under the shoulders if it helps. Gently suction the mouth and nostrils to remove debris. Choose a facemask that covers the baby's mouth and nose, but does not press on the eyes or overhang the chin (Figure 19.2a). Hold the mask over the baby's face with one hand, using some of the fingers of the same hand to lift the chin and support the jaw (jaw thrust; Figure 19.2b). Begin to ventilate the lungs with air using the source provided, but never connect a baby directly to the hospital gas supply without a suitable pressure-limiting device in the circuit. Medical gases are supplied at far too high a pressure for babies, who only need a pressure of about $30\,cmH_2O$ to expand their lungs. Make sure the chest is moving with the ventilator breaths and start with about five 'inflation breaths' of $30-35\,cmH_2O$ lasting for 1–2 seconds. Then reduce the pressure to that which is just sufficient to move the chest, usually about $20\,cmH_2O$, and continue to give about 30 breaths per minute.

Chest compression

Babies whose heart rate fails to rise above 60 bpm after a minute or two of effective ventilation should be given chest compression. Seize the baby's thorax with both hands, and place both thumbs over the lower

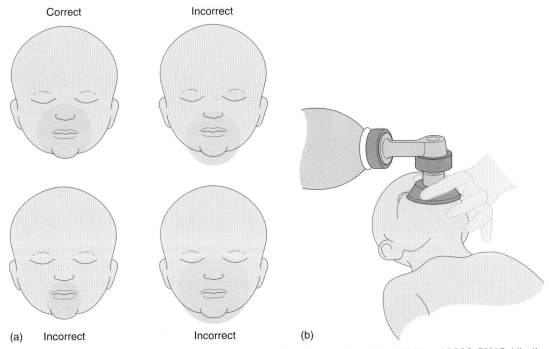

Figure 19.2 Correct use of the facemask. (From *Resuscitation of newborn babies*, 1998. RCPCH and RCOG, BMJ Publications, with permission.)

sternum, just below an imaginary line joining the baby's nipples. Encircle the baby's chest with the rest of both your hands, supporting the spine with your fingers. Press down on the lower sternum sufficiently hard to depress it about one-third of the depth of the baby's chest. Coordinate chest compression with ventilatory breaths and give about 90 compressions to 30 breaths per minute (a ratio of 3:1).

Use of drugs during resuscitation

Drugs are very rarely required during neonatal resuscitation and deciding to use them is a job for an experienced operator. Very occasionally, a baby has depressed respiration because the mother was given pethidine between 1 and 6 hours prior to delivery, and these babies can remain sleepy and reluctant to feed for 24–48 hours. Naloxone (Narcan) is a specific opiate antagonist which can reverse the effects of pethidine and should be given in a dose of 100 mg/kg, which is 0.25 mL/kg of the standard-strength solution. 'Neonatal' Narcan has a concentration of 20 mg/mL and should no longer be used. Naloxone is specifically contraindicated in babies born to drug-abusing mothers.

Failure to respond to resuscitation

Most babies who are depressed at birth respond readily to resuscitative efforts. Before considering whether to abandon resuscitation, check the equipment: check the position and size of the endotracheal tube; give intravenous adrenaline twice and consider giving bicarbonate and glucose. Exclude a pneumothorax, if necessary by needling the chest. Consider giving uncrossmatched O-negative blood if the baby looks pale, because massive feto-maternal haemorrhage, blood loss at delivery or a failure of an adequate placental transfusion due to extreme cord compression can be a reason for birth depression. If there is no cardiac output after about 20 minutes of adequate cardiopulmonary resuscitation, the prognosis for intact survival is grim, and the most senior person present should consider discontinuing resuscitation. If the baby has a heart rate but is not breathing, intensive care should be offered until more information is available.

Ethical issues surrounding resuscitation

This is an area which generates a great deal of anxiety. A junior doctor suddenly faced with a very preterm or abnormal baby is not in the right place at the right time, nor is he or she sufficiently experienced to make a value judgement about the resuscitation of a very preterm or malformed baby. Ideally, this situation should be avoided by prior warning, so that a discussion can be held between the most senior paediatrician available, a senior obstetrician and the parents and, if possible, the staff who will be present at the delivery. After being informed of the chance of intact survival, if the parents do not wish active resuscitation of their baby who will be born at 22 or 23 weeks gestation, or of a severely malformed baby, most neonatologists would support their decision and offer 'comfort care' only. Experience teaches that it is wise to warn the parents beforehand that sometimes there is a surprise and the baby is bigger and more mature than expected, in which case it may be appropriate to offer intensive care on a 'wait and see' basis. If there is not time to consult with the parents beforehand, or there is any conflict or doubt, full resuscitation should be offered. Most tiny babies who die do so very quickly, within 24 hours, and a period of intensive care allows time for the parents to take in the situation and to grieve afterwards because they are certain that 'everything has been done'. This course of action avoids the possibility of anger developing because of doubt about viability remaining in the parents' minds.

Care after resuscitation

Effective resuscitation does not stop once the baby is pink and crying lustily. No matter how well you think the resuscitation has gone, the parents will fear the worst and a full explanation is crucial. Consider whether the baby needs admission to the neonatal unit for observation, or further investigation and treatment for possible sepsis. Use all available information such as the cardiotocogram (CTG), the cord pH, the maternal history and a history of the labour to make a decision about further management. The first seizure in hypoxic–ischaemic encephalopathy often occurs after 12 hours, which makes early discharge risky after resuscitation has been required.

Care of the normal term newborn baby

Examination

A thorough physical examination of every neonate is accepted as good practice and forms a core item of

Table 19.4 Prevalence of serious congenital malformations per 1000 live births in England and Wales

Malformation	Prevalence
Congenital heart disease	6–8
Developmental dysplasia of the hip	1.5
Talipes	1.5
Down's syndrome	1.5
Cleft lip and/or palate	1.2
Urogenital (hypospadias, undescended testes)	1.2
Spina bifida/anencephaly	0.5

Source: Office for National Statistics.

the child health surveillance programme in the United Kingdom. There are national minimum standards for the newborn physical examination, which should be performed within 72 hours of birth. The aims of the neonatal examination are:

- diagnosis of congenital malformations (present in about 10–15 per 1000 babies; see Table 19.4);
- diagnosis of common minor problems, with advice about management or appropriate reassurance if no intervention is indicated (e.g. Mongolian blue spots, jaundice, naevi);
- continuing screening, begun antenatally, to identify those babies who should be offered specific intervention, e.g. hepatitis vaccination;
- health education advice, e.g. regarding breastfeeding, cot death prevention, immunization, safe transport in cars;
- general parental reassurance.

For some babies, early diagnosis may make an enormous difference to their subsequent health, for example in congenital cataract and urethral valves. For others, parental reassurance that their infant is normal and general advice are all that is required. Every newborn baby deserves at least one full examination. At present, this is usually carried out by a doctor, although in some areas midwives are being trained to perform this task. For recording purposes, it is useful to have a checklist printed or stamped in the baby's notes to serve as an aide-memoire. Items are merely ticked if normal, but any abnormalities are marked distinctively and a full description written out. The examination should be dated and signed. A suggested order for the examination is as follows:

- Introduce yourself to the mother, ask her about any antenatally diagnosed problems that may need follow up, and any family problems (deafness, dislocation of hips). Check for risk factors that predispose to neonatal sepsis, such as pyrexia in labour.
- Remove the baby's clothes except the nappy; look at the skin.
- Feel the anterior fontanelle for tension (leave until later if the baby is crying!); palpate the sutures (craniosynostosis is a disorder with premature fusion of the sutures); check the scalp for swellings (a cephalhaematoma is the most common).
- Measure the head circumference.
- Look at the face for colour (cyanosis/pallor/jaundice) or any peculiarities.
- Listen to the heart and estimate the heart rate – normally 110–150 bpm, but can drop to 80 bpm in sleep.
- Count the respiratory rate – normally less than 60 breaths per minute. The lungs can also be auscultated, but this is seldom informative.
- Palpate the abdomen, feeling for masses, including large bladder or kidneys.
- Examine the eyes, checking that it is possible to obtain a red reflex using an ophthalmoscope to exclude cataract. Fundal examination is not routine.
- Examine the ears, nose and mouth (cleft palate).
- Examine the neck, including the clavicles.
- Examine the arms, hands, legs and feet.
- Remove the nappy.
- Feel for the femoral pulses.
- Examine the genitalia and anus.
- Turn the baby to the prone position and examine his back and spine; assess tone.
- Return the infant to the supine position and evaluate the central nervous system.
- Examine the hips.
- Make sure you have not omitted anything.

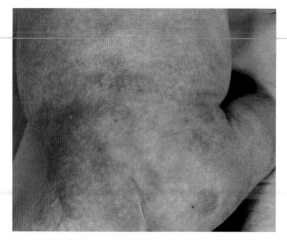

Figure 19.3 Erythema toxicum

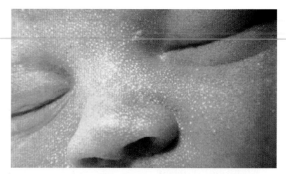

Figure 19.4 Milia. (From *A colour atlas of the newborn*, Milner RDS, Herber SM, 1994. Wolfe Medical Publications, with permission.)

Diagnosis of common minor problems

Erythema toxicum

Erythema toxicum (Figure 19.3) is a common rash which usually appears on the second or third day, and takes the form of a white pinpoint 'head' on an oval erythematous base. If the spots are biopsied, massive numbers of eosinophils are found. The rash rarely lasts for more than a few days and is harmless.

Transient neonatal pustular melanosis

This disorder is common in Afro-Caribbean babies. The eruption starts with small, pustule-like spots present soon after birth, which rapidly progress to a hyperpigmented macule resembling a freckle, which fades in a few weeks.

Milia

Milia (Figure 19.4) are tiny, yellowish-white spots, especially common on the nose and elsewhere on the face, which disappear spontaneously over a month or two. They represent retention cysts of the pilosebaceous follicles.

Mongolian blue spots

Blue spots are blue-black macular lesions, usually situated over the base of the spine and commoner in Afro-Carribean or Asian infants (Figure 19.5). They fade slowly over the first few years.

Port wine stains

Port wine stains are due to a malformation of the capillaries within the dermis. Port wine stains in

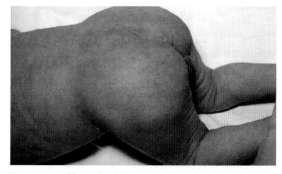

Figure 19.5 Mongolian blue spot. (From *A colour atlas of the newborn*, Milner RDS, Herber SM, 1994. Wolfe Medical Publications, with permission.)

the region of the trigeminal nerve are sometimes associated with intracranial vascular abnormalities (Sturge–Weber syndrome). Laser therapy can now produce an excellent cosmetic improvement for large facial lesions.

Skin tags/extra digits

These should be surgically removed; the old practice of tying a silk thread around them produces a cosmetically inferior result. As these are often familial, examination of the parents may provide proof of this.

Spinal birthmarks and sacral pits

Simple midline dimples are common and are not associated with spinal abnormalities. About 5 per cent of babies have some sort of dorsal cutaneous stigmata. Dimples that are large (>5 mm diameter) or high on the back (more than 2.5 cm from the anus) or that occur in combination with other lesions, such as haemangiomas, skin tags, hairy patches or subcutaneous masses, should arouse suspicion and are an indication for further investigation with ultrasound and/or magnetic resonance imaging (MRI) of the spinal cord. The consequences of missing a lesion that will cause cord tethering or infection can be disastrous.

Genitalia

The foreskin of a male baby cannot be retracted, and it is normal for it to remain non-retractile for up to four years. Both testes are usually in the scrotum at term, but it is common for them to be retractile. Bilateral undescended testes is an indication for review by a senior paediatrician; babies with a unilateral undescended testis can be reviewed at the 6-week check.

Scrotal swelling can be due to a hydrocele, inguinal hernia, trauma following breech delivery or torsion of the testis. Neonatal torsion is usually a prenatal event, and emergency surgery cannot save testicular function. However, many paediatric surgeons believe that it is important to fix the contralateral testis in this situation. If no gonads can be felt in the inguinal region, and the phallus is small (the usual neonatal penis is 3 cm stretched length), the baby may be a female baby with congenital adrenal hyperplasia and urgent investigation is vital to avoid a collapse due to salt loss. If there are palpable gonads and there is a small phallus, the baby is likely to be an under-virilized male wherever the urethral opening is, but it is best not to make any assumptions prior to full investigation.

In female babies, hymenal tags and small amounts of vaginal bleeding are common.

Danger signs in the well-baby nursery

The vast majority of normal babies remain perfectly well and establish feeds, while their mothers quickly take on full responsibility for their care. The challenge for healthcare professionals is to spot the baby who is developing a serious illness in order to try to avert a collapse. This can be difficult: the baby who is passed as fit for discharge in the morning can deteriorate so rapidly that he requires ventilation and inotropic support by tea-time. Conditions that can cause such a dramatic deterioration include congenital heart disease (coarctation or hypoplastic left heart

syndrome), sepsis, inborn error of metabolism, necrotizing enterocolitis or a gut volvulus, and intracranial haemorrhage.

Danger signs include:

- temperature instability;
- a change in activity, including refusal of feed or having to be wakened for feeds;
- unusual skin colour, mottling, extreme pallor, jaundice on the first day;
- an abnormal heart rate or respiratory rate, including grunting or fast breathing;
- apnoea;
- excessive jitteriness or abnormal stereotyped, repetitive movement patterns;
- delayed stooling (beyond 48 hours) or completely dry nappies;
- abdominal distension, green vomit (bilious until proved otherwise);
- odd lumps or swellings;
- lethargy, floppiness; paucity of movement, excessive sleeping.

Any of these should prompt a thorough re-examination of the baby, and if a deviation from normality is confirmed, the safest course of action is to admit the baby to the neonatal unit and initiate investigation and treatment, including a screen for infection and antibiotic treatment, without delay.

Screening for important neonatal conditions

Developmental dysplasia of the hip

The incidence of developmental dysplasia of the hip (DDH) is about 1–2 per 1000 births, but about 5–20 per 1000 babies have unstable hips in the neonatal period. Girls are affected more often than boys, in a ratio of 5:1. Expert management of DDH diagnosed in the neonatal period can be expected to produce a normal hip, while treatment initiated after the first six months of life undoubtedly gives much worse results, even after prolonged and aggressive surgical treatment. While it is not possible to detect all cases using the current screening methods, this should not be used as an excuse for a poor-quality screening programme. The cornerstone of the screening strategy for DDH remains a careful history and clinical examination, using the Ortolani–Barlow manoeuvres. These tests are difficult to describe in words and are best taught by demonstration. Unfortunately, despite initial confidence in the ability of the Ortolani and Barlow tests to detect DDH, the number of cases diagnosed late (0.2 per 1000) has not reduced. Some dislocated hips are not detectable with clinical examination in the newborn period and others may dislocate later, perhaps due to a shallow acetabulum which progresses to dislocation when weight-bearing begins.

Ultrasonography can now be added to clinical examination as a further tool for detecting DDH. Ultrasound can detect clinically stable but anatomically abnormal hips, and show normality in clinically suspect hips. Developmental dysplasia of the hip is more common following breech presentation, in females, if there is oligohydramnios, and in those with a positive family history. The NIPE (newborn and infant physical examination) programme recommends ultrasound at 6 weeks for babies with a positive Ortolani–Barlow test, or a positive family history or who were a breech presentation. Some hospitals offer hip ultrasound examinations to other selected high-risk groups (Table 19.5); few have the manpower for universal screening.

Hypoglycaemia

Healthy term babies of appropriate weight who are breastfed have lower blood glucose concentrations than formula-fed babies in the first 2–3 days of life. They also have raised ketone body concentrations and the neonatal brain can use ketone bodies as an alternative fuel. Healthy, normally grown term babies who are breastfeeding well do not need to have their blood glucose concentrations measured for screening purposes. There is no agreement on the lower limit of the normal range in this situation, bedside testing with reagent strips is notoriously inaccurate, and there is no evidence that a lower limit exists below which asymptomatic 'hypoglycaemia' is damaging. Recognition of these facts makes the use of supplementary feeding less likely and encourages breastfeeding.

However, there are undoubtedly babies who are at high risk of developing symptomatic hypoglycaemia and for whom screening is appropriate (Table 19.6). Babies who are at the highest risk are those whose growth has been restricted *in utero* and those born to diabetic mothers. Occasionally, an apparently healthy term baby has a rare condition such as idiopathic hyperinsulinaemic hypoglycaemia of infancy (formerly called neisidioblastosis) or medium chain acyl coenzyme A dehydrogenase (MCADD) deficiency, which will manifest as symptomatic hypoglycaemia in the first days of life. Very rarely, a healthy baby becomes hypoglycaemic from breast milk insufficiency. In these situations, prolonged symptomatic hypoglycaemia can occur, and this can be brain damaging (see the case history below). A balance needs to struck between screening for and prevention of symptomatic hypoglycaemia in at-risk infants with recognition of symptomatic hypoglycaemia in infants who are ill, while avoiding

Table 19.5 Screening strategy for using ultrasound in the detection of developmental dysplasia of the hip

- Breech presentation (whether delivered by Caesarean section or vaginally)
- Family history of dysplastic hip
- Any deformity suggesting intrauterine compression, or oligohydramnios
- Clicky hip on clinical examination, or one with restricted abduction
- If sufficient manpower is available, consider firstborn females

Table 19.6 Infants at risk of developing symptomatic hypoglycaemia

Infants with fetal growth restriction
Infants of diabetic mothers
Preterm infants
Infants who have experienced significant hypoxia in labour
Infants who are 'large for dates' – possibility of undiagnosed maternal gestational diabetes

CASE HISTORY

Baby John was born at term to a 35-year-old primigravida who went into spontaneous labour. The admission CTG was normal, but later showed reduced baseline variability, and an emergency Caesarean section was carried out. John weighed 2.76 kg (third centile) and was in good condition, with Apgar scores of 7[1] and 9[5]. He was transferred to the post-natal ward.

He fed hungrily at first, taking both breast and formula feeds. At the age of about 55 hours, John refused a feed and became floppy. His temperature had fallen to 35.5°C. He was placed in an incubator, but took only 15 mL of formula and remained floppy. His dextrostix was low, and overnight he remained floppy, cyanosed and intermittently jittery; a 10 per cent dextrose infusion was in place at a rate equivalent to 6 mg/kg per minute. John then developed seizures and required increased amounts of dextrose to maintain his glucose levels.

He has significant disability at follow up, with visual impairment and developmental delay. MRI of his brain showed changes considered to be characteristic of those seen as a result of hypoglycaemic damage at term. John's parents recently succeeded in obtaining substantial damages on his behalf.

Signs of hypoglycaemia in the newborn are vague and include apathy/floppiness, apnoea and excessive jitteriness (see above under Danger signs in the well-baby nursery, p. 289). These non-specific signs can also be due to sepsis. A term baby of normal weight who is sleepy needs help to feed directly from the breast or to be given expressed breast milk or formula from a cup or bottle. However, if the signs are more than just sleepiness, worsen or persist, the baby must be examined fully by a paediatrician, and investigations to exclude sepsis and/or hypoglycaemia should be considered. Checking a glucose level in this situation is not an excuse for omitting a proper examination. Early jaundice, fever, marked floppiness, tachypnoea and poor capillary refill are indications for investigation and treatment. If a low glucose is confirmed, the diagnosis is symptomatic hypoglycaemia until proven otherwise. This is an emergency, and intravenous glucose must be given without delay. Blood samples for true glucose, insulin and ketone body levels should be collected at the same time as commencing an intravenous infusion of 10 per cent dextrose. Boluses of dextrose should be avoided, and restricted to 'mini-boluses' of 3 mL/kg of 10 per cent dextrose to avoid rebound hypoglycaemia.

Hypoglycaemia in at-risk babies (see Table 19.6) should be prevented by screening and supplementary feeding. Small-for-dates babies can require as much as 12 mg/kg per minute to maintain glucose levels. Asymptomatic hypoglycaemia is managed with an increase in feeds in the first instance, with recourse to intravenous treatment only if the baby cannot tolerate feeds, symptoms develop or the hypoglycaemia persists.

over-investigation and over-treatment in the normal term baby whose mother is trying to establish breastfeeding.

Phenylketonuria

Screening for phenylketonuria (1 in 13 000 infants) using dried blood spots collected on to filter paper (the Guthrie test) was introduced in 1969. Milk feeds need to be established first, and midwives collect blood by heel prick on the 5th–9th day of life, posting the cards to the laboratory.

Hypothyroidism

The same system was expanded to include a screen for congenital hypothyroidism (1 in 3000) from 1981. Audit of the programme shows that it has been extremely successful and picks up far more cases then were suspected clinically at a much earlier stage in life. Virtually all infants with congenital hypothyroidism now start treatment by 28 days of age, and have a better IQ as a result.

Cystic fibrosis and other screens

All babies born in England are now screened for cystic fibrosis, which affects around 1 in 2500. The screen uses immunoreactive trypsin (IRT). There are over 1000 different mutations identified, but the most common genetic defect in the UK is DF508, which is present in over 90 per cent of cases. All newborn babies are now also offered hearing screening. Screening for sickle-cell disease and MCADD is now universal (www.screening.nhs.uk).

Specific geographical areas offer screening for haemoglobinopathies such a thalassaemia. Tests are also available for a host of other rare conditions, including maple syrup urine disease, homocystinuria, tyrosinaemia, biotinidase deficiency, galactosaemia, MCADD, Duchenne muscular dystrophy, fragile X syndrome and congenital adrenal hyperplasia, but none has been implemented in the UK. Widespread screening for neonatal neuroblastoma using VMA levels in urine did not prove cost effective in Canada and seems unlikely to be introduced worldwide, apart from in Japan, where the incidence is particularly high. Useful information on the UK screening programme is available on the following website: www.screening.nhs.uk.

Prophylaxis and prevention of disease in the well newborn

Prevention of vitamin K deficiency bleeding (haemorrhagic disease of the newborn)

Vitamin K deficiency bleeding (VKDB) occurs in three forms:

1. Very early VKDB: this is limited to babies whose mothers have taken drugs that interfere with the manufacture of vitamin K-dependent clotting factors, such as antituberculous or anticonvulsant drugs.

2. Classical VKDB presents on days 2–7 of life, with bleeding from the umbilical stump, bruising or melaena. The mortality of classical VKDB is low, and the disorder can be prevented by a single dose of vitamin K, given to the baby by any route.

3. Late VKDB occurs virtually exclusively in babies who are breastfed, unless they have liver disease. Small warning bleeds from the gum are a common feature, but the worst problems are associated with the high (50 per cent) chance of intracranial haemorrhage, which can cause permanent neurological handicap.

Late-onset VKDB can be prevented by a single intramuscular dose of vitamin K given at birth, but a single oral dose is ineffective. The UK Department of Health has recently endorsed two alternative regimens: either a single dose of intramuscular vitamin K (Konakion MM) or repeated oral doses. If oral vitamin K is chosen, the Department of Health recommends that two doses of Konakion MM be given orally in the first week, with a third dose at a month if the baby is breastfed. What is clear is that all infants must be offered vitamin K prophylaxis and there is no longer any place for selective regimens. If parents refuse vitamin K for their baby after counselling, the reasons for the refusal should be clearly documented.

Confirmation of the diagnosis of VKDB is obtained from coagulation tests, which show a normal platelet count and prolonged thrombin and prothrombin times. Treatment is with intravenous vitamin K and fresh frozen plasma.

Screening for group B streptococcus to prevent early-onset disease

Group B streptococcus (GBS) is the most frequent cause of severe early-onset infection in newborn babies, with a 10 per cent mortality and a risk of deafness or cerebral palsy in survivors that may be as high as 40–50 per cent. Early-onset GBS disease is often preventable. There can be no doubt about the effectiveness of intrapartum prophylaxis with high-dose intravenous penicillin (3 g).

The incidence of early-onset GBS disease has declined from about 1.5 to 0.5 cases per 1000 in the United States since the adoption of guidelines proposed by the Communicable Disease Center (CDC; Figure 19.6). Two alternative strategies exist. In the first, intrapartum antibiotic prophylaxis is offered to women identified as GBS carriers through prenatal screening cultures collected at 35–37 weeks gestation, and to women who develop premature onset of labour or rupture of membranes before the screening is done. In the second, intrapartum

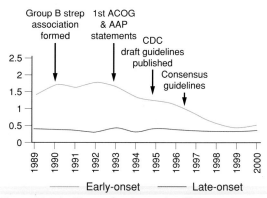

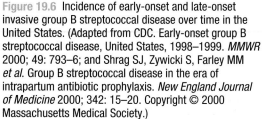

Figure 19.6 Incidence of early-onset and late-onset invasive group B streptococcal disease over time in the United States. (Adapted from CDC. Early-onset group B streptococcal disease, United States, 1998–1999. *MMWR* 2000; 49: 793–6; and Shrag SJ, Zywicki S, Farley MM *et al.* Group B streptococcal disease in the era of intrapartum antibiotic prophylaxis. *New England Journal of Medicine* 2000; 342: 15–20. Copyright © 2000 Massachusetts Medical Society.)

antibiotic prophylaxis is provided to women who have one or more risk conditions at the time of labour or membrane rupture. Screening is not done. Both are in use in different parts of the world, although the US CDC now firmly recommends screening. In the UK, the Royal College of Obstetricians and Gynaecologists (RCOG) has issued a guideline recommending that intrapartum antibiotic prophylaxis is offered to women with risk factors.

Jaundice and prevention of kernicterus

At least two-thirds of all babies develop visible jaundice in the first week of life, and jaundice is a common reason for readmission to hospital at this time. Jaundice in this group reflects the immaturity of the liver's excretory pathway for bilirubin at a time of heightened production. In healthy term infants, bilirubin rises over the first few days, and jaundice is not apparent on the first day of life. Any visible jaundice in the first 24 hours must be urgently investigated, and assumed to be due to haemolysis (rhesus incompatibility, ABO incompatibility, glucose 6-phosphate dehydrogenase (G6PD) deficiency) until proved otherwise. Neonatal 'physiological' jaundice is contributed to by a high neonatal haematocrit, short red cell survival, breastfeeding and an initial absence of gut bacteria. Although neonatal jaundice is usually benign, it is a dangerous fallacy to assume that healthy term newborns are immune from kernicterus (yellow staining of the basal ganglia by bilirubin; Figure 19.7). Survivors are severely handicapped by athetoid cerebral palsy, classically with accompanying sensorineural deafness, paralysis of up-gaze and dental enamel dysplasia. The level of unconjugated bilirubin at which kernicterus can occur in well term infants is not known with certainty, but appears to lie somewhere between 425 and 600 μmol/L. A level above 425 μmol/L is reached by only 1 in 770 normal term infants. The risk of kernicterus is probably greater for an infant of 37 weeks compared to one of 41 weeks gestation (see the case history below).

The key to successful kernicterus prevention lies in detecting the very few healthy (usually breastfed) babies who are likely to develop a serum unconjugated bilirubin of more than 425 mmol/L, and in paying careful attention to bilirubin levels in moderately preterm babies (34–36 weeks). Babies

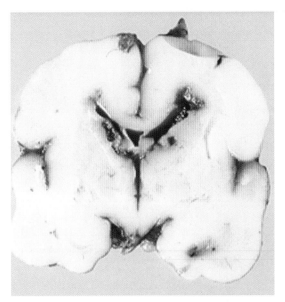

Figure 19.7 Autopsy specimen showing the yellow staining of kernicterus in the basal ganglia of the brain of a baby

'track' for serum bilirubin, so that an infant who is on the 50th centile at 48 hours (136 μmol/L) will not develop a 'dangerous level unless a new complication develops or he has an undiagnosed haemolytic disease (Figure 19.8). However, a baby with a similar level at 24 hours is already tracking along the 95th centile and needs a repeat estimation. Such a baby is not suitable for early discharge unless the parents are willing to return to the hospital for a check to be done.

All those who come into contact with babies in the first week of life need education about the assessment of jaundice. All too often, the early signs of bilirubin encephalopathy (lethargy, irritability, poor suck, shrill cry) are ignored. Assessing the level of jaundice from clinical examination can be difficult, especially in Afro-Caribbean and Asian babies. Various transcutaneous bilirubinometers are available and these devices assist in reducing the traffic of blood samples (and babies) to and from maternity hospitals. Phototherapy, used correctly, is a remarkably effective treatment and is capable of converting a fifth of the circulating unconjugated bilirubin to harmless photoisomers within a few hours. The National Institute for Health and Clinical Excellence (NICE) has developed a guideline for the management of neonatal jaundice which is available from their website.

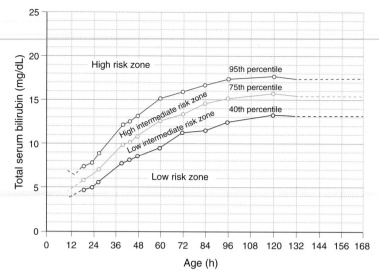

Figure 19.8 Hour specific bilirubin values from more than 13 000 healthy babies. Conversion of mg/dL to mmol/L requires multiplication by 17.1. (From Bhutani VK, Honson L, Sivieri MS, 1999. Predictive ability of a predischarge hour specific serum bilirubin for subsequent significant hyperbilirubinemia in healthy term and near term newborns. Reproduced with permission from *Pediatrics*, vol. 103, pages 6–14, copyright 1999.)

CASE HISTORY

Baby Kieran was born normally at 35 weeks gestation weighing 2.7 kg. His mother had gone into labour following preterm rupture of the membranes. He was in excellent condition at birth, with Apgar scores of 9[1] and 9[5] and a cord pH of 7.34. He required no resuscitation and went to the post-natal ward with his mother.

The midwives noticed jaundice for the first time when he was about 28 hours old. The bilirubin was checked 24 hours later and was 279 mmol/L. On the following day, Kieran was examined by the same doctor, who thought the jaundice was unchanged and discharged him home.

Kieran and his mother were visited at home by midwives, who reassured his young, first-time mother that his jaundice was not serious and no further bilirubin levels were measured. On the 8th day, his concerned parents took him to the local paediatric casualty department, where he was noted to be very jaundiced, cool and feeding poorly. Blood was taken in the accident and emergency department, which revealed a serum bilirubin level of 570 mmol/L. Kieran was admitted to the ward, where the following morning he was noted to be irritable, tense on handling and to be extending his neck (opisthotonus). An exchange transfusion was performed, but Kieran is disabled with deafness and athetoid cerebral palsy. He was awarded substantial damages after a successful claim of medical negligence.

Screening for cardiac disease

Early diagnosis of congenital heart disease is important because many of these lesions are now amenable to surgery, and because prostaglandin infusion can be used to keep the ductus arteriosus patent in babies whose lesion is duct dependent. The detection of significant cardiac disease is, like many other screening procedures, bedevilled by false-negative and false-positive results. Innocent murmurs are very common in babies, and yet many babies with seriously malformed hearts have no murmur at all.

Screening begins in the antenatal period, with increasing use of a four-chamber view of the heart as standard at 18–20 weeks. The fetus whose scan is abnormal is referred for detailed specialized scanning, and many diagnoses are now made this way. However, it is not possible to detect all congenital heart disease with antenatal scanning.

Heart disease in the neonate presents as cyanosis, shock, heart failure, or with the finding of a murmur or absent femoral pulses. Cyanosis can be surprisingly easy to miss, and recently it has been suggested that all babies could be 'screened' with pulse oximetry. While this is not yet of proven value, pulse oximetry is easy to use and should be carried out if there is any doubt

Table 19.7 The WHO ten steps to successful breastfeeding

1. Have a written breastfeeding policy that is routinely communicated to all healthcare staff
2. Train all healthcare staff in the skills necessary to implement this policy
3. Inform all pregnant women about the benefits and management of breastfeeding
4. Help mothers initiate breastfeeding within half an hour of birth
5. Show mothers how to breastfeed and how to maintain lactation even if they are separated from their infants
6. Give newborn infants no food or drink other than breast milk unless medically indicated
7. Practise rooming-in (allow mothers and infants to stay together) 24 hours a day
8. Encourage breastfeeding on demand
9. Give no artificial teats or pacifiers (also called dummies or soothers) to breastfeeding infants
10. Foster the establishment of breastfeeding support groups and refer mothers to them on discharge from the hospital or clinic

about the baby's colour. Innocent murmurs have several features.

- The murmur is mid-systolic, grade 1–2/6 and best heard at the left sternal edge.
- There are no audible clicks.
- The pulses are normal.
- The baby is otherwise well.

Suspicious features mean that the baby should remain in hospital and an early opinion from an expert should be sought. Neither a chest x-ray nor an electrocardiogram (ECG) assists in distinguishing an innocent murmur from one caused by significant heart disease, and they are no longer routinely performed in all babies with murmurs. Slow feeding, grunting, sweatiness and poor weight gain in spite of adequate feeding suggest heart failure and the baby must not be discharged.

Infant feeding

Breastfeeding

Breast milk is the ideal food for babies for the first 4–6 months of life. Human milk contains the carbohydrate lactose, and the proteins casein, alpha-lactalbumin, immunoglobulin and lactoferrin. Human milk is whey predominant (60:40 whey:casein ratio) and is easily digested. Lactoferrin combines with other anti-infective agents such as lysozyme, and the overall effect is to ensure that breastfed babies are well protected from gastrointestinal and other infections. The fat in human milk is predominantly unsaturated and there are long-chain polyunsaturated fatty acids that may provide important precursors for the infant's nervous system. Cow's milk contains much more protein than human milk (3.5 versus 1 g/dL), the protein is casein predominant and the whey protein differs from that of human milk (beta-lactoglobulin not alpha-lactalbumin). Casein is the constituent of milk that forms a curd precipitate with acid.

There is a delay of 48 hours before copious milk secretion begins in women. This is unusual; in all animals except guinea-pigs, lactogenesis takes place within hours of parturition. Lactogenesis is initiated by the slowly falling progesterone levels in the presence of a high prolactin concentration. In an attempt to reverse the trend away from breastfeeding, the World Health Organization (WHO) has proposed 'ten steps' as a core item of its Baby Friendly Hospital Initiative (Table 19.7). This programme has been very successful; for example, neonatal infection was reduced from 23 to 3.4 per cent in one Romanian hospital. In the United Kingdom, the latest national infant feeding survey was conducted in 2005, and found that only 35 per cent of UK babies were exclusively breastfed at a week of age. There is still a clear association with socioeconomic status, with 88 per cent of mothers in professional or managerial occupations initiating breastfeeding compared to

65 per cent of those in routine or manual occupations. Only 51 per cent of mothers aged less than 20 initiated breastfeeding. There is still a high drop-out rate, with a fifth giving up within a fortnight, citing painful nipples and the baby rejecting the breast as reasons.

Formula feeding

Modern formula milks are adjusted (humanized) so that the protein content and the whey:casein ratio are nearer those of human milk. Manufacturers do this by adding demineralized whey (from cheese production) and lactose, but differences in the fatty acid and amino acid composition remain, and formula milk cannot contain any of the anti-infective agents. There is no evidence to support the claim that formulae with a higher casein content are more 'satisfying' for 'the hungry and demanding baby'. Additives are required to emulsify and thicken the milk. Water is required to reconstitute milk powder. Some products sold as 'natural mineral water' contain unacceptably high levels of sodium and nitrate for babies and are unsuitable for rehydrating dried formula milk.

Unmodified 'doorstep' cow's milk, sheep's and goat's milk are completely unsuitable foods for babies less than a year old. The electrolyte composition is vastly different from that of human milk and they are highly allergenic. Soy formulae have no lactose, the carbohydrate being derived from corn syrup and sucrose. Soy protein is nutritionally inferior to human milk protein and infants grow less well on soy milk. The only reason to use soy formula is if the infant has a cow's milk allergy or requires a lactose-free formula.

Care of the ill term newborn baby

A brief description of a few of the more common and serious illnesses that afflict term newborns follows. For more detail, consult standard texts.

Birth trauma

Birth trauma is fortunately rare in modern neonatal practice, but occasional cases are still encountered.

Brachial plexus palsy (Erb's palsy)

Brachial plexus palsy is caused by damage to the brachial plexus, which does not always occur during

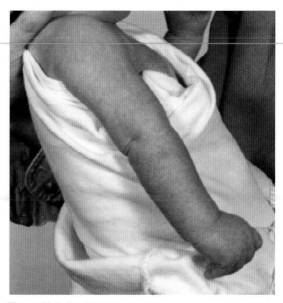

Figure 19.9 Brachial plexus palsy.

birth; cases have been described in babies born by Caesarean section. However, it is more common in large babies, particularly those whose delivery is complicated by shoulder dystocia. A brachial plexus lesion is revealed by lack of movement in the arm; initially the arm is flaccid. After 48 hours, an upper palsy can be distinguished from a complete palsy. In an upper root palsy (C5, C6, sometimes C7) the arm is internally rotated and pronated, there is no active abduction or elbow flexion (the waiter's tip position; Figure 19.9). In a complete palsy of upper and lower roots, the arm is flail; there may be a ptosis and a Horner's syndrome due to damage to the stellate ganglion adjacent to C8 and T1. Phrenic nerve palsy should be considered in these cases. While the prognosis of brachial plexus lesions is generally good, with most series reporting an initial recovery rate of 75–95 per cent, a recent study of the long-term effects revealed a surprisingly high incidence of later problems in childhood. The results of surgical nerve repair have improved markedly since the early days, and babies who have no recovery in biceps function by three months should be referred to a specialist.

Subgaleal (subaponeurotic) haemorrhage

The subaponeurotic space is potentially very large, lying as it does outside the skull and below the scalp. Babies who bleed into this space can become shocked, and there is a mortality of 20 per cent. The condition is fortunately rare after normal vertex vaginal delivery, but is reported in as many as 6 per 1000 babies delivered by the ventouse. Increasing use of the ventouse apparatus means that early recognition of subgaleal haemorrhage has become more important. The clue to the diagnosis is a boggy swelling of the scalp that crosses suture lines. The baby's head circumference will have increased at least 1 cm from the birth measurement if there is a sizeable subaponeurotic collection. When appropriately recognized and treated with blood transfusion, the long-term prognosis is good.

Transient tachypnoea of the newborn

Transient tachypnoea of the newborn (TTN) is the most common respiratory disease of term infants, occurring in 4 per 1000. The disease is due to delayed clearance of lung liquid and is much more common after Caesarean section delivery, particularly without labour. At term, the incidence falls between 37 and 40 weeks (Figure 19.10), and this finding has implications for the timing of elective Caesarean section at term. Fortunately, the disease is usually mild, but sometimes requires intubation and ventilation, with the associated risk of complications.

Meconium aspiration syndrome

Meconium aspiration syndrome (MAS) is a disease of post-term pregnancies, with an incidence of about 1:1000 total births in Europe and 2–6 per 1000 in the United States. Meconium can be aspirated before or after birth. The coexistence of asphyxia is the main determining factor in MAS; asphyxia exerts its own detrimental effect on lung function and is associated with the development of persistent pulmonary hypertension, which complicates the treatment of MAS still further. These problems, together with a pre-existing aspiration of meconium into the airway that is not amenable to even the most aggressive suctioning at delivery, combine to make MAS a very serious neonatal illness.

The fact that some cases cannot be prevented by tracheal toilet should not discourage attempts at preventing meconium entering the airway at birth. Suctioning of the baby's oropharynx when only the head has been delivered is no longer recommended, but the airways should be cleared of meconium after birth. Meconium in the airway creates a ball-valve effect in which air can be sucked past the obstruction

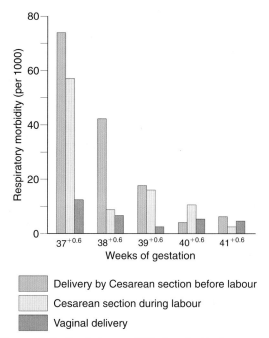

Figure 19.10 Respiratory morbidity (transient tachypnoea of the newborn plus respiratory distress syndrome) at term in infants admitted to the Neonatal Intensive Care Unit, Rosie Maternity Hospital, Cambridge, by each week of gestation and mode of delivery. (From Morrison JJ, Rennie JM, Milton P, 1995. Neonatal respiratory morbidity and mode of delivery at term: influence of timing of elective caesarean section. *British Journal of Obstetrics and Gynaecology* 102: 101–6, with permission.)

but not exhaled past it, and the substance acts as a chemical irritant to the airways.

Persistent pulmonary hypertension

The term persistent pulmonary hypertension of the newborn (PPHN) is preferable to that of persistent fetal circulation, because the placenta is no longer in the circuit. In this disorder, the baby is cyanosed because there is a failure of the usual rapid post-natal fall in pulmonary vascular resistance. There is no parenchymal lung disease, but the pulmonary capillaries are structurally abnormal, possessing excess smooth muscle that persists into smaller branches than usual. PPHN can occur as a primary disorder or as a complication of asphyxia, infection (such as GBS) or pulmonary hypoplasia. The diagnosis should be suspected in a baby who remains hypoxic in 100 per cent oxygen and whose chest x-ray is normal. Echocardiography confirms the right-to-left shunt at atrial and/or ductal level and excludes congenital heart disease from the differential diagnosis. Nitric oxide has recently been confirmed as effective treatment for PPHN and is now the therapy of choice if warmth, artificial ventilation, oxygen and/or alkali therapy do not succeed in correcting the acidosis.

Hypoxic–ischaemic encephalopathy

Seizures are the hallmark of this condition, and hypoxic–ischaemic encephalopathy (HIE) is the most common cause of early-onset seizures in a term baby. There are many other causes of neonatal seizure, for example meningitis, stroke and hypoglycaemia. A diagnosis of HIE should be considered when there is a combination of:

- fetal distress;
- birth depression (low Apgar score requiring resuscitation);
- metabolic acidosis on cord pH or an early neonatal sample;
- seizures;
- renal impairment (blood in the urine and a low urine output);
- alteration of central nervous system state – the baby is not normally conscious between seizures, but is irritable or lethargic with abnormal primitive reflexes.

The diagnosis should be supported by checking serum creatinine, calcium and glucose, performing a lumbar puncture to exclude meningitis, and carrying out a cranial ultrasound scan. This scan may be normal or show a loss of the gyral pattern with obliterated ventricles, suggesting cerebral oedema. Early electroencephalography (EEG) often confirms electrical seizure activity, and the background pattern can help in prognosis: a normal background, even in the presence of frequent seizures, is reassuring, whereas a very depressed or deteriorating background is an indication of a poor prognosis. An MRI scan, if available, is another investigation that confirms the diagnosis and helps in prognostication. Babies who are depressed at birth and who remain encephalopathic can be referred to a specialist centre for consideration of therapeutic hypothermia. Hypothermia has to be initiated within 6 hours to be effective, and is not yet a standard of care – results of several large trials are awaited.

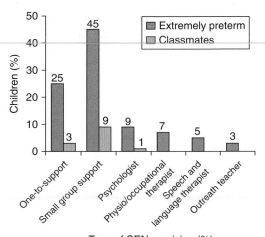

Figure 19.11   Special educational needs of the EPICURE cohort (courtesy of Professor Neil Marlow). (From Johnson S et al. 2009. *Archives of Disease in Childhood. Fetal and Neonatal edition* 94: F283–9, with permission.)

Management of the preterm infant

The prognosis for preterm infants has improved dramatically over the last 30 years, with survival rates for infants delivered beyond 30 weeks now over 95 per cent. Neurological handicap, predominantly cerebral palsy, is a serious problem in 10 per cent of survivors below 30 weeks. Cognitive impairment or behavioural difficulties, such as attention deficit hyperactivity disorder, is more common; around 10 per cent have a DQ less than 55, and a further 30 per cent have less severe learning difficulties. Less than a third of the EPICURE cohort of children born below 26 weeks gestation in 1995 had an IQ above 85 at the age of 11. The children were particularly poor at mathematics, and of those in mainstream school 55 per cent had special educational needs (Figure 19.11).

The management of many of the complications of prematurity (Table 19.8) is beyond the scope of this chapter, and the reader is directed to standard textbooks. A few of the major conditions are discussed below.

Respiratory distress syndrome, chronic lung disease

The incidence of respiratory distress syndrome (RDS) is strongly related to gestational age, occurring

Table 19.8 Main problems of prematurity

Respiratory distress syndrome
Chronic lung disease
Intraventricular haemorrhage, parenchymal cerebral haemorrhage
Periventricular leukomalacia
Infection
Hypoglycaemia
Necrotizing enterocolitis
Patent ductus arteriosus
Jaundice

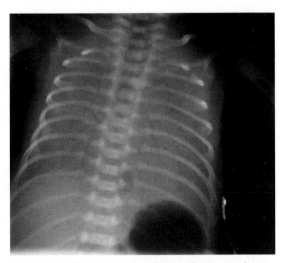

Figure 19.12 Chest x-ray in respiratory distress syndrome

in virtually 100 per cent of infants delivered at 26 weeks gestation, 40–50 per cent at 30–31 weeks and about 5 per cent at 35 weeks. RDS is a condition of increasing respiratory distress, commencing at, or shortly after, birth and increasing in severity until progressive resolution occurs among the survivors, usually between the 2nd and 4th day. It is due, at least in part, to insufficiency of pulmonary surfactant. RDS is manifest by respiratory distress (cyanosis, tachypnoea, grunting and recession), and respiratory failure is diagnosed by blood-gas analysis. Diagnosis can be confirmed by an x-ray film showing a ground-glass appearance and air bronchograms, although these radiological features are not pathognomonic of RDS (Figure 19.12). Antenatal steroids and post-natal surfactant are beneficial. Artificial ventilation remains the mainstay of management, although the modern trend is for 'gentle ventilation', aiming to reduce barotrauma and minimize the risk of chronic lung disease. Chronic lung disease still afflicts as many as 50 per cent of babies weighing <1 kg at birth, and these infants spend many months in oxygen, sometimes only to succumb later to winter viral infections or cor pulmonale.

Preterm brain injury

The neonatal brain is vulnerable to injury, and both intracranial parenchymal haemorrhage and periventricular leukomalacia (PVL) are associated with handicap in childhood. Intracranial haemorrhage is common in preterm infants, and occurs in the germinal matrix region. The germinal matrix is situated in the floor of the lateral ventricle. Bleeding into the germinal matrix often extends into the lateral ventricle of the brain (germinal matrix-intraventricular haemorrhage, GMH-IVH). GMH-IVH can resolve, but is sometimes complicated by persisting enlargement of the lateral ventricles or even progressive hydrocephalus. In these cases, the risk of handicap is more than 50 per cent. GMH-IVH can be diagnosed with ultrasound imaging via the fontanelle (Figure 19.13). Uncomplicated GMH-IVH – that is, bleeding not followed by ventricular dilatation or accompanied by a parenchymal lesion – carries a good prognosis. Only about 4 per cent of ex-preterm infants with no GMH-IVH or an uncomplicated GMH-IVH will develop major neurodevelopmental sequelae. Ventricular enlargement is often a sign of periventricular myelin loss and brain shrinkage, rather than raised intracranial pressure hydrocephalus. Brain growth is an important differentiating feature. The presence of progressive hydrocephalus requiring treatment increases the risk of serious sequelae in preterm infants to about 75 per cent.

Bleeding into the substance of the brain is usually followed by breakdown of tissue into a porencephalic cyst (Figure 19.13). The outlook for infants with such a cyst can be surprisingly good, but many have a hemiplegia. 'Periventricular leukomalacia' is the term used to describe multiple small cysts that are visualized within the periventricular white matter. MRI scanning later in childhood shows a paucity of myelin in such cases, and the lesion is a very reliable predictor of later cerebral palsy. Cerebral palsy is almost universal in cases with bilateral occipital PVL. Factors that predispose to PVL include prolonged rupture of membranes, chorioamnionitis and neonatal hypocarbia.

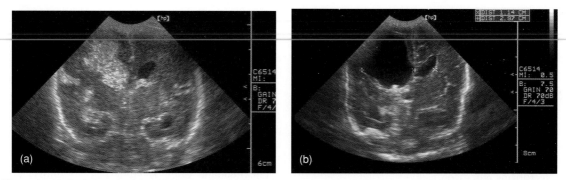

Figure 19.13 Evolution of a right-sided parenchymal lesion (a) into a porencephalic cyst (b) seen on a coronal ultrasound scan. The time interval between the scans was two months

Necrotizing enterocolitis

Necrotizing enterocolitis is a serious gastrointestinal disease affecting 2–5 per cent of preterm infants. Babies who have reversed end-diastolic flow in the umbilical artery and who are growth restricted are at particular risk. The characteristic clinical presentation is of a preterm infant less than 7 days old in whom enteral formula feeding has been commenced. Feeding is accompanied by abdominal distension, increased volume of gastric aspirate, which may be bile-stained or blood-stained, and a tender abdomen. Abdominal x-ray may reveal the characteristic signs of intramural gas, a sentinel loop or even gas in the portal tract. Treatment involves omission of enteral feeds and surgery for perforation or failure to respond to medical management. Mortality is about 10–20 per cent and is highest in very preterm infants who develop necrotizing enterocolitis in the first week of life. Long-term complications include stoma requirement, short bowel syndrome and nocturnal diarrhoea.

Key points

- Ten per cent of all babies require admission to neonatal units, but only 1 per cent require full intensive care.
- All those who attend deliveries should be able to initiate resuscitation with a bag and mask system.
- Survival rates for babies born after 29 weeks gestation are now over 95 per cent and most will grow and develop normally, but the outcome for those born at less than 26 weeks gestation includes cognitive impairment sufficient to require special educational resource in over half.

Additional reading and website resources

American Academy of Pediatrics and American College of Obstetricians and Gynecologists. Guidelines for perinatal care, 5th edn. Washington DC: AAP and ACOG, 2002.

Department of Health. Report of DH Expert Working Group on Neonatal Intensive Care Services. London: DOH, 2003.

Department of Health. National Service Framework for Children, Young People and Maternity Services. London: DOH, 2004.

Rennie JM (ed.). *Roberton's textbook of neonatology*, 4th edn. London: Churchill Livingstone, 2004.

Rennie JM, Roberton NRC. *A manual of neonatal intensive care*, 4th edn. London: Arnold, 2002.

Royal College of Paediatrics and Child Health/Royal College of Obstetricians and Gynaecologists. *Resuscitation of babies at birth*. London: BMJ Publishing Group, 1997.

Website resources

AIDS/HIV treatment information: www.hivatis.org.

Baby Life Support charity (support for parents): www.bliss.org.uk.

British Association of Perinatal Medicine: www.bapm.org.

Center for Disease Control and Prevention (USA): www.cdc.gov.

Confidential Enquiry into Maternal and Child Health: www.cemach.org.uk.

Contact a Family (information on specific disorders): www.cafamily.org.uk.

Department of Health (UK Government): www.doh.gov.uk.

Group B streptococcus support: www.gbss.org.uk.

Health Protection Agency (public health, UK): www.phls.co.uk.

National Institutes of Health (US Government): www.nih.gov.

National Institute for Health and Clinical Excellence: www.nice.org.uk.

National Neonatal audit programme (UK): www.rcpch.ac.uk/nnap.

Newborn Physical Examination: http://nipe.screening.nhs.uk.

OMIM – genetic diagnosis search site: www.ncbi.nlm.nih.gov/Omim.

Resuscitation Council (UK): www.resus.org.uk.

Statistics (UK Government): www.statistics.gov.uk.

Stillbirth and Neonatal Death Society: www.uk-sands.org.

Screening – UK national programme: www.nsc.nhs.uk; www.screening.nhs.uk.

UNICEF, world statistics: www.unicef.org.

CHAPTER 20

ETHICAL AND MEDICOLEGAL ISSUES IN OBSTETRIC PRACTICE

Philip N Baker

OVERVIEW

Obstetrics is a unique speciality, characterized by rapidly evolving clinical situations and full of ethical dilemmas. The importance of both ethical and medicolegal issues is arguably greater than in any other branch of medicine.

Ethics in obstetric practice

Declare the past, diagnose the present, foretell the future; practice these acts. As to disease, make a habit of two things – to help or at least do no harm.

Hippocrates

Obstetrics is full of ethical dilemmas; from genetic diagnosis to fetal therapy, there are issues of extreme complexity. Physicians need a sound knowledge of ethical principles, in order to ensure that their decisions are defensible to their peers, their patients and in a Court of Law. Obstetrics is unique in that the practitioner is often dealing with two patients, both inextricably linked, and whose interests usually but not invariably, coincide.

Obstetricians are bound by the duties of a doctor, as laid down by the General Medical Council, as for all other aspects of clinical practice. These principles of good practice bear repetition here:

- Make the care of your patient your first concern.
- Treat every patient politely and with consideration.
- Respect patients' dignity and privacy.
- Listen to patients and respect their views.
- Give patients information in a way they can understand.
- Respect the right of patients to be fully involved in decisions about their care.
- Keep your professional knowledge and skills up to date.

- Recognize the limits of your professional competence.
- Be honest and trustworthy.
- Respect and protect confidential information.
- Make sure that your personal beliefs do not prejudice your patients' care.
- Act quickly to protect patients from risk if you have good reason to believe that you or a colleague may not be fit to practice.
- Avoid abusing your position as a doctor.
- Work with colleagues in the ways that best serve patients' interests.

The principle of 'beneficence' is fundamental to the doctor–patient relationship. This requires the practitioner to objectively assess the different diagnostic and therapeutic options, and then to implement those that protect the interests of the patients by securing the greatest clinical benefits over harm. For centuries, this principle of beneficence guided clinical decision-making. However, over the past 100 years, it became increasingly apparent that beneficence alone was not enough; too often it led to paternalism, or the practitioner overriding a patient's wishes. Beneficence must be balanced by a respect for 'autonomy', which accepts that patients have their own perspectives on health-related interests, and thus have the right to make decisions based on their values and beliefs. In most situations, beneficence-based and autonomy-based obligations coincide. If there is conflict, patient autonomy should prevail, unless in the opinion of the practitioner, the course of action requested by the patient offends the practitioner's conscience. In such circumstances, the practitioner must refuse to accede to the patient's request. Private conscience does not justify the practitioner being judgemental or denying transfer of a patient to a colleague whose conscience is not affected by the issue.

The care of pregnant women involves an additional ethical issue peculiar to obstetrics, namely the status of the fetus. The fetus is not a person and has no rights in law. It could thus be argued that the fetus does not have moral status, however, this concept is increasingly being challenged, especially after 24 weeks gestation when the fetus is independently viable, albeit with technical support. Bioethicists contend that the independently viable fetus should be afforded moral status, i.e. that both the practitioner and the pregnant woman have beneficence-based moral obligations to the fetus. This means that obstetricians and midwives should regard the viable fetus as their patient. On rare occasions, there are conflicts between the autonomy-based decision of the mother regarding her viable fetus, and the professional judgement of the practitioner.

CASE HISTORY

A 32-year-old woman attended for a midtrimester detailed ultrasound scan in her third pregnancy (her previous pregnancies were uncomplicated and culminated in the vaginal delivery of term infants). The fetus was diagnosed as having a lumbosacral spina bifida. After extensive counselling, including advice from a paediatric neurosurgeon, the woman requested a termination of pregnancy. The obstetrician responsible for her care had strong religious beliefs that a termination of pregnancy was wrong.

Abortion is legal in the United Kingdom if two doctors decide in good faith that a particular pregnancy is associated with factors that satisfy one or more of five grounds specified in the Regulations of the Abortion Act and Section 37 of the Human Fertilisation and Embryology Act:

A. The continuance of the pregnancy would involve risk to the life of the pregnant woman greater than if the pregnancy were terminated.

B. The termination is necessary to prevent grave permanent injury to the physical or mental health of the pregnant woman.

C. The pregnancy has not exceeded its 24th week and the continuance of the pregnancy would involve risk, greater than if the pregnancy

were terminated, of injury to the physical or mental health of the pregnant woman.

D. The pregnancy has not exceeded its 24th week and the continuance of the pregnancy would involve risk, greater than if the pregnancy were terminated, of injury to the physical or mental health of the existing child(ren) of the family of the pregnant woman.

E. There is a substantial risk that if the child were born it would suffer from such physical or mental abnormalities as to be seriously handicapped.

The Regulations also permit abortion to be performed in an emergency on the basis of the signature of the doctor performing the procedure, which may be provided up to 24 hours after the termination. The emergency grounds are:

F. To save the life of the pregnant woman.

G. To prevent grave permanent injury to the physical or mental health of the pregnant woman.

Spina bifida is associated with a high risk of infant death or serious handicap. Although most abortions are undertaken on grounds C or D, the woman had the right to ask for termination of pregnancy under Section E of the Abortion Act (only 1 per cent of terminations are performed under these grounds). Furthermore, as the fetus was less than 24 weeks gestation, it was considered pre-viable and did not have the moral status of being a patient unless the woman conferred that status, something she was free to withhold. A decision to terminate the pregnancy was justified in respect of her autonomy-based decision.

The obstetrician declined to carry out the procedure as a matter of personal conscience. However, the woman was referred to another practitioner who had no objection to performing the termination of pregnancy.

CASE HISTORY

A 23-year-old woman in her second pregnancy underwent an ultrasound scan at 34 weeks gestation in order to assess fetal size; her first pregnancy had been complicated by fetal growth restriction. Ultrasound biometry was within the normal range, however, the fetus was found to have the 'double bubble' sign of duodenal atresia. A fetal blood sample was obtained by cordocentesis (see Chapter 7, Prenatal diagnosis) and rapid karyotyping revealed that the fetus had trisomy 21. Both the woman and her partner requested a termination of pregnancy.

A fetus at 34 weeks gestation has no legal rights. However, the fetus is viable and has therefore acquired the moral status of being a fetal patient. Duodenal atresia, a rare condition which occurs in about one in 10 000 births, is usually cured by surgery; one-third of children with duodenal atresia have Down's syndrome. Although Down's syndrome is associated with a low IQ, the child usually has a normal but dependent life.

Under Section E of the Abortion Act, there is no definition of 'serious abnormality'. To some obstetricians, this case would fit the description of 'serious abnormality'; they would recommend that a termination of pregnancy would be permitted under the Abortion Act and justified on the basis of maternal autonomy. However, Down's syndrome does not necessarily result in a life not worth living, and on ethical grounds, other practitioners would find it difficult to agree to a termination of pregnancy. Beneficence-based obligations to the fetus would not justify causing its death. On this basis, it would be ethically reasonable to deny maternal autonomy in this case.

The obstetricians responsible for the care of this case declined the woman's request for a termination of pregnancy. The pregnancy proceeded to a term delivery of a male infant with Down's syndrome and with duodenal atresia, but no other apparent abnormalities.

Consent

An adult patient who suffers from no mental incapacity has an absolute right to choose whether to consent to medical treatment, to refuse it or to choose one rather than another of the treatments being offered. . . . This right of choice is not limited to decisions which others might regard as sensible. It exists not withstanding that the reasons for making the choice are rational, irrational, unknown or even non-existent.

Lord Donaldson in the Court of Appeal

The law requires that the practitioner must obtain valid consent from the patient; all patients undergoing treatment should be given appropriate information on the nature and purpose of the treatment. Patients must be both capable and competent. The emphasis should be on consent as a process, not merely obtaining the patient's signature on a consent form. All too often clinicians equate consent with the signing of a form or consider consent primarily as protection against litigation. The signatures on a form are not a substitute for a proper discussion of the proposed intervention and engaging the patient in decision-making about her own care.

The law of consent is complex and is evolving in favour of providing patients with comprehensive information about the benefits and risk of treatments and procedures, including alternative management and the consequences of no treatment. Particular care must be taken when the benefits and risk of a treatment are unclear.

CASE HISTORY

A 34-year-old nulliparous women was admitted at 39 weeks gestation after the community midwife recorded that her blood pressure was 144/94 mmHg in the presence of + + + proteinuria. The fetal lie was longitudinal with a cephalic presenting part noted to be 4/5th palpable on abdominal examination. On vaginal examination, the cervix was found to be long and closed. When a cardiotocography (CTG) was commenced, the baseline fetal heart rate was normal; however, variability was reduced and there were unprovoked decelerations. The attending obstetric registrar made a diagnosis of pre-eclampsia (see Chapter 10, Pre-eclampsia and other disorders of placentation) and recommended Caesarean section on the basis of the pathological fetal heart rate allied to a cervix which was unfavourable for induction of labour. However, the woman and her partner refused to accept this advice. The obstetrician had to determine whether the woman was competent to give consent, i.e. that she was able to:

- comprehend and retain the treatment information;
- weigh that information in the balance to arrive at a choice.

A small minority of the population lack the necessary mental capacity to give consent, due to mental illness or retarded development. However, if she was deemed to be competent and the obstetrician proceeded with the Caesarean section, the operation would be performed against the express wishes of the woman, with the possible accusation that an assault on her body was being carried out. A competent adult has the right to refuse treatment, even if others, including health carers, believe that the refusal is neither in his or her best interests.

In this case, the solution was to persuade the prospective parents of the wisdom of performing the Caesarean section for the safety of the woman and her unborn child. In addition to benefits for the baby, delivery by Caesarean section will reduce the likelihood of maternal complications from pre-eclampsia. Persuasion should not be strident or threatening, but respectful and carefully reasoned.

Medicolegal issues

The nature of obstetrics is characterized by rapidly evolving clinical situations; risks to the mother and fetus are considerable and the potential for misjudgement or mismanagement by the attending doctors and midwives is ever present. Sometimes, patients suffer harm, physical or psychological, from care that was intended to heal them. In some cases, this is due to human error or to defects in the organization and delivery of care. In other cases, the harm is attributable to substandard care associated with technical incompetence, poor decision-making or departure from accepted clinical practice. Whatever the underlying cause, litigation may follow.

Some mistakes in clinical practice are obvious – such as leaving a swab inside the abdomen at Caesarean section. In contrast, most medicolegal issues are much more contentious. The most significant claims arise from brain damage and cerebral palsy; these are based on the allegation that negligent management resulted in fetal asphyxia and this resulted in brain damage.

As with all medicolegal cases, for the claimant to be successful it needs to be established that:

- There was a *breach of duty*. This means that the attending staff owed the patient a duty of care and that the standard of care afforded to the patient was below a standard which she could reasonably have expected. To determine this, the court relies on the evidence of expert witnesses. In turn, expert witnesses will take account of national and local evidence-based guidelines and conventional practice when advising on the standard of care

provided. The courts will apply the principle which states that a doctor is not negligent if he/she acts in accordance with accepted medical practice at the time, even though there may be doctors who hold a contrary opinion (the Bolam test), but the court must be satisfied that exponents of that practice could demonstrate that their opinion had a logical basis (the Bolitho test).

- There was *causation*, i.e. that the injury sustained was caused by the substandard care. A breach of duty, while regrettable and unacceptable, will not in itself be enough to establish a case of clinical negligence. The claimant has to show that the breach caused an injury; in other words, it must be shown that but for the breach of duty the injury would not have occurred (or would not have been as severe). If causation is established, the court will grant compensation for losses which the claimant has suffered as a result of the injury, provided that such losses are recognized by the court as deserving of compensation. The compensation comprises a sum for the 'pain, suffering and loss of amenity' caused by the injury and another sum covering the financial losses and extra expenses caused by the injury.

The litigation pathway

Obstetricians working under a contract of employment with the National Health Service (NHS) in the United Kingdom, unlike those working in the private sector or in countries like the United States, cannot be sued in their personal capacity. This is because they are indemnified by their employer for any alleged negligence in the course of their employment. This indemnity has implications for pattern of care because clinicians working under the fear of litigation are often accused of practising 'defensive medicine' – that is, practising an interventionist style of medicine in a bid to avert litigation.

In the United Kingdom, claims against the NHS are handled by the NHS Litigation Authority (NHSLA). Between 2001 and 2007, the NHSLA received 5691 new obstetric claims and the total amount paid out on obstetric claims was £1592 million. Apart from handling claims, the NHSLA has a statutory duty to help improve the quality of patient care by assisting NHS bodies with risk management. It does this largely through the Clinical Negligence Scheme for Trusts (CNST). This scheme, funded by member trusts, provides an indemnity to members and their employees in respect of clinical negligence claims. The CNST provides incentives for trusts to reduce patient safety incidents and litigation through attainment of risk management standards.

Most obstetricians have to address a complaint filed by a patient, at some point in their career. Sometimes, it is anticipated that this complaint will be followed by litigation. At other times, the complaints route is not followed and the first indication of imminent litigation is a letter from a solicitor requesting the patient's medical records. The solicitor passes the records to an expert witness (instructed on behalf of the claimant: either or both of the mother and baby) for a report on breach of duty and causation. If the report suggests that there is a claim, the solicitor writes a Letter of Claim setting out the facts of the case, the alleged substandard care and the resultant injury. The NHSLA obtains reports from the clinicians who looked after the patient, and then solicitors commissioned by the NHSLA instruct an expert witness (instructed on behalf of the defendant) to write a report on the case. On the basis of these reports, a letter of response is drafted, which sets out which aspects of the claim are agreed and which ones are repudiated. Negotiations and mediation sometimes follow; in many cases, it is apparent from initial investigations that the likelihood of a successful claim is very low and the claim is thus discontinued. In the cases where contentious issues remain unresolved, formal legal proceedings start and the processes can be very lengthy. A series of medicolegal multidisciplinary case conferences may be required; the claimant files Particulars of Claim and the NHSLA files a defence. Statements of witnesses of fact and reports of expert witnesses are exchanged between both parties, as are a schedule of the financial losses sustained as a result of the injury and the defendant's counter-schedule. Meetings of expert witnesses may be needed before a consensus is reached. In the small number of cases that remain unresolved at this stage, trial begins, but only a minority of cases reach the courts.

Medicolegal cases can be particularly distressing for all involved; all staff involved in the case must endeavour to respond to requests for information in as timely, as honest and as objective a manner as is possible.

CASE HISTORY

A 22-year-old nulliparous woman was admitted in spontaneous labour at term following an uncomplicated pregnancy. After several hours in labour, the attending midwife artificially ruptured the membranes and the liquor was noted to be meconium stained. Thereafter, there were persistent references to difficulty in obtaining an adequate CTG tracing; the attending midwife described 'artefactual judder' and loss of contact. Fetal heart rate decelerations were also noted and the duty obstetric registrar reviewed the CTG tracing on several occasions. When delay in the first stage of labour was identified, an intravenous oxytocin infusion was commenced. Shortly after, the midwife performed vaginal examination and identified that the cervix was 8 cm dilated, the obstetric registrar was asked to attend in order to assess the CTG tracing. The CTG tracing was described as showing reduced variability and the presence of late fetal heart rate decelerations. The initial management plan was merely to observe the fetal heart rate pattern, however, when the CTG tracing was identified as unchanged 30 minutes later, a decision to expedite the delivery by emergency Caesarean section was taken. A female infant weighing 3.54 kg was delivered; Apgar scores were 3 at 1 minute and 6 at 5 minutes. The pH values of paired umbilical cord blood samples were 7.13 and 7.19. The neonatal course was largely uncomplicated, although there was an equivocal episode on the post-natal ward which may have represented a neonatal seizure. The baby was discharged home with her mother 5 days following her Caesarean section. Thereafter, the health visitor raised concerns regarding delayed development. The child was subsequently found to have an evolving picture of cerebral palsy.

The allegations in the Letter of Claim related to the intrapartum care, and included the following:

- Fetal heart rate recordings throughout much of the labour were inadequate.
- The degree and significance of the fetal heart rate abnormalities were not recognized by attending staff.
- The instigation of an oxytocin infusion was inappropriate in the presence of fetal heart rate abnormalities.
- The fetal heart rate abnormalities should have led to earlier investigations or intervention.
- The decision to perform a Caesarean section was inappropriately delayed.
- Once the decision to perform a Caesarean section had been taken, the decision–delivery interval was excessive.

This case is typical of the most significant claims in obstetrics, which arise from brain damage and cerebral palsy; such claims are based on the allegation that negligent management resulted in fetal asphyxia and in brain damage.

Cases often revolve around the interpretation of intrapartum CTG tracings. It is important to obtain good quality CTG tracings; if the recordings are inadequate, every effort should be made to rectify this. It was agreed by the experts instructed by the claimant and by the defendant, that fetal heart rate monitoring in the early part of the labour was inadequate, and that a fetal scalp electrode should have been applied. However, it was also agreed that this deficiency in the care afforded was unlikely to have altered the outcome of the case, as during the time of the inadequate fetal monitoring there were unlikely to have been fetal heart rate abnormalities which mandated intervention.

When reviewing CTG tracings, it is important to avoid retrospective over-interpretations of the changes in the fetal heart rate pattern. For this reason, it is helpful to refer to recognized, published guidelines, such as the NICE (National Institute for Health and Clinical Excellence) guidelines. Using such guidelines, fetal heart rate patterns are described as normal, suspicious or pathological (see Chapter 6, Antenatal imaging and assessment of fetal well-being). The experts agreed that both the midwifery and the obstetric staff had underestimated the degree of abnormality that was apparent from the CTG tracing. The attending midwife should have alerted the duty obstetrician at an earlier time.

Good medical practice is based on careful assessment of the clinical situation, followed by instigation of an appropriate management plan. Both the assessment and the management plan should have been documented. When a fetal heart rate pattern deviated from normal, the nature of the abnormality should have been detailed. The management plan consequent upon the fetal heart rate pattern should also have been stated. There is little point performing an investigation, such as the CTG tracing, if recognized abnormalities are then ignored. Management options might include continued observation of the fetal heart rate pattern for evidence of further deterioration (either in the baseline rate or in the decelerative pattern), fetal blood sampling or an emergency Caesarean section. The experts deemed that fetal blood sampling should have been performed, particularly as meconium-stained liquor was present. Meconium-stained liquor is associated with up to a two-fold increase in perinatal complications. In the absence of fetal heart rate abnormalities, meconium staining of liquor is not an indication for additional investigation or intervention. However, in this case, with fetal heart rate abnormalities also present, meconium was associated with an increased likelihood of aberrant fetal acid-base balance and low Apgar scores.

Although the instigation of an oxytocin infusion was also criticized, it was felt that this did not have an adverse effect on the outcome of the case. In the presence of fetal heart rate abnormalities, the oxytocin infusion should have been discontinued or reduced, and the instigation of an infusion when fetal heart rate abnormalities were present, was inappropriate. However, in this case, the oxytocin infusion was assessed as having little if any effect on the frequency of uterine contractions. Moreover, there was no associated deterioration in the pattern of the fetal heart rate decelerations.

On the balance of probabilities, it was agreed that timely fetal blood sampling would have resulted in the decision to perform an emergency Caesarean section being taken approximately 13 minutes earlier. In addition, it was agreed that there was no justification for the decision–delivery interval exceeding the standard 30-minute medicolegal threshold. Allegations of breach of duty were not contested by the defendant trust; it was agreed that substandard care inappropriately delayed the delivery by 40 minutes.

The claim then focused on issues of causation. In many cases where a child suffers brain damage and develops cerebral palsy, it is accepted that the care afforded was substandard. The argument is then one of the causation, i.e. whether the substandard care caused or contributed to the disability. The situation is influenced by evidence that <15 per cent of infants born with significant brain damage acquire this disability consequent upon the events of labour and delivery. The problem faced by all obstetricians is that parents who give birth to a child with neurodevelopmental handicap will seek to ascribe the handicap to issues of intrapartum care. The American College of Obstetricians and Gynaecologists Taskforce on Neonatal and Encephalopathy and Cerebral Palsy have published the criteria to define an event in labour/delivery sufficient to cause cerebral palsy:

- Essential criteria:
  - Evidence of a metabolic acidosis in the fetal umbilical cord arterial blood obtained at delivery. Ideally, samples are taken from both the umbilical artery and vein. In this situation, metabolic acidosis is defined as a pH <7 and a base deficit of 12 mmol/L.
  - Early onset of severe or moderate neonatal encephalopathy in infants; this is characterized by an altered level of consciousness and often by seizures. (This criterion applies to babies born at 34 or more weeks gestation.)
  - The type of cerebral palsy that results from the events of the labour/delivery is spastic quadriplegic or dyskinetic cerebral palsy.
  - Other causes of neurodevelopmental handicap, such as trauma, genetic disorders, infectious conditions and coagulation disorders, need to be excluded.

continued ≫

- Criteria that suggests that the timing of any injury is close to labour and delivery (within 48 hours):
  - The hypoxic event occurring immediately prior to delivery or during labour.
  - A sudden and sustained fetal heart rate bradycardia or the absence of fetal heart rate variability in the presence of persistent late/variable decelerations. For this criterion to be met, the fetal heart rate abnormality must follow the hypoxic event and have been preceded by a normal fetal heart rate pattern.
  - Apgar scores of 0–3 beyond 5 minutes. A low Apgar score after 5 minutes indicates an infant who needs continued resuscitative efforts.
  - Onset of multisystem involvement within 72 hours of birth. In many cases, organ damage such as that to the neonatal kidney may be temporary.

- An early imaging study showing evidence of acute non-focal cerebral abnormalities. Ultrasound and magnetic resonance imaging (MRI) scans of the baby's head, performed after delivery, can aid assessment of the timing of any injury.

In this case, it was apparent that many of the above criteria were not met. Different medicolegal opinions were obtained, from neonatologists, paediatric neurologists and neuroradiologists. It was eventually agreed that the nature of the neurodevelopmental handicap, allied to the MRI findings, suggested that on the balance of probabilities, the damaging insult was unlikely to have occurred in the 40 minutes prior to the delivery.

Despite the criticisms of the attending midwifery and obstetric staff, and the establishment of a clear breach of duty, the case was successfully defended on grounds of causation.

Key points

- Case records should be as clear, concise and accurate as possible.
- The reason for deviating from any protocol or guideline should be clearly stated within the medical records.
- Cardiotocography interpretation should be consistent with recognized, published guidelines.
- Staff involved in any medicolegal case must endeavour to respond to requests for information in as timely, as honest and as objective a manner as is possible.

Additional reading

General Medical Council. *Maintaining good medical practice*. London: GMC, 1998.

Royal College of Obstetricians and Gynaecologists. Clinical Governance Advice No. 6. Obtaining valid consent. Available from: www.rcog.org.uk.

NHS Litigation Authority (NHSLA). Available from: www.nhsla.com.

INDEX

Page numbers in *italic* refer to figures; those in **bold** to tables.